Informatik aktuell

Reihe herausgegeben von

Gesellschaft für Informatik e.V. (GI), Bonn, Deutschland

Ziel der Reihe ist die möglichst schnelle und weite Verbreitung neuer Forschungs- und Entwicklungsergebnisse, zusammenfassender Übersichtsberichte über den Stand eines Gebietes und von Materialien und Texten zur Weiterbildung. In erster Linie werden Tagungsberichte von Fachtagungen der Gesellschaft für Informatik veröffentlicht, die regelmäßig, oft in Zusammenarbeit mit anderen wissenschaftlichen Gesellschaften, von den Fachausschüssen der Gesellschaft für Informatik veranstaltet werden. Die Auswahl der Vorträge erfolgt im allgemeinen durch international zusammengesetzte Programmkomitees.

Andreas Maier · Thomas M. Deserno ·
Heinz Handels · Klaus Maier-Hein ·
Christoph Palm · Thomas Tolxdorff
(Hrsg.)

Bildverarbeitung für die Medizin 2024

Proceedings, German Conference on
Medical Image Computing, Erlangen,
March 10–12, 2024

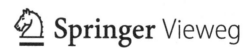

Hrsg.

Andreas Maier 🆔
Friedrich-Alexander-Universität
Erlangen-Nürnberg
Erlangen, Deutschland

Heinz Handels 🆔
Institut für Medizinische Informatik
Universität zu Lübeck
Lübeck, Deutschland

Christoph Palm 🆔
Informatik und Mathematik
OTH Regensburg
Regensburg, Deutschland

Thomas M. Deserno 🆔
Peter L. Reichertz Institut für Medizinische
Informatik
Technische Universität Braunschweig
Braunschweig, Deutschland

Klaus Maier-Hein 🆔
Medical Image Computing, E230
Deutsches Krebsforschungszentrum
(DKFZ)
Heidelberg, Deutschland

Thomas Tolxdorff 🆔
Institut für Medizinische Informatik
Charité - Universitätsmedizin Berlin
Berlin, Deutschland

ISSN 1431-472X   ISSN 2628-8958   (electronic)
Informatik aktuell
ISBN 978-3-658-44036-7   ISBN 978-3-658-44037-4   (eBook)
https://doi.org/10.1007/978-3-658-44037-4

Die Deutsche Nationalbibliothek verzeichnet diese Publikation in der Deutschen Nationalbibliografie;
detaillierte bibliografische Daten sind im Internet über http://dnb.d-nb.de abrufbar.

Planung/Lektorat: Petra Steinmueller
Springer Vieweg ist ein Imprint der eingetragenen Gesellschaft Springer Fachmedien Wiesbaden GmbH
und ist ein Teil von Springer Nature.
Die Anschrift der Gesellschaft ist: Abraham-Lincoln-Str. 46, 65189 Wiesbaden, Germany

Das Papier dieses Produkts ist recyclebar.

Bildverarbeitung für die Medizin 2024

Veranstalter

FAU   Friedrich-Alexander-Universität Erlangen-Nürnberg

Unterstützende Fachgesellschaften

BVMI   Berufsverband Medizinischer Informatiker
CURAC   Computer- und Roboterassistierte Chirurgie
DAGM   Deutsche Arbeitsgemeinschaft für Mustererkennung
DGBMT   Fachgruppe Medizinische Informatik der
             Deutschen Gesellschaft für Biomedizinische Technik im
             Verband Deutscher Elektrotechniker
GI   Gesellschaft für Informatik – Fachbereich Informatik
             in den Lebenswissenschaften
GMDS   Gesellschaft für Medizinische Informatik,
             Biometrie und Epidemiologie
IEEE   Joint Chapter Engineering in Medicine and Biology,
             German Section

Tagungsvorsitz

Prof. Dr.-Ing. habil. Andreas Maier
Lehrstuhl für Mustererkennung (Informatik 5)
Friedrich-Alexander-Universität Erlangen-Nürnberg

Tagungssekretariat

Dr.-Ing. Siming Bayer Lehrstuhl für Mustererkennung (Informatik 5)

Anschrift: Martensstr. 3, D-91058 Erlangen
Telefon: +49 9131 85 27775
Fax: +49 9131 85 27270
Email: orga-2024@bvm-workshop.org
Web: https://bvm-workshop.org

Lokale BVM-Organisation

Dr.-Ing. Siming Bayer, Dr.-Ing. Tomás Arias Vergara, Alexandra Hauske, u.a.

Verteilte BVM-Organisation

Begutachtung	Heinz Handels und Jan-Hinrich Wrage – Institut für Medizinische Informatik, Universität zu Lübeck
Mailingliste	Klaus Maier-Hein – Medical Image Computing, Deutsches Krebsforschungszentrum (DKFZ) Heidelberg
Special Issue	Andreas Maier – Lehrstuhl für Mustererkennung, Friedrich-Alexander Universität Erlangen-Nürnberg
Tagungsband	Thomas M. Deserno, Nico Baumann, Paula Lüpke – Peter L. Reichertz Institut für Medizinische Informatik, TU Braunschweig
Web & News	Christoph Palm, Leonard Klausmann, Alexander Leis und Sümeyye R. Yildiran – Regensburg Medical Image Computing (ReMIC), Ostbayerische Technische Hochschule Regensburg

BVM-Komitee

Prof. Dr. Thomas M. Deserno, Peter L. Reichertz Institut für Medizinische Informatik der TU Braunschweig und der Medizinischen Hochschule Hannover

Prof. Dr. Heinz Handels, Institut für Medizinische Informatik, Universität zu Lübeck

Prof. Dr. Andreas Maier, Lehrstuhl für Mustererkennung, Friedrich-Alexander-Universität Erlangen-Nürnberg

Prof. Dr. Klaus Maier-Hein, Medical Image Computing, Deutsches Krebsforschungszentrum Heidelberg

Prof. Dr. Christoph Palm, Regensburg Medical Image Computing (ReMIC), Ostbayerische Technische Hochschule Regensburg

Prof. Dr. Thomas Tolxdorff, Institut für Medizinische Informatik, Charité–Univer- sitätsmedizin Berlin

Programmkomitee

Jürgen Braun, Charité-Universitätsmedizin Berlin
Katharina Breininger, FAU Erlangen-Nürnberg
Thomas Deserno, TU Braunschweig
Jan Ehrhardt, Universität zu Lübeck
Sandy Engelhardt, Universitätsklinik Heidelberg
Ralf Floca, DKFZ Heidelberg
Nils Forkert, University of Calgary, Canada
Michael Götz Universitätsklinikum Ulm
Horst Hahn, Fraunhofer MEVIS, Bremen
Heinz Handels, Universität zu Lübeck

Tobias Heimann, Siemens Healthineers Erlangen
Mattias Heinrich, Universität zu Lübeck
Anja Hennemuth, Charité-Universitätsmedizin Berlin
Alexander Horsch, TU München und Uni Tromsö, Norwegen
Dagmar Kainmüller, MDC Berlin
Bernhard Kainz, FAU Erlangen-Nürnberg
Andreas Kist, FAU Erlangen-Nürnberg
Florian Knoll, FAU Erlangen-Nürnberg
Ron Kikinis, Harvard Medical School
Dagmar Krefting, Universität Göttingen
Andreas Maier, FAU Erlangen-Nürnberg
Klaus Maier-Hein, DKFZ Heidelberg
Lena Maier-Hein, DKFZ Heidelberg
Andre Mastmeyer, Hochschule Aalen
Dorit Merhof, Universität Regensburg
Jan Modersitzki, Fraunhofer MEVIS, Lübeck
Heinrich Müller, TU Dortmund
Nassir Navab, TU München
Marco Nolden, DKFZ Heidelberg
Christoph Palm, OTH Regensburg
Bernhard Preim, Universität Magdeburg
Petra Ritter, BIH Berlin
Karl Rohr, Universität Heidelberg
Daniel Rückert, TU München
Sylvia Saalfeld, Universität Magdeburg
Dennis Säring, FH Wedel
Julia Schnabel, Helmholtz München, TU München
Ingrid Scholl, FH Aachen
Stefanie Speidel, HZDR/NCT Dresden
Nicolai Spicher, Universität Göttingen
Thomas Tolxdorff, Charité-Universitätsmedizin Berlin
Klaus Tönnies, Universität Magdeburg
Gudrun Wagenknecht, Forschungszentrum Jülich
René Werner, UKE Hamburg
Thomas Wittenberg, Fraunhofer IIS, Erlangen
Ivo Wolf, Hochschule Mannheim
Moritz Zaiß, Universitätsklinikum Erlangen

Preisträger der BVM 2022 in Heidelberg

BVM Award CHILI

Anna-Maria Wölfl
(Artificial Intelligence in Biomedical Engineering, FAU Erlangen-Nürnberg)
Pitch Detection in Endoscopic Images – Masterarbeit
Dr. Lasse Hansen (Institut für Medizinische Informatik, Universität zu Lübeck)
Point Clouds and Keypoint Graphs in 3D Deep Learning for Medical Image Analysis –
Doktorarbeit

Beste wissenschaftliche Arbeiten

1. **Jonathan Ganz**
   (Technische Hochschule Ingolstadt)
   Ganz J, Lipnik K, Ammeling J, Richter B, Puget C, Parlak E, Diehl L, Klopfleisch L, Donovan TA, Kiupel M, Bertram CA, Breininger K, Aubreville M
   Deep Learning-based Automatic Assessment of AgNOR-scores in Histopathology Images
2. **Marcel Ganß**
   (Chair for Computer Aided Medical Procedures and Augmented Reality, Technical University Munich)
   Ganß M, De Benetti F, Brosch-Lenz J, Uribe-Munoz C, Shi K, Eiber M, Navab N, Wendler T
   Deep Learning Approaches for Contrast Removal from Contrast-enhanced CT
3. **Marc K. Ickler**
   (Division of Medical Image Computing, German Cancer Research Center, Heidelberg)
   Ickler MK, Baumgartner M, Roy S, Wald T, Maier-Hein KH
   Taming Detection Transformers for Medical Object Detection

Bester Vortrag

Fabian Wagner
(Pattern Recognition Lab, FAU Erlangen-Nürnberg)
Wagner F, Thies M, Denzinger F, Gu M, Patwari M, Ploner S, Maul N, Pfaff L, Huang Y, Maier A
Trainable Joint Bilateral Filters for Enhanced Prediction Stability in Low-dose CT

Bestes Poster

Robert Mendel
(Regensburg Medical Image Computing (ReMIC), OTH Regensburg)
Mendel R, Rauber D, Palm C
Exploring the Effects of Contrastive Learning on Homogeneous Medical Image Data

Vorwort

Die Tagung Bildverarbeitung für die Medizin (BVM) wird seit weit mehr als 20 Jahren an wechselnden Orten Deutschlands veranstaltet. Inhaltlich fokussiert sich die BVM dabei auf die computergestützte Analyse medizinischer Bilddaten, die Anwendungsgebiete sind vielfältig, z.B. im Bereich der Bildgebung, der Diagnostik, der Operationsplanung, der computerunterstützten Intervention und der Visualisierung.

In dieser Zeit hat es bemerkenswerte methodische Weiterentwicklungen und Umbrüche gegeben, wie zum Beispiel im Bereich des maschinellen Lernens, an denen die BVM-Community intensiv mitgearbeitet hat. In der Folge dominieren inzwischen Arbeiten im Zusammenhang mit Deep Learning die BVM. Auch diese Entwicklungen haben dazu beigetragen, dass die Medizinische Bildverarbeitung an der Schnittstelle zwischen Informatik und Medizin als eine Schlüsseltechnologie zur Digitalisierung des Gesundheitswesens etabliert ist.

Zentraler Aspekt der BVM ist neben der Darstellung aktueller Forschungsergebnisse schwerpunktmäßig aus der vielfältigen, deutschlandübergreifenden BVM-Community insbesondere die Forderung des wissenschaftlichen Nachwuchses. Die Tagung dient vor allem Promovierenden aber auch Studierenden mit hervorragenden Abschlussarbeiten als Plattform, um ihre Ergebnisse zu präsentieren, dabei in den fachlichen Diskurs mit der Community zu treten und Netzwerke mit anderen Forschenden zu knüpfen. Trotz der vielen Tagungen und Kongresse, die auch für die Medizinische Bildverarbeitung relevant sind, hat die BVM deshalb nichts von ihrer Bedeutung und Anziehungskraft eingebüßt.

Inhaltlich kann auch bei der BVM 2024 wieder ein attraktives und hochklassiges Programm geboten werden. Es wurden aus 91 Einreichungen über ein anonymisiertes Review-Verfahren mit jeweils drei Reviews 28 Vorträge, 59 Posterbeiträge und vier Softwaredemonstrationen angenommen. Die besten Arbeiten werden auch in diesem Jahr mit Preisen ausgezeichnet.

Die Webseite des Workshops findet sich unter:

https://www.bvm-workshop.org

Das Programm wird durch Tutorials und zwei eingeladene Vorträge ergänzt, für die wir uns herzlich bedanken. Als Referenten fur die Vorträge begruüßen wir herzlich:

- Prof. Sophia Bano, PhD, UCL East Robotics, Department of Computer Science & Wellcome / EPSRC Centre for Interventional and Surgical Sciences (WEISS) University College London,
- Prof. Dr.-Ing. Silke Christiansen, Fraunhofer-Institut für Keramische Technologien und Systeme IKTS, Forchheim.

An dieser Stelle möchten wir allen, die bei den umfangreichen Vorbereitungen zum Gelingen des Workshops beigetragen haben, unseren herzlichen Dank für ihr Engagement aussprechen: den Vortragenden der Gastvorträge, den Verfassenden der Beiträge, den Lehrenden der Tutorien, den Industrievertretenden, dem Programmkomitee, den Fachgesellschaften, den Mitgliedern des BVM-Organisationsteams und allen Mitarbeitenden des Lehrstuhls für Mustererkennung der Friedrich-Alexander-Universität Erlangen-Nürnberg.

Wir wünschen allen Teilnehmenden des Workshops BVM 2024 spannende neue Kontakte und inspirierende Eindrücke aus der Welt der medizinischen Bildverarbeitung.

Januar 2024

Andreas Maier (Erlangen)
Thomas M. Deserno (Braunschweig)
Heinz Handels (Lübeck)
Klaus Maier-Hein (Heidelberg)
Christoph Palm (Regensburg)

Thomas Tolxdorff (Berlin)

Inhaltsverzeichnis

Die fortlaufende Nummer am linken Seitenrand entspricht den Beitragsnummern, wie sie im endgültigen Programm des Workshops zu finden sind. Dabei steht V für Vortrag, P für Poster und S für Softwaredemonstration.

Keynotes

Session 1: Computer-aided Diagnosis

Session 2: Convolutional Neural Networks and Deep Learning

Session 3: Image Registration and Fusion

Session 4: Image Segmentation and Image Analysis

Session 5: Machine Learning and Artificial Intelligence

Postersession 1: Computer-aided Diagnosis

Postersession 2: Convolutional Neural Networks and Deep Learning

Postersession 3: Image Registration and Fusion

Postersession 4: Image Segmentation and Image Analysis

Postersession 5: Imaging and Acquisition

Postersession 6: Machine Learning and Artificial Intelligence

Keynote: Recent Advances in Surgical AI for Next Generation Interventions

Sophia Bano

UCL East Robotics, Department of Computer Science & Wellcome
EPSRC Centre for Interventional and Surgical Sciences (WEISS)
University College London
sophia.bano@ucl.ac.uk

Recent trends in Artificial Intelligence (AI) and surgical science have revolutionized the field of surgery, paving the way for a new era of AI-assisted robotic interventions. These cutting-edge technologies offer tremendous potential to enhance imaging, surgical navigation, and robotic interventions, ultimately reducing cognitive load on surgeons and optimizing procedural efficiency. This talk will highlight AI applications in different surgical procedures and where we stand in terms of their clinical translation for moving towards next generation of surgical intervention. [1].

References

1. Github: https://sophiabano.github.io/.

Keynote: 4-D+ nanoSCOPE Project

Silke Christiansen

Fraunhofer-Institut für Keramische Technologien und Systeme (IKTS), Forchheim, Germany
silke.christiansen@ikts.fraunhofer.de

The number of elderly and very elderly people is increasing worldwide, and so is the number of patients suffering from osteoporosis. This disease significantly impairs the quality of life and leads to high social costs. Nevertheless, the origin and course of osteoporosis are still not sufficiently understood. This is because methods for an in-depth analysis of the fine bone structure over time in living individuals are not yet available, especially those that also allow large matrix studies with statistical significance. An interdisciplinary research project now wants to change this. The 4-D+ nanoSCOPE project is developing a groundbreaking X-ray microscope (image acquisition with submicron resolution over a hundred times faster than is currently possible). An interdisciplinary team intend to enable X-ray microscopy studies in living creatures for the very first time. They plan to do so by combining state-of-the-art imaging techniques with innovative precision learning software and a novel Xray microscope. Their method has the potential to revolutionize our understanding of bone structure and improve bone remodelling, by enabling an effective assessment of the effects on bone of age, hormones, inflammation and treatment. [1].

References

1. Web: https://www.4dnanoscope.de.

A. Maier et al. (Hrsg.), *Bildverarbeitung für die Medizin 2024*,
Informatik aktuell, https://doi.org/10.1007/978-3-658-44037-4_2

Improving Hybrid Quantum Annealing Tomographic Image Reconstruction with Regularization Strategies

Merlin A. Nau[1,2], A. Hans Vija[3], Maximilian P. Reymann[1,2], Wesley Gohn[3], Andreas K. Maier[5]

[1] Pattern Recognition Lab, Department of Computer Science, Friedrich-Alexander Universität Erlangen-Nürnberg, Germany
[2] Siemens Healthineers GmbH, Forchheim, Germany
[3] Siemens Medical Solutions USA, Inc., Hoffman Estates, USA
merlin.nau@fau.de

Abstract. Quantum computing and quantum annealing present promising avenues for addressing complex problems in various fields, including tomographic image reconstruction. This study investigates the application of hybrid quantum annealing in the context of tomographic image reconstruction, focusing on the formulation of compatible conventional image regularization strategies: L2 and total variation. Using a Shepp-Logan phantom of image size 32×32 with 4-bit grayscale encoding, we study the effect of the regularization techniques under the influence of their parameters and the runtime of the hybrid quantum annealer. The study reveals, that L2 regularization effectively enhances the obtained image reconstructions and total variation can further improve them. Despite efforts to employ regularized hybrid quantum annealing reconstructions, they still fall short in comparison to traditional reconstruction techniques.

1 Introduction

Tomographic image reconstruction is a challenging inverse problem in medical imaging, complicated by noise and ill-posedness. As quantum computing (QC) technologies inch closer to practical application, there is growing interest in applying QC to problem settings in medical imaging [1]. In QC, gate-based approaches are currently the prevailing approach, but quantum annealing (QA) methods are actively explored. In this manuscript, we aim to apply regularization techniques to perform emission tomography reconstruction on a toy problem using a QA-compatible formulation. The tomographic imaging process is commonly dealt with in a discrete-to-discrete linear imaging model:

$$\mathbf{g} = \mathbf{H}\mathbf{f} \qquad (1)$$

Here $\mathbf{g} \in \mathbb{R}^K$ represents the measurements obtained from the imaging system. $\mathbf{H} \in \mathbb{R}^{K \times N}$ is the system matrix that models our imaging system and $\mathbf{f} \in \mathbb{R}^N$ is our measured object, we try to recover during image reconstruction.

Tomographic image reconstruction methods often fall into two categories. The first relies on integral-transforms and requires the inversion of a physical transform, e.g. the Radon transform. One common approach to solve this is the Filtered Backprojection (FBP) algorithm, that involves the Fourier transform. Algorithmic approaches for

© Der/die Autor(en), exklusiv lizenziert an
Springer Fachmedien Wiesbaden GmbH, ein Teil von Springer Nature 2024
A. Maier et al. (Hrsg.), *Bildverarbeitung für die Medizin 2024*,
Informatik aktuell, https://doi.org/10.1007/978-3-658-44037-4_3

implementing the Fourier transform on gate-based QC have been proposed, showing theoretical potential for exponential speedup compared to classical methods [2]. The first notable proposal of QC for medical image reconstruction focuses on replacing the Fourier transform in FBP with its quantum counterpart [3]. While this is an intriguing finding, this work primarily delves into theory and lacks practical examples and limitations.

The second category involves image reconstruction using linear algebra methods, typically solved iteratively. The core step of solving linear systems of equations, is theoretically faster on a gate-based quantum computer, as exemplified by the HHL algorithm [4]. Despite recent developments, the HHL-algorithm still faces hardware constraints and data loading constraints [5].

QA is another avenue in near-term QC that focuses on finding better solutions to optimization problems in particular. QA, and associated hybrid systems, have demonstrated the ability to solve linear systems of equations [6], in particular ill-posed ones [7, 8], and have been proposed for tomographic image reconstruction [9–11].

In this work, we extend the approach presented by Nau et al. [9] to reconstruct tomographic images using a hybrid QC platform from D-Wave utilizing quantum annealers, referred to as QA reconstruction. Previous experiments were restricted to small pixel value ranges, mainly binary images. As the pixel value range expands to 4-bit range, reconstruction quality deteriorates as one approaches the current limitation of 32×32 pixels. To improve these reconstructions, we introduce conventional L2 and total variation (TV) regularization terms to the optimization objective. We assess the regularization performance under the influence of their parameters λ_{L2} and λ_{TV} as well as the timing parameter of the hybrid solver.

2   Materials and methods

QA is a class of QC that relies on the principles of the adiabatic theorem. The adiabatic theorem states that a quantum system, over time, will evolve to its lowest energy state. This lowest energy state corresponds to a minimum in an energy landscape, making it well-suited for optimization problems. QA is primarily employed to solve combinatorial optimization problems, with a key focus on quadratic unconstrained binary optimization (QUBO)

$$\min(\text{QUBO}(\mathbf{x}))_{\mathbf{x} \in \{0,1\}^n} = \sum_{i=0}^{N-1} \mathbf{Q}_{i,i}\mathbf{x}_i + \sum_{i=0}^{N-1}\sum_{j=i+1}^{N-1} \mathbf{Q}_{i,j}\mathbf{x}_i\mathbf{x}_j = \mathbf{x}^T\mathbf{Q}\mathbf{x} \qquad (2)$$

The QUBO formulation is defined by the solution vector $\mathbf{x} \in \{0,1\}^N$ and the matrix $\mathbf{Q} \in \mathbb{R}^{N \times N}$ and is composed of linear bias terms on the matrix diagonal and the quadratic coupling value between variables on the upper-triangular matrix. The QA system of a D-Wave annealer is composed of a topology of interconnected superconducting qubits, which can be initialized with the linear bias terms and quadratic couplings of the QUBO matrix $\mathbf{Q}$. This problem is then encoded on the quantum processing unit (QPU) of the quantum annealer, where one qubit corresponds to one variable.

Despite the fact that quantum annealers have up to 5000 qubits, the restricted qubit connectivity on the QPU currently hinders their applicability to problems where many quadratic interaction are present in $\mathbf{Q}$. Specifically densely-connected problems, like the one encountered in image reconstruction, are challenging to solve. One approach to embed larger problems on the QPU involves using multiple physical qubits, so called chains, to represent a single logical qubit and expand the connectivity. However, this method is still only feasible for relatively small problem sizes, limited around 100 fully-connected binary variables [9]. This limitation becomes even more pronounced when we want to encode integer pixel values using multiple qubits as proposed in [10].

To mitigate these current limitations of quantum annealers, D-Wave has introduced a hybrid solver [12]. This solver mimics the solution on a quantum annealer classically, and efficiently offloads sub-problems to run on the quantum annealer. This hybrid solver also extends the binary variables $\mathbf{x}$ in Equation (2) to integer variables, opening a new class of solvable problems: constrained quadratic models (CQM). Our solution vector $\mathbf{x}$ can now take on 4-bit integer values $\mathbb{Z}_{4-bit}$ with a minimum value of 0 and a maximum value of 15. The least-squares optimization objective of tomographic image reconstruction can then be translated to a CQM fomulation to obtain a reconstructed image

$$\text{CQM}(\mathbf{f}) = \|\mathbf{Hf} - \mathbf{g}\|_2^2 = \mathbf{f}^T\mathbf{H}^T\mathbf{Hf} - \mathbf{f}^T\mathbf{H}^T\mathbf{g} - \mathbf{g}^T\mathbf{Hf} + \mathbf{g}^T\mathbf{g} \qquad (3)$$

In the following subsections, we show that we can introduce common additive quadratic regularization terms to the CQM optimization objective.

2.1 L2 regularization

L2 regularization adds a penalty to the cost function that controls the magnitude of the reconstructed pixel values. Because it is a qudratic formulation it can be incorporated into the CQM. In particular, L2 regularization, can provide smoother and more stable solutions at reduced noise.

$$\text{CQM}(\mathbf{f}) = \|\mathbf{Hf} - \mathbf{g}\|_2^2 + \lambda_{L2}\|\mathbf{f}\|_2^2 \qquad (4)$$

The first part in this equation resembles the reconstruction term from Equation (3) followed by the L2 regularization term, controlled by λ_{L2}.

2.2 Total variation regularization

TV regularization is commonly used in image reconstruction and denoising. The TV of an image measures the sum of the gradients in horizontal and vertical direction. For clarification we reshape $\mathbf{f}$ to the 2D image dimension. We remove the square root of the sum of differences from the original TV equation to adjust the regularizer for the CQM

$$\text{TV}(\mathbf{f}) = \sum_{i=0}^{N-1}\sum_{j=0}^{N-1}(\mathbf{f}_{i,j} - \mathbf{f}_{i,j+1})^2 + (\mathbf{f}_{i,j} - \mathbf{f}_{i+1,j})^2 \qquad (5)$$

Unlike L2 regularization, TV encourages piece-wise smoothness in the reconstructed image by penalizing large gradients in the image. It is especially effective at preserving edges and fine details while reducing noise [13]. The amount of TV regularization is controlled by the parameter λ_{TV}

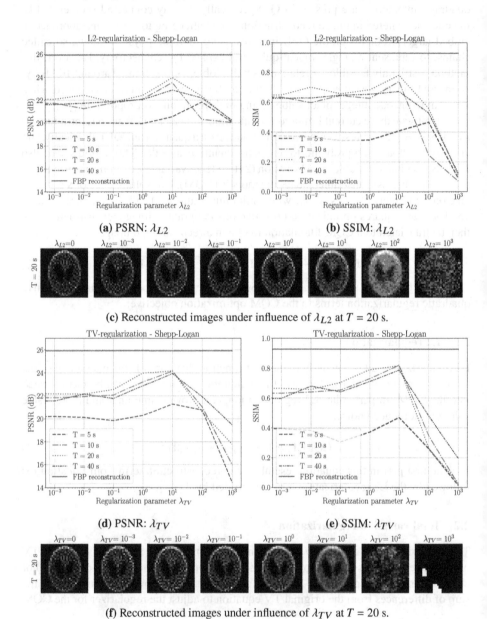

(a) PSRN: λ_{L2} (b) SSIM: λ_{L2}

(c) Reconstructed images under influence of λ_{L2} at $T = 20$ s.

(d) PSNR: λ_{TV} (e) SSIM: λ_{TV}

(f) Reconstructed images under influence of λ_{TV} at $T = 20$ s.

Fig. 1. Shepp Logan image reconstructions computed with a hybrid solver. L2 and TV-regularization PSNR (a) and (d), SSIM (b) and (e) under influence of timing paramter T and regularization parameter λ_{L2} and λ_{TV}, respectively. The reconstructed images are shown for regularization parameter λ_{L2} in (c) and λ_{TV} in (f) at $T = 20$ s.

$$\text{CQM}(\mathbf{f}) = |\mathbf{Hf} - \mathbf{g}|_2^2 + \lambda_{TV} \cdot \text{TV}(\mathbf{f}) \tag{6}$$

3 Results

We conduct our experiment on a Shepp-Logan phantom of size $N = 32 \times 32$ with 4-bit grayscale pixel range that is simulated in *scikit-image* using the provided *radon* function to model the imaging process of 32 views. We compare our regularized QA reconstruction with the conventional FBP using a ramp filter implemented in the *iradon* function. The QA reconstruction is carried out on a quantum-annealing based hybrid solver with a tuneable parameter of the maximum solving time T. In contrast to previous papers [9–11], we investigate the effect of this parameter by performing a trial over four different values $T \in \{5, 10, 20, 40\}$ s. The hybrid solver, mimics a quantum annealer, and returns a sampleset of solutions, each associated with a corresponding energy. We always choose the solutions corresponding to the lowest energy, which is correlated with the optimum value found for the objective function. We introduce L2 and TV regularization in the objective function using *SymPy* and investigate the performance of the parameters on a grid search of $\lambda_{L2}, \lambda_{TV} \in \{0, 10^{-3}, 10^{-2}, 10^{-1}, 10^0, 10^1, 10^2, 10^3\}$ for the test image. For quantitative evaluation of L2 regularization, we plot the peak signal to noise ratio (PSNR) and structural similarity index measure (SSIM) for the different values of λ_{L2} and T in Figure 1a and 1b and compare the influence of the parameters for the phantom. We further show the reconstructed images, at time $T = 20$ s, that has achieved the overall best reconstruction performance in Figure 1c. The plots of PSNR and SSIM for TV-regularization are shown in Figure 1d and 1e. The corresponding reconstructions at $T = 20$ s is in Figure 1f. Finally, we show the reconstruction obtained with L2- and TV-regularization for $T = 20$ s and $\lambda_{L2}, \lambda_{TV} = 10^1$, that yielded the best performance for PSNR, along with a FBP reconstruction and the ground truth in Figure 2.

4 Discussion

In this manuscript we have shown, that it is possible to formulate conventional image regularization in the objective function for an image reconstruction problem solved with a hybrid quantum annealer. We have shown that the incorporation of L2 and TV regularization can enhance the solution quality of QA reconstructions.

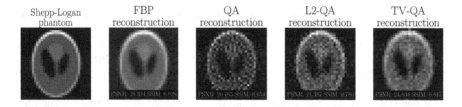

Fig. 2. Comparison of Shepp-Logan phantom with a FBP reconstruction, QA reconstruction, QA with L2 regularization ($\lambda_{L2} = 10, T = 20$ s) and with TV regularization ($\lambda_{TV} = 10, T = 20$ s).

Figure 1a and 1b show that the introduction of an L2 regularization strategy enhances the quality of solutions in hybrid image reconstruction. This improvement is observed across different values of T, with the most pronounced effect occurring at $T = 20$ s and $\lambda_{L2} = 10^1$, shown in Figure 1c. Despite the improvement, the reconstructions under L2 regularization still exhibit an undesirable level of noise. To address this, we explored the application of a TV regularizer, which outperforms the L2 regularizer in terms of PSNR and SSIM, see Figure 1d and 1e. It results in further improved images, see Figure 1f. Finally, we compare the best QA reconstructions, considering PSNR with no, L2, and TV regularization to conventional FBP reconstruction, see Figure 2. FBP still outperforms all regularized QA reconstructions, even in this simulated setting, where algebraic reconstruction techniques could lead to even better reconstructions.

Our findings suggest that the incorporation of regularization functions into optimization objectives has the potential to enhance the quality of solutions on hybrid QA solvers and reduce noise in the image. At this point it is important to note that the reconstructed image size is inherently limited by the growing matrix size classically. We also did not discuss runtime, projection noise, or the discretized nature of the QA reconstruction, which cannot compete with conventional image reconstruction algorithms currently.

References

1. Flöther FF. The state of quantum computing applications in health and medicine. arXiv preprint arXiv:2301.09106. 2023.
2. Coppersmith D. An approximate fourier transform useful in quantum factoring. arXiv preprint quant-ph/0201067. 2002.
3. Kiani BT, Villanyi A, Lloyd S. Quantum medical imaging algorithms. arXiv preprint arXiv:2004.02036. 2020.
4. Harrow AW, Hassidim A, Lloyd S. Quantum algorithm for linear systems of equations. Phys Rev Lett. 2009;103(15):150502.
5. Aaronson S. Read the fine print. Nat Phys. 2015;11(4):291–3.
6. Chang CC, Gambhir A, Humble TS, Sota S. Quantum annealing for systems of polynomial equations. Sci Rep. 2019;9(1):10258.
7. Borle A, Lomonaco SJ. How viable is quantum annealing for solving linear algebra problems? arXiv preprint arXiv:2206.10576. 2022.
8. Choong HY, Kumar S, Van Gool L. Quantum annealing for single image super-resolution. Proc IEEE CVF. 2023:1150–9.
9. Nau MA, Vija AH, Gohn W, Reymann MP, Maier AK. Exploring the limitations of hybrid adiabatic quantum computing for emission tomography reconstruction. J Imaging. 2023;9(10):221.
10. Jun K. A highly accurate quantum optimization algorithm for CT image reconstruction based on sinogram patterns. Sci Rep. 2023;13(1):14407.
11. Haga A. Quantum annealing-based computed tomography using variational approach for a real-number image reconstruction. arXiv preprint arXiv:2306.02214. 2023.
12. D-Wave. D-Wave Leap. https://cloud.dwavesys.com/leap/. Accessed: 2023-03-01. 2023.
13. Strong D, Chan T. Edge-preserving and scale-dependent properties of total variation regularization. Inverse Probl. 2003;19(6):S165.

Abstract: Deep Learning-based Detection of Vessel Occlusions on CT-Angiography in Patients with Suspected Acute Ischemic Stroke

Gianluca Brugnara[1,2], Michael Baumgartner[3,4,5], Edwin D. Scholze[1,2],
Katerina Deike-Hofmann[4,5], Klaus Kades[3,5], Jonas Scherer[3], Stefan Denner[3,8],
Hagen Meredig[1,2], Aditya Rastogi[1,2], Mustafa A. Mahmutoglu[1,2], Christian Ulfert[1],
Ulf Neuberger[1], Silvia Schönenberger[6], Kai Schlamp[7], Zeynep Bendella[4],
Thomas Pinetz[8], Carsten Schmeel[4,5], Wolfgang Wick[6], Peter A. Ringleb[6],
Ralf Floca[3,9], Markus Möhlenbruch[1], Alexander Radbruch[4,5], Martin Bendszus[1],
Klaus Maier-Hein[3,10], Philipp Vollmuth[1,2,3]

[1]Department of Neuroradiology, Heidelberg University Hospital, Heidelberg (HD)
[2]Section for Computational Neuroimaging, Department of Neuroradiology, Heidelberg
University Hospital, HD
[3]Division of Medical Image Computing, German Cancer Research Center (DKFZ), HD
[4]Department of Neuroradiology, Bonn University Hospital, Bonn
[5]Clinical Neuroimaging Group, German Center for Neurodegenerative Diseases, DZNE, Bonn
[6]Neurology Clinic, Heidelberg University Hospital, Heidelberg
[7]Dep. of Diagnostic and Interventional Radiology with Nuclear Medicine, Thoraxklinik, HD
[8]Institute for Applied Mathematics, University of Bonn
[9]Heidelberg Institute of Radiation Oncology (HIRO), National Center for Radiation Research in
Oncology (NCRO)
[10]Pattern Analysis and Learning Group, Heidelberg University Hospital
philipp.vollmuth@med.uni-heidelberg.de

Swift diagnosis and treatment play a decisive role in the clinical outcome of patients with acute ischemic stroke (AIS), and computer-aided diagnosis (CAD) systems can accelerate the underlying diagnostic processes. Here, we developed an artifical neural network (ANN) which allows automated detection of abnormal vessel findings. Pseudo-prospective external validation was performed in consecutive patients with suspected AIS from 4 different hospitals during a 6-month timeframe and demonstrated high sensitivity ($\geq 87\%$) and negative predictive value ($\geq 93\%$). Benchmarking against two CE- and FDA-approved software solutions showed significantly higher performance for our ANN with improvements of $25–45\%$ for sensitivity and $4–11\%$ for NPV. We provide an imaging platform (https://stroke.neuroAI-HD.org) for online processing of medical imaging data with the developed ANN, including provisions for data crowdsourcing. Notably, this work has previously been published in Nature Communications [1].

References

1. Brugnara G, Baumgartner M, Scholze ED, Deike-Hofmann K, Kades K, Scherer J et al. Deep-learning-based detection of vessel occlusions on CT-angiography in patients with suspected acute ischemic stroke. Nat Commun. 2023;14(1):4938.

Abstract: Cytologic Scoring of Equine Exercise-induced Pulmonary Hemorrhage
Performance of Human Experts and a Deep Learning

Christof A. Bertram[1], Christian Marzahl[2], Alexander Bartel[3], Jason Stayt[4],
Federico Bonsembiante[5], Janet Beeler-Marfisi[6], Ann K. Barton[3], Ginevra Brocca[5],
Maria E. Gelain[5], Agnes Gläsel[7], Kelly du Preez[8], Kristina Weiler[7],
Christiane Weissenbacher-Lang[1], Katharina Breininger[2], Marc Aubreville[9],
Andreas Maier[2], Robert Klopfl/-eisch[3], Jenny Hill[4]

[1]University of Veterinary Medicine Vienna, Vienna, Austria
[2]Friedrich-Alexander-Universität Erlangen-Nürnberg, Erlangen, Germany
[3]Freie Universität Berlin, Berlin, Germany
[4]Novavet Diagnostics, Bayswater, Western Australia
[5]University of Padova, Legnaro, Italy
[6]University of Guelph, Guelph, Ontario, Canada
[7]Justus-Liebig-Universität Giessen, Giessen, Germany
[8]University of Pretoria, Pretoria, South Africa
[9]Technische Hochschule Ingolstadt, Ingolstadt, Germany
christof.bertram@vetmeduni.ac.at

Exercise-induced pulmonary hemorrhage (EIPH) is a common respiratory condition in race horses with negative implications on performance. The gold standard diagnostic method is cytology of bronchoalveolar lavage fluid using the time-consuming total hemosiderin score (THS). For the routine THS, 300 alveolar macrophages are classified into 5 grades based on the amount of intracellular hemosiderin pigment (degradation product of heme iron of red blood cells). Besides the high time investment, there is notable inter-rater variability in assigning hemosiderin grades. Thus automated image analysis is of high interest to improve this diagnostic test. In this study [1] we validated a deep learning-based algorithm (RetinaNet) in 52 whole slide images (WSI) against the performance of 10 experts (each graded 300 cells per case) and a ground truth with labels for all macrophage in the WSI (range: 596 - 8954 macrophages). Compared to the ground truth reference, the algorithm had a diagnostic accuracy of 92.3%, while the 10 experts had an accuracy of 75.5% (range: 63.4 - 92.3%). Automated analysis of a single WSI took on average 1:37 minutes, while experts required an average of 14 minutes for 300 cells. In conclusion, the deep learning-based algorithm has a high diagnostic accuracy and is, therefore, a promising tool to reduce expert labor and to facilitate the routine use of the THS.

References

1. Bertram CA, Marzahl C, Bartel A, Stayt J, Bonsembiante F, Beeler-Marfisi J et al. Cytologic scoring of equine exercise-induced pulmonary hemorrhage: performance of human experts and a deep learning-based algorithm. Vet Pathol. 2023;60.

Abstract: Adaptive Region Selection for Active Learning in Whole Slide Image Semantic Segmentation

Jingna Qiu[1], Frauke Wilm[1,2], Mathias Öttl[2], Maja Schlereth[1], Chang Liu[2],
Tobias Heimann[3], Marc Aubreville[4], Katharina Breininger[1]

[1]Department AI in Biomedical Engineering, FAU Erlangen-Nürnberg, Erlangen, Germany
[2]Pattern Recognition Lab, FAU Erlangen-Nürnberg, Erlangen, Germany
[3]Digital Technology and Innovation, Siemens Healthineers, Erlangen, Germany
[4]Technische Hochschule Ingolstadt, Ingolstadt, Germany
jingna.qiu@fau.de

The annotation of gigapixel-sized whole slide images (WSI) in digital pathology can be time-intensive, especially when generating annotations for training deep segmentation models. Instead of requesting annotations for the full WSI, region-based active learning (AL) allows to specify selected regions for annotation in an iterative process, reducing annotation while maintaining segmentation performance. Existing methods for section selection on WSI evaluate the informativeness of a quadratic grid of a predefined size of $l \times l$ pixels according to a suitable informativeness criterion and then select the k most informative regions. Our experiments show that the benefit of this method strongly depends on the choice of these two hyperparameters, i.e., the AL step size, and that a suboptimal AL step size can result in uninformative or redundant annotation requests [1]. We evaluate our approach on the publicly available CAMELYON16 dataset and show that it consistently achieves higher sampling efficiency measured by annotated area compared to the reference approach across various AL step sizes. With only 2.6% of tissue area annotated, we achieve the same performance compared to a full annotation setting and thereby substantially reduce the costs of annotating a WSI dataset for the task of segmentation. Our approach can in theory be applied with any informativeness measure, with future work looking closer into an improved characterization of annotation effort. The source code is available at https://github.com/DeepMicroscopy/AdaptiveRegionSelection.

References

1. Qiu J, Wilm F, Öttl M, Schlereth M, Liu C, Heimann T et al. Adaptive region selection for active learning in whole slide image semantic segmentation. Proc MICCAI. Springer Nature Switzerland, 2023:90–100.

© Der/die Autor(en), exklusiv lizenziert an
Springer Fachmedien Wiesbaden GmbH, ein Teil von Springer Nature 2024
A. Maier et al. (Hrsg.), *Bildverarbeitung für die Medizin 2024*,
Informatik aktuell, https://doi.org/10.1007/978-3-658-44037-4_6

Abstract: Flexible Unfolding of Circular Structures for Rendering Textbook-style Cerebrovascular Maps

Leonhard Rist[1,2], Oliver Taubmann[2], Hendrik Ditt[2], Michael Sühling[2], Andreas Maier[1]

[1]Friedrich-Alexander-Universität Erlangen-Nürnberg, Erlangen, Germany
[2]CT R&D Image Analytics, Siemens Healthineers, Forchheim, Germany
leonhard.rist@fau.de

Comprehensive, contiguous visualizations of the main cerebral arteries and the surrounding parenchyma offer considerable potential for improving diagnostic workflows in cerebrovascular disease. Instead of manually navigating through Computer Tomography Angiography volumes, e.g. in time-critical stroke assessment, a 2D overview would allow for rapid examination of vascular topology and lumen. Unfolding the brain vasculature into a 2D vessel map is, however, infeasible using the common Curved Planar Reformation (CPR) due to the circular structure of the Circle of Willis (CoW). Additionally, the spatial configuration of the vessels typically renders them unsuitable for mapping onto simple geometric primitives. We propose CeVasMap [1], a flexible mesh-based solution for mapping multiple vascular structures, including circular ones, and their surroundings into a two-dimensional representation. It extends the As-Rigid-As-Possible (ARAP) deformation algorithm by a smart initialization of the required 3D readout mesh which is fitted to the CoW. Depending on the resulting degree of distortion, it is also possible to merge neighboring arteries directly into the same view. In cases of high distortion, these neighboring vessels are instead unfolded individually and attached to the main structure, creating a textbook-style overview image. An extensive distortion analysis is provided respectively for each vessel, comparing global and local gradient norms of the 2D-3D vector field of individual and merged unfoldings with their CPR representations. In addition to enabling the unfolding of circular structures and allowing more realistic curvature preservation, our method is on par in terms of incurred distortions to optimally oriented CPRs for individual vessel unfoldings and comparable to unfavorable CPR orientations when merging the complete CoW with a median distortion of 65 µm/mm. Compared to row-wise constant distortion in CPR, unfolding with CeVasMap results in a high ratio of distortion-free image parts whereas the occurring distortions are close to the centerlines.

References

1. Rist L, Taubmann O, Ditt H, Sühling M, Maier A. Flexible unfolding of circular structures for rendering textbook-style cerebrovascular maps. Proc MICCAI. 2023:737–46.

Springer Fachmedien Wiesbaden GmbH, ein Teil von Springer Nature 2024
A. Maier et al. (Hrsg.), *Bildverarbeitung für die Medizin 2024*,
Informatik aktuell, https://doi.org/10.1007/978-3-658-44037-4_7

Attention-guided Erasing

Novel Augmentation Method for Enhancing Downstream Breast Density Classification

Adarsh Bhandary Panambur[1,2], Hui Yu[2], Sheethal Bhat[1,2], Prathmesh Madhu[2],
Siming Bayer[1,2], Andreas Maier[2]

[1]Siemens Healthineers, Erlangen, Germany
[2]Pattern Recognition Lab, FAU Erlangen-Nürnberg, Erlangen, Germany
adarsh.bhandary.panambur@fau.de

Abstract. The assessment of breast density is crucial in the context of breast cancer screening, especially in populations with a higher percentage of dense breast tissues. This study introduces a novel data augmentation technique termed attention-guided erasing (AGE), devised to enhance the downstream classification of four distinct breast density categories in mammography following the BI-RADS recommendation in the Vietnamese cohort. The proposed method integrates supplementary information during transfer learning, utilizing visual attention maps derived from a vision transformer backbone trained using the self-supervised DINO method. These maps are utilized to erase background regions in the mammogram images, unveiling only the potential areas of dense breast tissues to the network. Through the incorporation of AGE during transfer learning with varying random probabilities, we consistently surpass classification performance compared to scenarios without AGE and the traditional random erasing transformation. We validate our methodology using the publicly available VinDr-Mammo dataset. Specifically, we attain a mean F1-score of 0.5910, outperforming values of 0.5594 and 0.5691 corresponding to scenarios without AGE and with random erasing (RE), respectively. This superiority is further substantiated by t-tests, revealing a p-value of $p<0.0001$, underscoring the statistical significance of our approach.

1 Introduction

With an estimated occurrence of 2.3 million cases worldwide each year, breast cancer stands as the most prevalent form of cancer among the adult population [1]. The screening of patients for cancer is conducted through gold-standard mammography. Breast density, denoting the quantity of fibroglandular tissue in the breast, is known to be linked with the risk of breast cancer. Following the breast imaging reporting and database system (BI-RADS) scoring system [2], breast density is categorized into four groups from A to D. Breast density A designates almost entirely fatty breast tissue, B corresponds to scattered fibroglandular tissues, C indicates heterogeneously dense tissue, and D denotes extremely dense tissue, as outlined by the BI-RADS classification [2]. In certain Asian populations such as Vietnam, women are recognized to exhibit dense breasts, a factor that is indicative of a higher risk of breast cancer [3]. This may also influence the screening performance of radiologists, as higher breast density can

© Der/die Autor(en), exklusiv lizenziert an
Springer Fachmedien Wiesbaden GmbH, ein Teil von Springer Nature 2024
A. Maier et al. (Hrsg.), *Bildverarbeitung für die Medizin 2024*,
Informatik aktuell, https://doi.org/10.1007/978-3-658-44037-4_8

Tab. 1. Class sample distribution in VinDr-Mammo dataset for breast density classification [9].

	Breast Density A	Breast Density B	Breast Density C	Breast Density D
Training	72	1,308	10,366	1,854
Validation	8	220	1,866	306
Test	20	380	3,060	540
Total	100	1,908	15,292	2,700

also result in obscuring of underlying lesions in the mammography images, resulting in decreased mammographic sensitivity. With the increase in the population eligible for mammographic screening, automated methods can support streamlining the radiologists' workflow. The methods for automated breast density assessment primarily involve traditional volumetric methodology [4], machine learning and deep learning-based approaches [5]. However, only a few research works have explored the task of automatically classifying breast density in populations with a very high percentage of individuals with extremely dense breasts, such as in Vietnam [6]. In this study, our goal is to classify breast density in mammogram images using a dataset from a Vietnamese screening population. Traditional deep learning methods typically employ separate networks to segment the background tissue or pectoralis muscle, especially in the case of mediolateral oblique (MLO) views at the pixel level, and subsequently classify the tissue into different density categories [7]. However, these methods rely on high-quality annotations provided either by radiologists or through traditional image processing techniques. Self-supervised learning (SSL) aims to learn robust lower-dimensional representations of images without using class information and has proven successful for downstream tasks such as classification. Recently proposed SSL techniques, leveraging vision transformers (ViT), have demonstrated robust localization capabilities [8].

In this work, we propose a novel data augmentation method called attention-guided erasing (AGE). AGE utilizes attention head visualizations extracted from a self-supervised ViT backbone trained using the DINO method [8]. These visualizations weakly localize the dense parts of the breast tissue. The generated maps are then employed to erase background regions, revealing only potential regions of dense breast tissues for the network to analyze. The proposed augmentation technique is specifically designed for use during the downstream transfer learning task of breast density classification. The main contributions of our research are as follows: (a) We introduce a novel augmentation technique called AGE for breast density classification in mammogram images, validated utilizing the VinDr-Mammo dataset [9]. (b) We conduct extensive quantitative experiments, comparing the results with the traditionally used random erasing (RE) augmentation. Our findings demonstrate significant improvements when employing the AGE augmentation with varying random probabilities during training. (c) We present state-of-the-art results on the VinDr-Mammo test dataset [9]. The paper is structured with Section 2 providing an overview of the data and methods, and Section 3 presenting the quantitative outcomes for breast density classification, along with an analysis and discussion of these results.

2   Materials and methods

2.1   Data

We utilize the publicly available VinDr-Mammo dataset, which comprises full-field digital mammography images obtained from Hospital 108 and Hanoi Medical University Hospital in Hanoi, Vietnam [9]. The dataset includes 20,000 images acquired from 5,000 patients, encompassing both craniocaudal (CC) and MLO views from both the right and left breasts of each patient. Three experienced radiologists reached a consensus in analyzing the dataset to annotate the BI-RADS and breast density [2]. The distribution of class samples utilized in this work is depicted in Table 1. We employed the original distribution of the training set released by the authors of VinDr-Mammo [9] to split the training and validation datasets. The patient-level split ensures equal class distribution and accounts for the variety of mammography systems used in data acquisition. We reused the original test split. In total, the training, validation, and test datasets consist of 13,600, 2,400, and 4,000 images, respectively.

2.2   Methodology

Figure 1 shows an overview of the proposed methodology. We use the training dataset to train a ViT based on the DINO self-supervised pretraining method [8]. Subsequently, we use the trained backbone to extract visualizations from the six attention heads of the pretrained backbone. We select the best attention head that potentially localizes dense breast tissue and then erase the background regions around the weakly localized breast tissue. This process is intended to encourage the network to focus more on the dense tissue than the surrounding regions in the breast during transfer learning. In order to train a robust backbone with localization capability for our classification network, we perform self-supervised pretraining on the VinDR-Mammo training dataset using the

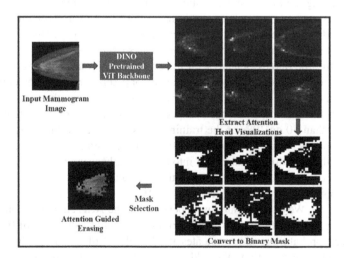

Fig. 1. Overview of the proposed methodology for the attention-guided erasing (AGE).

Tab. 2. Classification performance on the VinDr-Mammo test dataset. P indicates the probability of erasing augmentations on the inputs during training.

Model	Macro F1-Score
ResNet-34 [6]	0.504
EfficientNet-B2 [6]	0.5525
DINO (No Erasing)	0.5594 (0.026)
DINO (RE, $P = 0.2$)	0.5691 (0.020)
DINO (AGE, $P = 0.6$)	*0.5910 (0.017)*
DINO (RE, P = 0.2)	0.5691 (0.020)
DINO (AGE, P = 0.6)	0.5910 (0.017)

DINO method [8]. DINO employs a knowledge distillation approach where a student network learns to predict the teacher network outputs by utilizing a cross-entropy loss to match the softmax probabilities of the student and teacher outputs [8]. Two views consisting of different random transformations of the input image are fed into the same architecture-based student and teacher networks with different parameters [8]. The exponential moving average of the student network's parameters is used to update the teacher network to avoid the model collapse [8]. We reuse the implementation as suggested in the original work in this stage, including the ImageNet pretrained DeiT-small ViT and the standard set of randomly applied data augmentations including horizontal flip, colour jitter, gaussian blur, and solarization [8]. For input preparation, a random resized crop was applied at both global (0.4, 1.0) and local scales (0.05, 0.4) to the 224×224 resolution of the full-resolution mammogram image, with a patch size of 16 serving as the input to the network [8]. During pretraining, we employed a modest batch size of 32 to conform to the limitations of single GPU memory, leveraging a Quadro RTX 5000. The networks were trained for 300 epochs to facilitate thorough learning, with the final model being saved at the point of least training loss [8].

After training the model in a self-supervised manner, we analyze the self-attention exhibited by six attention heads focused on the [CLS] token in the final layer. Visual inspection indicated that each attention head concentrated on a distinct region of the image. By analyzing the activation patterns of these attention heads, we were able to weakly identify the one associated with breast density. In our study, we hypothesized that the attention head with activations, typically for pixels numbering fewer than 50 but not exclusively, is likely representative of breast tissue. This hypothesis was formulated by analyzing the maximum number of pixel counts in each of the attention heads, which is less than 50 on 10% of the training dataset. Based on this analysis, the sixth attention head was selected which mostly concentrates on the dense breast tissue. We then convert the attention visualization into binary masks using thresholding. Based on the binary mask, erasing is employed for the surrounding regions around the weakly localized dense tissues, a strategy termed the AGE data augmentation during transfer learning (Fig. 1). We experimented with performing the AGE augmentation during the downstream transfer learning task with various probability values (P) of 0.2, 0.4, 0.6, and 0.8. The probability value indicates the likelihood of an image during training undergoing the augmentation. We added a classification layer on top of the DINO

Tab. 3. Comparison of RE and AGE at different probabilities using mean and standard deviations (in brackets) of the Macro F1-scores. The best results are in *italics*.

Random Probability	Random Erasing	Attention-Guided Erasing (Ours)
$P = 0.2$	0.5691 (0.020)	0.5774 (0.024)
$P = 0.4$	0.5617 (0.034)*	0.5731 (0.017)
$P = 0.6$	0.5522 (0.014)*	*0.5910 (0.017)*
$P = 0.8$	0.5503 (0.009)*	0.5747 (0.025)

pretrained DeiT-small ViT for the four-class classification task. All experiments were trained for 50 epochs with a batch size of 8 and early stopping. A binary cross-entropy loss function was optimized using a standard Adam optimizer with a learning rate of $5e^{-6}$ and a weight decay of $1e^{-4}$. We utilized a standard set of data augmentations as reported in [10].

3 Results and discussion

Table 2 presents the classification performance using the mean macro F1-scores on the test dataset computed over five runs. We use the macro F1-score reported in [6] for comparison, where the authors achieve scores of 0.504 and 0.5525 using single-view ResNet-34 and EfficientNet-B2, respectively. In comparison, DINO-based transfer learning without any erasing augmentation achieves a mean F1-score of 0.5594. We then experiment by adding RE [11] and AGE augmentations ($P = 0.2, 0.4, 0.6$ and 0.8). We observe an increase of almost 1% with a score of 0.5691 when using the RE augmentation with a P value of 0.2. With the motivation to keep the class-specific features intact while erasing the background regions, we use our proposed AGE augmentation with various random probabilities. We observe a significant gain of more than 3.5% in mean macro F1-score while using AGE compared to not using the AGE augmentation. We achieve a mean macro F1-score of 0.5910 in comparison to 0.5594 (No erasing) and 0.5691 (RE). This increase in gain suggests that AGE provides a better diversity of transformations during training, resulting in a more robust classification backbone. Particularly, AGE method improved mean F1-scores for densities A (0.0847 to 0.2158) and B (0.6566 to 0.6684), while it slightly reduced the scores for densities C (0.8672 to 0.8610) and D (0.6290 to 0.6187) compared to the baseline model with no erasing. Moreover, we observe increased stability in the reported standard deviations (Tab. 2), indicating a regularization effect while using the proposed AGE augmentation. We also employ a two-tailed unpaired t-test to assess the statistical significance of the classification performances. We achieve a p-value of $p<0.0001$ emphasizing the statistical significance of our AGE approach. Table 3 further depicts the ablation study with mean macro F1 scores for each of the probability values for RE and AGE augmentations. The asterisk represents statistically worse results than the best method. It can be seen that the AGE augmentation consistently outperforms the classification performance of models trained without erasing and with RE. This is indicative of the fact that only the breast tissue is the class representative feature for density estimation, and the background regions of the breast can impact the classification performance. For example, the presence of pectoralis muscle and dense skin folds in MLO views, and the presence of suspicious regions of interest near the skin surface can potentially result in difficulty in the classification of breast density, especially in the case of high-class imbalance observed due to the higher percentage of dense breasts in the Vietnamese cohort. In the case of RE, we observe consistent performance drops, potentially due to erasing the class-relevant features in the majority of training samples with increasing probabilities. In future work, we aim to perform a comprehensive ablation study to investigate the impact of various data augmentation strategies in combination with AGE for breast density estimation. Furthermore, we plan to use AGE for other medical imaging modalities to check its generalization capabilities to more complex classification problems.

Disclaimer. The methods described in this paper are currently not available for commercial use, and there is no assurance of their future availability.

References

1. Sung H, Ferlay J, Siegel RL, Laversanne M, Soerjomataram I, Jemal A et al. Global cancer statistics 2020: GLOBOCAN estimates of incidence and mortality worldwide for 36 cancers in 185 countries. CA Cancer J Clin. 2021;71(3):209–49.
2. Sickles EA, D'Orsi CJ, Bassett LW et al. ACR BI-RADS® Mammography. ACR BI-RADS® Atlas, Breast Imaging Reporting and Data System. Reston, VA, American College of Radiology, 2013:121–40.
3. Trieu PDY, Mello-Thoms C, Peat JK, Do TD, Brennan PC. Risk factors of female breast cancer in Vietnam: a case-control study. Cancer Res Treat. 2017;49(4):990–1000.
4. Brandt KR, Scott CG, Ma L, Mahmoudzadeh AP, Jensen MR, Whaley DH et al. Comparison of clinical and automated breast density measurements: implications for risk prediction and supplemental screening. Radiology. 2016;279(3):710–9.
5. Gardezi SJS, Elazab A, Lei B, Wang T. Breast cancer detection and diagnosis using mammographic data: systematic review. J Med Internet Res. 2019;21(7):e14464.
6. Nguyen HTX, Tran SB, Nguyen DB, Pham HH, Nguyen HQ. A novel multi-view deep learning approach for BI-RADS and density assessment of mammograms. IEEE EMBC. 2022:2144–8.
7. Maghsoudi OH, Gastounioti A, Scott C, Pantalone L, Wu FF, Cohen EA et al. Deep-LIBRA: an artificial-intelligence method for robust quantification of breast density with independent validation in breast cancer risk assessment. Med Image Anal. 2021;73:102138.
8. Caron M, Touvron H, Misra I, Jégou H, Mairal J, Bojanowski P et al. Emerging properties in self-supervised vision transformers. Proc ICCV. 2021.
9. Nguyen HT, Nguyen HQ, Pham HH, Lam K, Le LT, Dao M et al. VinDr-Mammo: a large-scale benchmark dataset for computer-aided diagnosis in full-field digital mammography. Sci Data. 2023;10(1):277.
10. Panambur AB, Madhu P, Maier A. Effect of random histogram equalization on breast calcification analysis using deep learning. Proc BVM. Springer. 2022:173–8.
11. Zhong Z, Zheng L, Kang G, Li S, Yang Y. Proc AAAI. Vol. 34. (07). 2020:13001–8.

Appearance-based Debiasing of Deep Learning Models in Medical Imaging

Frauke Wilm[1,2], Marcel Reimann[1,3], Oliver Taubmann[3], Alexander Mühlberg[3],
Katharina Breininger[1]

[1]Department Artificial Intelligence in Biomedical Engineering, Friedrich-Alexander-Universität
Erlangen-Nürnberg, Germany
[2]Pattern Recognition Lab, Friedrich-Alexander-Universität Erlangen-Nünberg, Germany
[3]CT R&D Image Analytics, Siemens Healthineers, Forchheim, Germany
reimann.marcel@outlook.com

Abstract. Out-of-distribution data can substantially impede the performance of deep learning models. In medical imaging, domain shifts can, for instance, be caused by different image acquisition protocols. To address these domain shifts, domain adversarial training can be employed to constrain a model to domain-agnostic features. This, however, requires prior knowledge about the domain variable, which might not always be accessible. Recent approaches make use of control regions to guide the training process and thereby alleviate the need for prior domain knowledge. In this work, we combine these approaches with traditional domain adversarial training to exploit the benefits of both methods. We test the proposed method on two medical datasets and demonstrate performance increases of up to 10 %, compared to a baseline trained without debiasing.

1 Introduction

Deep learning-based image analysis algorithms have demonstrated outstanding performance for many clinical applications, often reaching the performance of trained medical experts [1]. However, their performance can substantially be affected by out-of-distribution (OOD) data. These OOD data can, for instance, originate from different hospitals with different image acquisition systems or from changing the imaging protocol within one hospital. If the origin of this domain shift is known, measures to compensate for this known bias can already be undertaken during model development. Domain adversarial training [2], for instance, has previously demonstrated good performance for medical image segmentation in the presence of domain shifts introduced during image acquisition [3]. Most of these approaches require the bias to be known before model development. Some variables, however, can manifest as unknown biases, e. g., patient anatomy or scanner calibration [4]. Previous work by Langer et al. [5] has made use of so-called control region (CR) to mitigate these unknown biases. These CRs were selected based on their information content. The idea was to select scan regions that do not carry any task-related biological information but capture potential technical variations. For standard computed tomography (CT) scans, this could, e. g., be air in the periphery of the scanned volume. The authors showed that the robustness against domain shifts could be increased by dropping highly correlated activations from the embedded features of the original samples and the embedding of the extracted CRs. In this work, we build upon the work of Langer et al. [5] and combine the proposed appearance-based debiasing with advanced training methods, i. e., domain adversarial training [2], to best utilize the benefits of both methods. We alleviate the need for explicitly knowing the domain label by extracting PyRadiomics [6] features of the control region as a domain proxy and re-formulating the adversarial task as a domain regression.

2 Materials and methods

For this work, two medical datasets were utilized, focusing on technical variations in the context of two imaging modalities-CT and histopathology.

2.1 CT-COPD dataset

The first dataset comprises a subset of a non-public dataset on chronic obstructive pulmonary disease (COPD), presented at the Annual Meeting of Radiological Society of North America (RSNA) in 2018 [7]. The dataset contains volumetric CT scans of 827 patients with a random patient-level split into training, validation, and testing folds (495:166:166). According to the medical records, a third of the patients was diagnosed with the presence of centrilobular emphysema (CLE), which was used as a class label for the prediction task (CLE vs. non-CLE). The study received approval from the local ethics committee. No informed consent was required, as the CT images were acquired during routine clinical examination. For each patient, two reconstructions (B157d3 and Br36d3) were considered, resulting in a total of 1,654 scans. All reconstructed volumes were pre-processed following the work of Langer et al. [5]. Using a pre-trained segmentation algorithm, lung masks were extracted for each volume. Afterward, five evenly-spaced concentric image slices of size 192×192 pixels were extracted around each lung lobe. Random flipping and translations were applied with a probability of 0.1, before center-cropping the volumes to spatial dimensions of 128×128. To ensure comparability across the scans, all slices were normalized to a value range close to $[0, 1]$ by dividing them by 3,072 (a value empirically defined by Langer et al. [5]).

2.2 MS-SCC dataset

The second dataset comprises a multi-scanner histopathology dataset, published by Wilm et al. [8]. The dataset is composed of 44 canine tissue samples with a random patient-level split into training, validation, and testing folds (30:5:9). Each sample was digitized with five different scanning systems, but to simplify the bias experiments (Sec. 2.3) only four scanning systems were selected for this work (Leica Aperio ScanScope CS2, Hamamatsu NanoZoomer S210, Hamamatsu NanoZoomer 2.0-HT, Leica Aperio GT450). From each whole slide image (WSI), seven tumor and seven non-tumor patches (128×128 pixels) were sampled, guided by the annotation database. In total, this resulted in 2,464 patches (44 WSIs $\times$ 14 patches $\times$ four scanners).

2.3 Bias experiments

Figure 1 illustrates the dataset composition for modeling different biases for the CT-COPD dataset. All dataset compositions retained the same ratio of CLE ($\sim 1/3$) and non-CLE patients ($\sim 2/3$). In the balanced training setup, half of the CLE scans were reconstructed with the Br36d3 kernel and the other half with the Bl57d3 kernel. The same applied to the non-CLE scans. For the biased training set, the majority of CLE scans were reconstructed with the Br36d3 kernel, whereas the majority of non-CLE with the Bl57d3 kernel. The validation and test set remained balanced.

2.4 Appearance-based domain adversarial debiasing using control regions

Figure 2 visualizes the proposed architecture of the domain adversarial training setups using a domain vector derived from the selected CRs. First, the region of interest (ROI) containing the biologically relevant information was encoded using a standard encoder architecture. The embedded features were passed through two network heads—one for predicting the medical class label and one for regressing a domain vector. By using a gradient reversal layer in between the encoder and the domain regressor, the network could be trained in an adversarial fashion, i. e., to extract features that impede the domain prediction and are thereby more domain-invariant. Instead of using the domain label and training the domain adversarial branch with a classification-based loss, we derived a domain vector from the CR and designed the prediction task as a domain regression. Thereby, the architecture could be trained solely appearance-based without explicit knowledge of the target domain label. For the ground-truth domain vector, we computed the PyRadiomics [6] features of the CRs and scaled them to unit variance. Using a two-tailed t-test for the CT-COPD dataset and a one-way ANOVA for the histopathology dataset, the PyRadiomics features were evaluated for significant differences between the kernel or scanner domains, and the domain vector was defined by selecting 20 significant features ($p \ll 0.05$). We compared the proposed method to three training setups: a baseline trained without debiasing (baseline), standard domain adversarial training with the known domain label (adversarial), and the DecorreLayer presented by Langer et al. [5] (decorrel). For each method, automatic hyperparameter optimization was used for tuning the optimizer, learning rate, weight decay, and momentum.

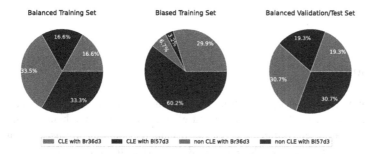

Fig. 1. Dataset compositions for bias modeling, illustrated for the CT-COPD dataset. The biased training set introduces a bias towards the Br36d3 reconstruction kernel for CLE patients.

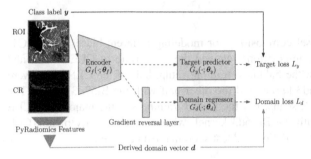

Fig. 2. Architecture for appearance-based domain adversarial training using a region of interest (ROI) and a control region (CR) to derive the domain vector. For better visualization, ROI and CR are displayed using a linear window with a width of 1500 HU, centered at -300 HU.

2.5 Control region selection

For the CT-COPD dataset, the control region was selected as patches of air close to the selected ROI and at the same z-axis positions as the sampled image slices. This definition follows the original implementation by Langer et al. [5]. For the MS-SCC dataset, a similar approach was followed by placing the control region outside of the tissue sample on the white slide background. However, an intermediate analysis of different background regions on the same slide revealed color shifts between the regions, potentially due to different lighting conditions or out-of-focus artifacts. Therefore we decided to partition the WSI into six equally sized areas and randomly select a background patch from each area. The concatenated background patches were then converted to grayscale to enable the use of PyRadiomics for feature extraction.

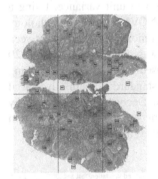

Fig. 3. Patch selection for MS-SCC dataset. Red patches correspond to tumor tissue, green patches to non-tumor tissue, and blue patches were used as control regions (CRs). For CR extraction, the slide was partitioned into six parts to compensate for non-homogeneous lightning conditions across the slide. Patches are indexed based on a grid.

3 Results

During hyperparameter optimization, we used the validation splits to evaluate the performance difference when training the baseline architecture on a balanced training set compared to a biased training set. For performance evaluation, we used the area under the receiver operating characteristic (AUROC). When training on the balanced subset of the CT-COPD dataset, the model achieved a maximum validation AUROC of 0.80, compared to a maximum AUROC of 0.76 for the biased training set. On the MS-SCC dataset, the balanced training resulted in a maximum class-averaged validation AUROC of 0.84 compared to 0.76 for the biased training.

Table 1 summarizes the test performance for all tested architectures and both datasets, achieved by the best hyperparameter configuration optimized on the validation set. All values are reported as AUROC on the balanced test set when training on the biased training set. For the CT-COPD dataset, the standard adversarial training with a known class label achieved the best performance with a maximum AUROC of 0.80. For the MS-SCC dataset, the proposed appearance-based debiasing method with multiple CRs achieved the highest performance with a class-averaged AUROC of 0.79. After testing, we used the CT-COPD dataset for preliminary experiments for hyperparameter robustness. For these experiments, we varied the learning rate and weight decay on a logarithmic scale around the optimally found values (factors 0.1, 0.5, 1, 2, and 10) and measured the median performance of all approaches (reported in parentheses in Tab. 1).

	CT-COPD	MS-SCC
baseline	0.79 (0.71)	0.69
adversarial	0.80 (0.76)	0.77
decorrel (single CR)	0.77 (0.70)	0.68
decorrel (multi CRs)	-	0.71
ours (single CR)	0.79 (0.72)	-
ours (multi CRs)	-	0.79

Tab. 1. Area under the receiver operating characteristic (AUROC) on the balanced test set. *Ours* refers to the proposed appearance-based adversarial debiasing, with a single control region (CR) for the CT-COPD dataset and additionally multiple CRs for the MS-SCC dataset. Values in parenthesis report the median performance when changing the optimally found hyperparameters to test for hyperparameter robustness.

4 Discussion and outlook

The presented work proposed a debiasing technique that combines traditional adversarial debiasing with appearance-based methods, utilizing control regions. When comparing the performance of the baseline trained on the balanced dataset to the unbalanced dataset, the hidden bias resulted in a performance decrease of 4 % on the CT-COPD dataset and 8 % on the MS-SCC dataset. Contrary to previous results by Langer et al. [5], our baseline trained without debiasing achieved good results for the CT-COPD dataset, suggesting no substantial benefits for any of the debiasing methods. For the experiments presented in this work, however, we used extensive hyperparameter tuning to optimize all architectures and used a balanced validation set for model selection. Our preliminary experiments on hyperparameter robustness demonstrated a substantially higher robustness of the adversarial debiasing, compared to our baseline (median performances of 0.76 and 0.71). Future work could further study these effects, given a non-balanced validation set. On the MS-SCC dataset, the traditional adversarial debiasing with a known domain label did not perform as well. This could be related to the increased number of domains (four scanners), which makes the optimization task more difficult. For the MS-SCC dataset, the proposed appearance-based debiasing with multiple CRs outperformed all other debiasing methods with a maximum class-averaged AUROC of

0.79. Furthermore, using multiple CRs benefited the model in the DecorreLayer setting, which is assumed to be related to uneven illumination across the WSI. Compared to the traditional adversarial debiasing, the proposed method is independent of a known domain label. The use of control regions facilitates debiasing against hidden biases, which can extend beyond technical variations that are introduced by acquisition parameters, e. g., patient anatomy, or demographics. Additional experiments on modeling various bias strengths did not show relevant changes in the performance of the evaluated architectures and are therefore not reported here. A current limitation of the proposed method is the use of PyRadiomics features to generate the domain vector. For simplicity, the domain vector has been limited to 20 PyRadiomics features that exhibited significant differences between the domains. This approach cannot be followed when the domain label is unknown. This limitation could be addressed by training an autoencoder to extract the domain vector from the CR, or by directly replacing the domain regressor with a decoder that reconstructs the CR. The domain adversarial branch could then be trained using a structural similarity loss. First experiments along these lines have been conducted but did not yet exhibit robust training curves and will therefore be considered ground for future work.

Acknowledgement. K. Breininger gratefully acknowledges support by d.hip campus - Bavarian aim in form of a faculty endowment. F. Wilm and K. Breininger acknowledge support by the Deutsche Forschungsgemeinschaft (DFG, German Research Foundation) project number 460333672–CRC 1540 Exploring Brain Mechanics (subproject X02).

References

1. Aubreville M, Bertram CA, Marzahl C, Gurtner C, Dettwiler M, Schmidt A et al. Deep learning algorithms out-perform veterinary pathologists in detecting the mitotically most active tumor region. Sci Rep. 2020;10(1):16447.
2. Ganin Y, Ustinova E, Ajakan H, Germain P, Larochelle H, Laviolette F et al. Domain-adversarial training of neural networks. J Mach Learn Res. 2016;17(59):1–35.
3. Wilm F, Marzahl C, Breininger K, Aubreville M. Domain adversarial RetinaNet as a reference algorithm for the mitosis domain generalization challenge. Proc MICCAI. 2022:5–13.
4. Mühlberg A, Katzmann A, Heinemann V, Kärgel R, Wels M, Taubmann O et al. The technome-a predictive internal calibration approach for quantitative imaging biomarker research. Sci Rep. 2020;10(1):1103.
5. Langer S, Taubmann O, Denzinger F, Maier A, Mühlberg A. Mitigating unknown bias in deep learning-based assessment of CT images deep technome. Proc BVM. 2023:177–82.
6. Van Griethuysen JJ, Fedorov A, Parmar C, Hosny A, Aucoin N, Narayan V et al. Computational radiomics system to decode the radiographic phenotype. Cancer Res. 2017;77(21):e104–e107.
7. Remy-Jardin MJ, Kaergel R, Suehling M, Faivre JB, Flohr TG, Remy J. Detection and phenotyping of emphysema using a new machine learning method. Proc RSNA. 2018.
8. Wilm F, Fragoso M, Bertram CA, Stathonikos N, Öttl M, Qiu J et al. Multi-scanner canine cutaneous squamous cell carcinoma histopathology dataset. Proc BVM. 2023:206–11.

Abstract: Interpretable Medical Image Classification Using Prototype Learning and Privileged Information

Luisa Gallée[1], Meinrad Beer[2], Michael Götz[1,3]

[1]Experimental Radiology, University Hospital Ulm, Ulm, Germany
[2]Department of Diagnostic and Interventional Radiology, University Hospital Ulm, Ulm, Germany
[3]i2SoUl - Innovative Imaging in Surgical Oncology Ulm, University Hospital Ulm, Ulm, Germany
luisa.gallee@uni-ulm.de

Interpretability is often an essential requirement in medical imaging. Advanced deep learning methods are required to address this need for explainability and high performance. In this work, we investigate whether additional information available during the training process can be used to create an understandable and powerful model. We propose an innovative solution called Proto-Caps that leverages the benefits of capsule networks, prototype learning, and the use of privileged information [1]. This hierarchical architecture establishes a basis for inherent interpretability. The capsule layers allow for mapping human-defined visual attributes onto the encapsulated representation of the high-level features. Furthermore, an active prototype learning algorithm incorporates even more interpretability. As a result, Proto-Caps provides case-based reasoning with attribute-specific prototypes. Applied to the LIDC-IDRI dataset [2], Proto-Caps predicts the malignancy of lung nodules and also provides prototypical samples that are similar in regards to the nodules' spiculation, calcification, and six more visual features. Besides the additional interpretability, the proposed solution shows an above state-of-the-art prediction performance. Compared to the explainable baseline model, our method achieves more than 6 % higher accuracy in predicting both malignancy (93.0 %) and mean characteristic features of lung nodules. Relatively good results can be also achieved when using only 1 % of the attribute labels during the training. This result motivates further research as it shows that with Proto-Caps it only requires a few additional annotations of human-defined attributes resulting in an interpretable decision-making process. The code is publicly available at https://github.com/XRad-Ulm/Proto-Caps.

References

1. Gallée L, Beer M, Götz M. Interpretable medical image classification using prototype learning and privileged information. Int Conf on Medl Image Comput and Comput-Assist Interv. Springer. 2023:435–45.
2. Armato III SG, McLennan G, Bidaut L, McNitt-Gray MF, Meyer CR, Reeves AP et al. Data from LIDC-IDRI. The Cancer Imaging Arch. 2015. [Data set].

© Der/die Autor(en), exklusiv lizenziert an
Springer Fachmedien Wiesbaden GmbH, ein Teil von Springer Nature 2024
A. Maier et al. (Hrsg.), *Bildverarbeitung für die Medizin 2024*,
Informatik aktuell, https://doi.org/10.1007/978-3-658-44037-4_10

Abstract: Robust Multi-contrast MRI Denoising using Trainable Bilateral Filters without Noise-free Targets

Laura Pfaff[1,2], Fabian Wagner[1], Julian Hossbach[1,2], Elisabeth Preuhs[2], Mareike Thies[1], Felix Denzinger[1,2], Dominik Nickel[2], Tobias Wuerfl[2], Andreas Maier[1]

[1]Pattern Recognition Lab, Friedrich-Alexander-Universität, Erlangen-Nürnberg, Germany
[2]Siemens Healthineers AG, Erlangen, Germany
laura.pfaff@fau.de

Magnetic resonance imaging (MRI) is widely acknowledged as one of the most diagnostically valuable and versatile medical imaging techniques available today, characterized by its exceptional soft tissue contrast, the absence of ionizing radiation, and the capability to acquire multiple different image contrasts. However, low signal-to-noise ratio (SNR) is a common challenge, particularly in low-field MRI scans, leading to reduced image quality and impaired diagnostic value. The effectiveness of traditional denoising methods, such as bilateral filters (BFs), heavily relies on the choice of hyperparameters. In contrast, deep learning approaches like convolutional neural networks (CNNs) are computationally demanding, require paired noisy and noise-free data for supervised learning, and often struggle to generalize to different magnetic resonance (MR) image contrasts. To bridge the gap between traditional denoising methods and deep learning, we employ a novel approach that combines a neural network comprised of trainable BF layers. This network is trained using an extended version of Stein's unbiased risk estimator (SURE) as a self-supervised loss function, which estimates the mean squared error (MSE) between the denoised image and the unknown noise-free ground truth by incorporating a noise level map [1]. Our experiments demonstrate the effectiveness of our self-supervised approach, with the BF network outperforming the CNN by 14.7% in terms of peak signal-to-noise ratio (PSNR) when tested on unseen MR image contrasts. In conclusion, our research introduces a novel approach to address noise reduction challenges in MRI, particularly in low-SNR scenarios and across different MR image contrasts. The combination of trainable BF layers and SURE-based model supervision holds potential for future research in medical imaging, as it eliminates the dependency on noise-free training data, demonstrating parameter-efficiency, robustness and enhanced diagnostic outcomes even in the presence of unseen MR image features.

References

1. Pfaff L, Wagner F, Hossbach J, Preuhs E, Maul N, Thies M et al. Robust multi-contrast MRI: denoising using trainable bilateral filters without noise-free targets. Proc ISBI. IEEE. 2023:1–5.

Privacy-enhancing Image Sampling for the Synthesis of High-quality Anonymous Chest Radiographs

Kai Packhäuser[1], Lukas Folle[1], Tri-Thien Nguyen[2], Florian Thamm[1], Andreas Maier[1]

[1]Pattern Recognition Lab, Friedrich-Alexander-Universität Erlangen-Nürnberg, Germany
[2]Institut für Radiologie und Neuroradiologie, Klinikum Fürth, Germany
kai.packhaeuser@fau.de

Abstract. The development of well-performing deep learning-based algorithms for thoracic abnormality detection and classification relies on access to large-scale chest X-ray datasets. However, the presence of patient-specific biometric information in chest radiographs impedes direct and public sharing of such data for research purposes due to the potential risk of patient re-identification. In this context, synthetic data generation emerges as a solution for anonymizing medical images. In this study, we utilize a privacy-enhancing sampling strategy within a latent diffusion model to generate fully anonymous chest radiographs. We conduct a comprehensive analysis of the employed method and examine the impact of different privacy degrees. For each configuration, the resulting synthetic images exhibit a substantial level of data utility, with only a marginal gap compared to real data. Qualitatively, a Turing test conducted with six radiologists confirms the high and realistic appearance of the generated chest radiographs, achieving an average classification accuracy of 55 % across 50 images (25 real, 25 synthetic).

1 Introduction

Chest radiographs inherently contain biometric information (similar to a fingerprint), posing a potential risk for successful patient re-identification through a linkage attack [1]. Therefore, to be able to securely release such data for research purposes, there is an urgent need for robust and reliable anonymization techniques. While perturbation-based anonymization approaches – such as PriCheXy-Net [2] – represent one possibility to remove the biometric fingerprint from chest radiographs, the generation of entirely synthetic medical images has attracted attention as a promising solution for anonymization and addressing data-sharing limitations. However, state-of-the-art generative models, e. g., latent diffusion models (LDMs) [3], are characterized by the memorization effect [4], which occurs when patient-specific biometric patterns from the original training data are replicated in synthetic scans. To avoid this issue, Packhäuser et al. [5] proposed a privacy-enhancing image sampling strategy to be able to generate fully anonymous chest radiographs using a trained LDM. During inference, this strategy acts as a filtering technique, excluding synthetic images, provided a specific patient identity has been reproduced. As demonstrated by the authors, this approach guarantees a high degree of data utility, with only a marginal gap compared to real data. Nevertheless, the study did not explore whether the observed gap in data utility arises from the proposed sampling strategy or the intrinsic quality of the trained generative model. Hence, further research is required to attain a more holistic understanding of this

© Der/die Autor(en), exklusiv lizenziert an
Springer Fachmedien Wiesbaden GmbH, ein Teil von Springer Nature 2024
A. Maier et al. (Hrsg.), *Bildverarbeitung für die Medizin 2024*,
Informatik aktuell, https://doi.org/10.1007/978-3-658-44037-4_12

method. In this work, we provide a comprehensive analysis of the previously proposed privacy-enhancing sampling strategy [5]. Given an LDM which is trained to generate class-conditional chest radiographs, we sample synthetic images with varying privacy degrees. For each configuration, we evaluate both the filtering ratio and the extent of data utility. Furthermore, to clinically assess the visual quality of the resulting synthetic chest radiographs, we conduct a Turing test with six experienced radiologists.

2 Materials and methods

2.1 Dataset

We leverage the public ChestX-ray14 dataset [6], which comprises 112,120 chest radiographs derived from 30,805 individual patients. Each image is associated with a set of 14 labels, indicating the presence or absence of specific thoracic abnormalities, such as Atelectasis, Cardiomegaly, Consolidation, Edema, Effusion, Emphysema, Fibrosis, Hernia, Infiltration, Mass, Nodule, Pleural Thickening, Pneumonia, and Pneumothorax. Healthy subjects are assigned an additional class, denoting the absence of any of the aforementioned abnormalities. To streamline the task of class-conditional image synthesis, we implement certain data exclusion criteria in this study. Firstly, we only focus on chest radiographs that carry a single abnormality label. Additionally, we impose a constraint that permits a maximum number of 5 follow-up scans per patient, aiming to prevent the generative model from capturing patient-specific patterns that could arise from overly represented individuals. Lastly, we solely incorporate images from patients aged 21 years and older, as the anatomical development of younger patients may not be complete. This data reduction procedure results in a total of 56,352 remaining images that are split into a training, validation, and test set by a ratio of 70:10:20. For this, we use a patient-wise splitting strategy while maintaining the overall class distribution.

2.2 Latent diffusion model

For the task of class-conditional image generation, we employ an LDM, as originally proposed by Rombach et al. [3]. This approach utilizes the encoder of a vector-quantized variational autoencoder (VQ-VAE) to create lower-dimensional latent representations of the input data. Operating in this latent space, the model leverages the concept of diffusion processes which are realized by performing multiple denoising steps with a U-Net. Lastly, the decoder of the autoencoder performs a transformation from the latent space back to the image domain. This process allows for the generation of complex and realistic images with fine-grained details. The integration of class-conditional information is achieved through the utilization of a trainable lookup table. The conditioning entails the fusion of class embeddings with the diffusion process using cross-attention in the U-Net. We closely adhered to the implementation by Rombach et al. [3]. In this work, synthetic images are generated with a resolution of 256×256 pixels. The training process for the LDM involves the following details: First, the autoencoder is trained over 100 epochs at a learning rate of $4.5 \cdot 10^{-6}$ with a combination of the perceptual loss [7] and a patch-based adversarial objective [8]. Training of the underlying diffusion model is performed by optimizing for the L1 loss at a learning rate of 10^{-6} until the validation loss no longer shows noticeable improvements (250 epochs).

2.3 Privacy-enhancing image sampling strategy

We employ the privacy-enhancing sampling strategy proposed by Packhäuser et al. [5], as illustrated in Fig. 1. This strategy acts as a filtering technique and excludes a synthetic image in case patient-specific biometric patterns have been replicated. To execute this image selection process, a patient retrieval network is applied for each generated chest radiograph to recognize its top-ranked image from the original training dataset in terms of patient identity. Then, a patient verification network performs a 1-to-1 matching step between the synthetic scan and the real scan, resulting in the patient similarity score s. A high similarity score s indicates a high probability that the recommended image pair belongs to the same patient. This approach leverages pre-trained retrieval and verification models introduced in prior research [1], performing with a top-1 precision of 99.6 % and an area under the receiver operating characteristic curve (AUC) of 99.4 %, respectively. Based on the similarity score s and a privacy threshold t, a synthetic image is excluded if $s > t$. In this context, a lower privacy threshold leads to higher privacy guarantees. Note that no images are excluded if the privacy threshold is set to $t = 1$. Given a set of N_s synthetic images, the filtering ratio can be computed according to $R = \frac{N_{ex}}{N_s}$, with N_{ex} being the number of excluded samples containing identifiable patterns that have been reproduced from the original training set.

2.4 Experiments

We followed the image generation pipeline according to Packhäuser et al. [5]. Using the trained LDM, we created a total of 10 independent synthetic chest X-ray datasets S_t by applying 10 different privacy thresholds $t \in \{0.1, 0.2, ..., 1.0\}$. For each considered privacy threshold, we analyzed the filtering ratio R during the dataset formation process. Note, for each configuration, image sampling was performed until the size and class distribution of the synthetic dataset matched the one of the original real dataset. Moreover, following the procedure in [5], image utility of each resulting synthetic dataset was measured on a downstream classification task, with the intention of analyzing how well synthetic data can convey relevant information during the training process of an abnormality classifier. For this, we trained different classification models using CheXNet [9] with exclusively synthetic training data. We adhered to the training details as outlined in the original paper [9]. Each individual classification model was evaluated on the same real test set. After performing 10 independent training and testing runs for each setting, we report the average of the resulting mean AUC values, respectively. Lastly, for

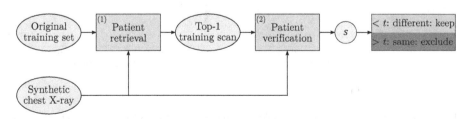

Fig. 1. Illustration of the privacy-enhancing image sampling strategy.

a privacy threshold of $t = 0.5$, we assessed the clinical quality of the resulting synthetic
chest radiographs by conducting a Turing test with six experienced radiologists. During
the first phase of the test, 50 individual images (25 real, 25 synthetic) were presented
to the subjects, who were tasked with classifying each image as either real or synthetic.
During the second phase, 25 pairs of images, each consisting of one real and one synthetic image, were presented side by side, and the subjects had to determine which of
the two images in each pair was synthetic. To avoid potential bias, no details regarding
the image generation process were provided to the subjects. In order to have the images
evaluated solely for the appearance of anatomical structure and abnormality patterns,
we only considered real and synthetic scans free from potential foreign material (e. g.,
implants) for the Turing test. Additionally, to maintain a standardized evaluation scheme,
page characters were obscured with black pixel boxes in both real and synthetic scans.

3   Results

The results of the performed quantitative experiments are visualized in Fig. 2. As shown
in Fig. 2a, the filtering ratio R continuously increases by lowering the privacy threshold t.
For instance, at $t = 0.1$, 52.7 % of generated chest radiographs are excluded during the
dataset formation process. In contrast, no synthetic images are eliminated when using
a privacy threshold of $t = 1$. Interestingly, as illustrated in Fig. 2b, the choice of the
privacy threshold t has no significant impact on image utility. This becomes apparent
by the consistently high classification results (mAUC) in the range of 77.6 % to 78.1 %.
Compared to a classifier trained on real data (visualized with the dotted line in Fig. 2b),
we only observe a marginal performance gap of 3.5 % to 4.0 %, depending on the
configuration. This suggests that the synthetic datasets are able to convey relevant class
information to a considerable extent regardless of the degree of privacy. Finally, for the
qualitative image assessment, the results of the conducted Turing test are summarized
in Tab. 1. It provides an overview of the individual performances of each radiologist,

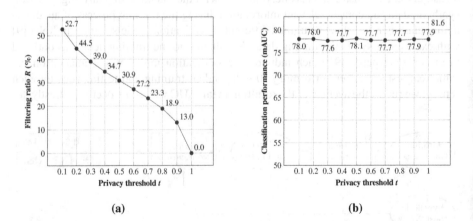

(a)   (b)

Fig. 2. Effect of varying privacy thresholds t on the filtering ratio R (a) and the data utility (b).
The dotted line in the right subplot indicates the performance of a classifier trained on real data.

Tab. 1. Results of the Turing test conducted with six experienced radiologists. In phase 1, synthetic images are encoded as the positive class. The accuracy is used to evaluate both test phases.

			Phase 1			Phase 2
	TP	TN	FP	FN	Accuracy	Accuracy
Radiologist 1	13	13	12	12	52 %	44 %
Radiologist 2	15	8	17	10	46 %	72 %
Radiologist 3	7	16	9	18	46 %	36 %
Radiologist 4	21	20	5	4	82 %	88 %
Radiologist 5	14	15	10	11	58 %	48 %
Radiologist 6	9	13	12	16	44 %	48 %
Average	-	-	-	-	55 %	56 %

along with the resulting average performance across all subjects. In the first phase, the radiologists correctly classified an average of 55 % of the shown cases. In the second phase, the radiologists attained an average task accuracy of 56 %. This indicates that even for experts, and despite direct comparisons, distinguishing the synthetic chest radiographs from real ones is a notably non-trivial task. Randomly selected images generated by the trained LDM are shown in Fig. 3. These examples clearly demonstrate the high and realistic image quality that has been achieved.

4 Discussion

In this paper, we leveraged an LDM to synthesize high-quality class-conditional chest radiographs. During inference, we applied the privacy-enhancing image sampling strategy proposed in prior research [5]. With our conducted experiments, we provided a more comprehensive analysis of this strategy, complementing the original paper. More precisely, we analyzed the effect of varying privacy thresholds t on the filtering ratio R and the utility of the resulting synthetic datasets. Moreover, for a privacy threshold of $t = 0.5$, we were able to confirm the quality of the resulting synthetic chest radiographs by conducting a Turing test with six experienced radiologists. Based on our

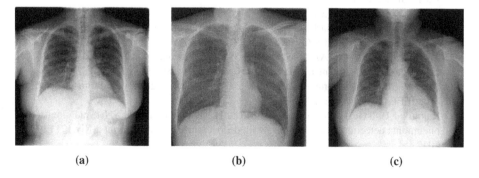

(a)   (b)   (c)

Fig. 3. Randomly selected images generated by the trained LDM at a privacy threshold of $t = 0.5$.

obtained results, we would like to emphasize again that synthetic chest radiographs are not anonymous per se. Instead, generative models tend to reproduce patient-specific biometric patterns during inference. The reported filtering ratio R (see Fig. 2a) clearly demonstrates how many images are affected during the sampling procedure, indicating the necessity of privacy-enhancing mechanisms for generative modeling. Furthermore, given the obtained classification results (see Fig. 2b), we identified that the applied privacy-enhancing sampling strategy itself has no negative impact on image utility. Thus, the resulting performance gap can be attributed solely to the trained LDM. Therefore, in future work, we aim to minimize this gap by further optimizing the quality of the trained LDM. Together with the application of rigorous privacy mechanisms, this could potentially allow for the mitigation of data sharing limitations in the future.

Acknowledgement. The authors gratefully acknowledge the scientific support and HPC resources provided by the Erlangen National High Performance Computing Center (NHR@FAU) of the Friedrich-Alexander-Universität Erlangen-Nürnberg (FAU). The hardware is funded by the German Research Foundation (DFG). The authors declare that they have no conflicts of interest.

References

1. Packhäuser K, Gündel S, Münster N, Syben C, Christlein V, Maier A. Deep learning-based patient re-identification is able to exploit the biometric nature of medical chest X-ray data. Sci Rep. 2022;12(1):1–13.
2. Packhäuser K, Gündel S, Thamm F, Denzinger F, Maier A. Deep learning-based anonymization of chest radiographs: a utility-preserving measure for patient privacy. Proc MICCAI. 2023:262–72.
3. Rombach R, Blattmann A, Lorenz D, Esser P, Ommer B. High-resolution image synthesis with latent diffusion models. Proc IEEE CVPR. 2022:10684–95.
4. Carlini N, Hayes J, Nasr M, Jagielski M, Sehwag V, Tramer F et al. Extracting training data from diffusion models. Proc USENIX Secur Symp. 2023:5253–70.
5. Packhäuser K, Folle L, Thamm F, Maier A. Generation of anonymous chest radiographs using latent diffusion models for training thoracic abnormality classification systems. Proc IEEE ISBI. 2023:1–5.
6. Wang X, Peng Y, Lu L, Lu Z, Bagheri M, Summers RM. ChestX-ray8: hospital-scale chest X-ray database and benchmarks on weakly-supervised classification and localization of common thorax diseases. Proc IEEE CVPR. 2017:2097–106.
7. Zhang R, Isola P, Efros AA, Shechtman E, Wang O. The unreasonable effectiveness of deep features as a perceptual metric. Proc IEEE CVPR. 2018:586–95.
8. Esser P, Rombach R, Ommer B. Taming transformers for high-resolution image synthesis. Proc IEEE CVPR. 2021:12873–83.
9. Rajpurkar P, Irvin J, Zhu K, Yang B, Mehta H, Duan T et al. CheXNet: radiologist-level pneumonia detection on chest X-rays with deep learning. arXiv preprint arXiv:1711.05225. 2017.

Segmentation-guided Medical Image Registration
Quality Awareness using Label Noise Correctionn

Varsha Raveendran[1,2], Veronika Spieker[1,2], Rickmer F. Braren[3],
Dimitrios C. Karampinos[3], Veronika A. Zimmer[1,2], Julia A. Schnabel[1,2,4]

[1]Institute of Machine Learning in Biomedical Imaging, Helmholtz Munich, Germany
[2]School of Computation, Information & Technology, Technical University of Munich, Germany
[3]School of Medicine & Health, Technical University of Munich, Germany
[4]School of Biomedical Engineering & Imaging Sciences, King's College London, UK
varsha.raveendran@tum.de

Abstract. Medical image registration methods can strongly benefit from anatomical labels, which can be provided by segmentation networks at reduced labeling effort. Yet, label noise may adversely affect registration performance. In this work, we propose a quality-aware segmentation-guided registration method that handles such noisy, i.e., low-quality, labels by self-correcting them using Confident Learning. Utilizing NLST and in-house acquired abdominal MR images, we show that our proposed quality-aware method effectively addresses the drop in registration performance observed in quality-unaware methods. Our findings demonstrate that incorporating an appropriate label-correction strategy during training can reduce labeling efforts, consequently enhancing the practicality of segmentation-guided registration.

1 Introduction

Medical image registration is essential in estimating organ motion for various medical imaging protocols, e.g. motion-corrected magnetic resonance imaging (MRI) [1]. Yet, non-rigid organ motion, such as induced by respiration in the abdomen, continues to pose a challenge for reliable motion estimates due to discontinuous deformations [2]. Segmentations offer valuable anatomical cues to guide learning-based registration models to focus optimization efforts on regions of interest. Previous works included segmentations to mask regions of interest [3] or within the loss function [4], resulting in improved registration accuracy. Nevertheless, obtaining high-quality (HQ) segmentations, i.e., annotated by experts, for every registration procedure is costly and impractical.

To overcome the labeling effort, methods using a reduced amount of HQ labels have been proposed. Missing labels are either predicted by a separate network [5] or using transfer learning with externally labeled datasets [6]. Yet, these "cheaper" segmentation predictions may be noisy or inaccurate, i.e., low-quality (LQ), thereby, reducing the final registration accuracy [7]. To the best of our knowledge, no segmentation-based registration considering such quality degradation of LQ labels has yet been proposed.

In this work, we present a novel segmentation-guided registration method that operates with fewer expensive HQ labels, simultaneously leveraging cheaper LQ labels. To avoid registration quality degradation, we employ self-correction of LQ labels based on confident learning (CL) [8, 9] and show the potential of our method on two datasets.

A. Maier et al. (Hrsg.), *Bildverarbeitung für die Medizin 2024*,
Informatik aktuell, https://doi.org/10.1007/978-3-658-44037-4_13

2   Materials and methods

2.1   Method

2.1.1   Network overview. Consider a set of n d-dimensional images $I_i : \Omega \subset \mathbb{R}^d \to R$, $i = 1, ..., n$ with corresponding binary labels $S_i : \Omega \subset \mathbb{R}^d \to [0, 1]$. Let I and S be further split into k images with HQ labels and $(n-k)$ images with LQ labels, I_{HQ}/S_{HQ} and I_{LQ}/S_{LQ}, respectively. Given a fixed I_f and a moving image I_m where $f \neq m$, image registration aims to find an optimal spatial transform $\phi : \mathbb{R}^d \to \mathbb{R}^d$ so that $I_m \circ \phi \approx I_f$. For our registration module (RegNet), we optimize a network M_R to predict ϕ based on a set of input images (I_m, I_f), as proposed in Voxelmorph [4]. The network M_R employs a U-Net and spatial transformation layers to obtain ϕ. For the segmentation module (SegNet), we follow a similar architecture as in [8] to leverage the available labels S and apply a mean teacher strategy to encounter over-fitting to S_{LQ} within S. The student network, M_S is trained with the entire set, (I_n, S_n). The teacher network, M_T is exclusively trained with images with low-quality labels, (I_{LQ}, S_{LQ}). While M_S and M_T have the same U-Net architecture, the student's weights are refined through back-propagation, and the teacher's weights are updated via the exponential moving average (EMA) of the student's weights at the end of every iteration.

2.1.2   Label correction. To obtain reliable segmentation predictions, a label correction process [8] is employed in training M_S, mitigating the impact of low-quality labels in the training data (marked in yellow in Fig. 1). The network M_T is adapted to provide

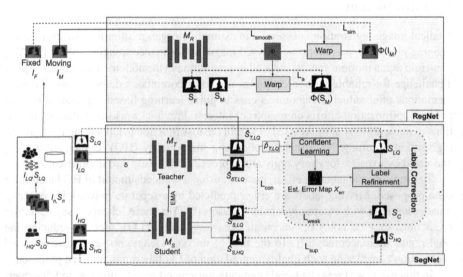

Fig. 1. Quality-aware segmentation (SegNet) and registration networks (RegNet): The student segmentation network is trained on both high (HQ) and low-quality (LQ) labels. The teacher uses LQ labels to provide weak supervision to SegNet (orange lines). The teacher's predictions are used to train RegNet when the input labels are of low quality (blue line).

predicted segmentation probabilities $\hat{p}_{T,LQ} : \Omega \subset \mathbb{R}^d \rightarrow [0,1]$ for images from I_{LQ}. Using $\hat{p}_{T,LQ}$ and the provided labels S_{LQ}, the CL module estimates label errors. Specifically, a binary error map $\mathcal{X}_{err}$ with label errors marked as "1" is created and further used to obtain the corrected label S_C as follows

$$S_C = S_{LQ} + \mathcal{X}_{err} \cdot (-1)^{S_{LQ}} \tag{1}$$

2.1.3 Training strategy. The proposed quality-aware network is trained by alternately optimizing the SegNet and RegNet modules while keeping the other fixed.

The network M_S is optimized with the following loss:

$$\mathcal{L}_{seg} = \mathcal{L}_{sup} + \lambda_{seg} * (\mathcal{L}_{con} + \beta_{weak} * \mathcal{L}_{weak}) \tag{2}$$

The supervised loss $\mathcal{L}_{sup}$ is the sum of cross entropy loss and Dice loss between the student's predictions $(\hat{S}_{S,HQ})$ on images I_{HQ}, and the ground truth S_{HQ}. The consistency loss $\mathcal{L}_{con}$ is computed with Dice between the student's predictions $(\hat{S}_{S,LQ})$ on images I_{LQ} and the teacher's predictions for the noise-added images $(\hat{S}_{\delta T,LQ})$. This ensures that even with perturbations, the predictions remain consistent [10]. $\mathcal{L}_{weak}$ is the Dice loss between $\hat{S}_{S,LQ}$ and the corrected label S_C. The network M_R is trained by optimizing the following loss

$$\mathcal{L}_{reg} = \mathcal{L}_{sim} + \lambda * \mathcal{L}_{smooth} + \gamma * \mathcal{L}_a \tag{3}$$

where $\mathcal{L}_{sim}$ is the NCC loss between I_f and $\phi(I_m)$, $\mathcal{L}_{smooth}$ uses the bending energy to regularize the deformation field, weighted by λ, and $\mathcal{L}_a$ is the anatomy loss between the warped label and target label, weighted by γ. $\mathcal{L}_a$ depends on the quality of the labels. If $S_i \in S_{LQ}$ then M_T's predictions $\hat{S}_{LQ}$ are used in the anatomy loss computation. Given fixed S_f and moving S_m labels, $\mathcal{L}_a$ is defined below

$$\mathcal{L}_a = \begin{cases} \mathcal{L}_a(S_f, \phi(S_m)) \text{ if } S_m \in S_{HQ} \text{ and } S_f \in S_{HQ} \\ \mathcal{L}_a(M_T(I_f), \phi(S_m)) \text{ if } S_m \in S_{HQ} \text{ and } S_f \in S_{LQ} \\ \mathcal{L}_a(S_f, \phi(M_T(I_m))) \text{ if } S_m \in S_{LQ} \text{ and } S_f \in S_{HQ} \\ \mathcal{L}_a(M_T(I_f), \phi(M_T(I_m))) \text{ if } S_m \in S_{LQ} \text{ and } S_f \in S_{LQ} \end{cases} \tag{4}$$

2.2 Experimental setup

2.2.1 Data. We evaluate the proposed quality-aware registration method on the public *NLST* data [11] from Learn2Reg [12] and an in-house acquired abdominal *MRI* dataset. *NLST* contains 3D CT volumes and corresponding follow-up scans done in 1, 2, or 3-year intervals as image pairs. The training and test set consists of 99 and 10 pairs of images with corresponding segmentations, respectively. *MRI* consists of a dynamic series of 2D images, acquired during free-breathing at 3T (Ingenia Elition X, Philips Healthcare) on six volunteers after obtaining ethics approval (FOV=300x550mm^2, TE/TR=2.1/0.95ms, spatial resolution=1.23x1.23mm^2, dynamic scan time=110ms). Image pairs were generated using combinations of different inhalation points with end-exhale phases from the first 150 temporal slices. The liver was chosen as the organ of interest and manually segmented for training/validation purposes.

2.2.2   Simulate low-quality labels. To validate the method in a controlled setting, low-quality labels (S_{LQ}) are simulated by randomly distorting the true segmentation boundary of the ground truth label (S_{HQ}) using a Markov process [13]. The number of Markov steps can be varied to control the noise introduced in the labels. The value is set to 150 in our experiments. The remaining S_{HQ} are considered true labels.

2.2.3   Training. Different datasets were created to experiment with varying ratios of HQ and LQ labels, i.e., [HQ/LQ] = [0/100], [30/70], [70/30], [100/0], where HQ refers to x% of labels from (I_{HQ}, S_{HQ}) and LQ to y% from (I_{LQ}, S_{LQ}). The ratio of epochs for training RegNet to SegNet is 5:1, since M_S converges early. After hyperparameter tuning, the weights for the anatomy loss, $\gamma = 10$, and regularization loss ($\lambda = 40$ for NLST, $\lambda = 10$ for MRI) resulting in the lowest number of folding were chosen. The learning rate for M_S was set to 1e-3 and M_R to 5e-4.

2.2.4   Experiments. For benchmarking, baseline models were trained with 0% labels (only Reg), 100% LQ labels (0/100 quality-unaware), and 100% HQ labels (100/0 only HQ). Evaluation was done on models with the lowest validation loss, using Dice and HD95 values between warped and target labels. In a modularized manner, the following models were trained:

- *Only HQ* without LQ labels (ablation): Models were trained only with S_{HQ} (30%, 70%, 100%), while I_{LQ} remained unlabeled. No label correction is applied.
- *Quality-unaware without* label correction (ablation): Models were trained with the defined splits of S_{HQ} and S_{LQ} without label correction. This configuration allowed us to explore the performance impact on RegNet when the networks were trained without differentiating label quality.
- *Quality-aware with* label correction (proposed): Separate models were trained on the defined data splits S_{HQ} and S_{LQ}. SegNet and RegNet were aware of the quality of the labels, and Confident Learning is included.

3   Results

As shown in Table 1, adding LQ labels without any form of correction (quality-unaware) results in degraded registration performance. This observation is consistent with re-sults obtained in [8]. The proposed quality-aware method addresses this performance decline and surpasses the quality-unaware method. It exhibits improved performance when higher percentages of HQ labels are utilized during training. Superior Dice and HD95 show the effectiveness of quality-aware training compared to 0% HQ and quality-unaware training. Additionally, it can be observed that the quality-aware method per-forms better than utilizing only 30% HQ labels. Qualitative analysis of the predicted motion fields in Fig. 2 shows reduced foldings (0.002 for 30% HQ compared to 0.014 with quality-unaware) and improved deformation fields with the quality-aware method.

Tab. 1. Quantitative results comparing the proposed method (Quality-aware) with models trained with only high-quality labels (Only HQ) and a mix of high-/low-quality labels without label correction (Quality-unaware). Italic values indicate the best model for each HQ/LQ split.

%HQ	%LQ	Models	NLST		MRI	
			Dice ↑	HD95 ↓	Dice ↑	HD95 ↓
0	0	Initial	0.91 (0.02)	7.86 (2.41)	0.92 (0.07)	7.97 (5.71)
0	0	Only Reg	0.97 (0.01)	3.85 (1.76)	*0.93* (0.06)	*7.14* (5.35)
	100	Quality-unaware	*0.97* (0.01)	*2.61* (1.08)	0.92 (0.03)	9.03 (2.75)
30	0	Only HQ	*0.97* (0.01)	*2.69* (1.09)	0.93 (0.05)	7.18 (4.40)
	70	Quality-unaware	0.96 (0.01)	3.39 (1.20)	0.93 (0.04)	7.98 (3.64)
	70	Quality-aware	0.97 (0.01)	2.72 (1.32)	*0.94* (0.04)	*6.83* (0.04)
70	0	Only HQ	*0.97* (0.01)	2.87 (1.35)	*0.94* (0.04)	6.46 (0.94)
	30	Quality-unaware	0.96 (0.01)	3.01 (1.31)	0.91 (0.04)	9.55 (0.02)
	30	Quality-aware	0.96 (0.01)	*2.85* (1.23)	*0.94* (0.03)	6.60 (3.34)
100	0	Only HQ	0.99 (0.00)	1.91 (0.79)	0.95 (0.03)	6.05 (4.20)

4 Discussion

We proposed a quality-aware segmentation-guided registration approach to leverage low-quality labels while reducing labeling efforts. Our experiments show that including large amounts of LQ labels to train quality-unaware models degrades registration performance. This can be attributed to the memorization power of neural networks and the dependency of the registration network performance on the segmentation networks [8]. Consequently, this may cause the registration network to learn label noise, leading to incorrect boundary-based transformations. Quality-aware training, employing Confident Learning, effectively mitigates the noise. This enables the use of inexpensive yet noisy labels to enhance registration accuracy. Notably, the quality-aware method shows more promise with the MRI dataset. The resulting deformation fields exhibit increased noise with quality-unaware models and are not constrained within the liver. Through label correction, the optimization process seems to prioritize the liver region, resulting in a more stable and smoother deformation field. The performance disparity of NLST compared to the MRI dataset could be due to the nature of the NLST dataset, where the RoI (lungs) occupies the entire volume. The contrast between the foreground (lungs) and background functioned similarly to a segmentation label. Therefore, even an improvement in the label quality did not make a significant performance difference. In contrast, the liver occupies a smaller region in the MRI images, and thus, reducing label noise en-

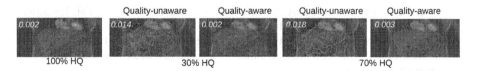

Fig. 2. Liver MRI: Deformation fields for models trained with 30% and 70% HQ labels. The remaining percentage of labels were of low quality. The percentage of foldings is shown in white.

abled the registration algorithm to focus on the targeted region. However, the proposed approach performed inferior to models trained on 100% LQ labels for NLST, which requires further investigation. The high dependency of the registration network on the segmentation model is a potential reason, motivating further hyperparameter tuning and loss strategy optimization. The target goal of the quality-aware approach is to achieve performance comparable to models trained with 100% HQ labels. Additionally, future work includes expansion to complex tasks, i.e. multi-label cases and even larger deformations. To conclude, the presented results encourage applying quality-aware methods to leverage segmentations for registration at reduced labeling efforts, thereby offering a more practical approach to segmentation-guided medical image registration.

Acknowledgement. V.R. and V.S. contributed equally to the work. V.S. is partially supported by the "Helmholtz Association - Munich School for Data Science (MUDS)".

References

1. Spieker V, Eichhorn H, Hammernik K, Rueckert D, Preibisch C, Karampinos DC et al. Deep learning for retrospective motion correction in MRI: a comprehensive review. IEEE Trans Med Imaging. 2023.
2. Heinrich MP, Papież BW. Image registration with sliding motion. Handbook of Medical Image Computing and Computer Assisted Intervention. Elsevier, 2020:293–318.
3. Ruhaak J, Polzin T, Heldmann S, Simpson IJA, Handels H, Modersitzki J et al. Estimation of large motion in lung CT by integrating regularized keypoint correspondences into dense deformable registration. IEEE Trans Med Imaging. 2017;36(8):1746–57.
4. Balakrishnan G, Zhao A, Sabuncu MR, Guttag J, Dalca AV. VoxelMorph: a learning framework for deformable medical image registration. 2018.
5. Xu Z, Niethammer M. DeepAtlas: joint semi-supervised learning of image registration and segmentation. 2019.
6. Karimi D, Dou H, Warfield SK, Gholipour A. Deep learning with noisy labels: exploring techniques and remedies in medical image analysis. Med Image Anal. 2020;65:101759.
7. Chen X, Xia Y, Ravikumar N, Frangi AF. Joint segmentation and discontinuity-preserving deformable registration: application to cardiac cine-MR images. 2022.
8. Xu Z, Lu D, Luo J, Wang Y, Yan J, Ma K et al. Anti-interference from noisy labels: mean-teacher-assisted confident learning for medical image segmentation. IEEE Trans Med Imaging. 2022.
9. Northcutt C, Jiang L, Chuang I. Confident learning: estimating uncertainty in dataset labels. J Artif Int Res. 2021;70:1373–411.
10. Luo Y, Zhu J, Li M, Ren Y, Zhang B. Smooth neighbors on teacher graphs for semi-supervised learning. PROC IEEE CVPR. 2018:8896–905.
11. Aberle DR, Berg CD, Black WC, Church TR, Fagerstrom RM, Galen B et al. The national lung screening trial: overview and study design. Radiol. 2011;258(1):243–53.
12. Hering A, Hansen L, Mok TCW, Chung ACS, Siebert H, Häger S et al. Learn2Reg: comprehensive multi-task medical image registration challenge, dataset and evaluation in the era of deep learning. 2022.
13. Yao J, Zhang Y, Zheng S, Goswami M, Prasanna P, Chen C. Learning to segment from noisy annotations: a spatial correction approach. Proc ICLR. 2023.

Displacement Representation for Conditional Point Cloud Registration

HeatReg Applied to 2D/3D Freehand Ultrasound Reconstruction

Lasse Hansen[1], Jürgen Lichtenstein[2], Mattias P. Heinrich[3]

[1]EchoScout GmbH, Lübeck
[2]Clinic of Oral and Maxillofacial Surgery, UKSH Campus Kiel
[3]Institute of Medical Informatics, Universität zu Lübeck
lasse@echoscout.ai

Abstract. In this work, we create a point cloud-based framework based on Free Point Transformers (FPTs) for 2D/3D registration of untracked ultrasound (US) sweeps. Applications include outpatient follow-up assessments and intraoperative scenarios like ultrasound-guided navigation. Through a simple modification in displacement prediction representation, we enhance registration results by more than 25% w.r.t. prior work while preserving the model-free paradigm, maintaining network parameters, and only marginally increasing computation time. Experiments on the SegThy dataset, featuring manually segmented anatomies on MR (magnetic resonance) scans in the thyroid gland area, demonstrate our method's effectiveness. We simulate numerous realistic ultrasound sweeps, aiming to register them back into the MR volume. Beyond methodological contributions, our fast registration framework strives to enable clinically capable systems, advancing ultrasound-guided surgery.

1 Introduction

Ultrasound is a medical imaging technology that provides the promise of ubiquitous visual access to internal anatomy for almost all medical professions and subsequently substantially improved patient care without inducing any ionising radiation . Due to its portability, high temporal resolution and low cost ultrasound is seen as a disrupting technology for point-of-care use and to improve access to high quality health care in lower income countries. However, the dynamic image interpretation is challenging and highly operator dependent hence pairing ultrasound with intelligent algorithms that aid intraoperative guidance is necessary.

1.1 Related work

To date most related work on 2D/3D freehand reconstruction relies on image registration, either for in-plane motion across subsequent temporal frames [1], inter-sweep registration [2], (sparse) 2D to 3D registration or point cloud alignment. To deal with both global 2D to 3D and local deformable in-plane motion an MRF (markov random field)-based discrete optimisation strategy was proposed in [3]. [4] describe a learned

© Der/die Autor(en), exklusiv lizenziert an
Springer Fachmedien Wiesbaden GmbH, ein Teil von Springer Nature 2024
A. Maier et al. (Hrsg.), *Bildverarbeitung für die Medizin 2024*,
Informatik aktuell, https://doi.org/10.1007/978-3-658-44037-4_14

local descriptor-based global alignment between 3D MRI and 2D US sequences based on ground truth pose supervision and pairwise keypoint matching. Due to the fact that image segmentation with deep learning networks has overcome previous limitations in accuracy and robustness of hand-crafted classical machine learning strategies the use of surface point clouds, which can be directly obtained from automatic U-Net predictions, becomes another interesting avenue. A robust free point transformer (FPT) was proposed in [5] for prostate US registration. FPT learns a global feature vector for a fixed and moving point cloud using a (shared) PointNet [6] and subsequent 1×1 convolutions (local multi-layer perceptron) to estimate a displacement vector for each point.

1.2 Contribution

The contributions of our work are twofold: (i) a point cloud-based 2D/3D registration framework for slice-to-volume alignment and evaluate it on a thyroidMRdataset, clearly identifying the importance of 1) simultaneous multi slice registration and 2) exploitation of multiple auxiliary structures in close proximity to the anatomical target region; (ii) a new displacement representation for deep learning-based point cloud registration. Instead of directly regressing the 3D displacement coordinates, the network predicts scalar weights on nearest neighbour points in the fixed cloud that indicate the direction of movement. A conceptual similarity exists to dense heatmap-based landmark localisation [7], which, the best of our knowledge, has not been proposed for displacement prediction in point cloud registration.

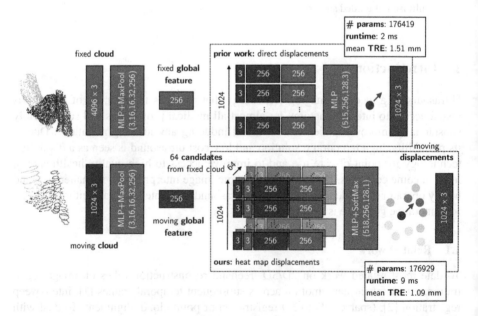

Fig. 1. Overview of the point cloud network used in this work applied to 2D/3D US to MR registration, and comparison of our proposed candidate based regression with prior work.

2 Methods

The goal of point cloud registration is to align a moving $P_m \in \mathbb{R}^{N_m \times 3}$ and fixed $P_f \in \mathbb{R}^{N_f \times 3}$ cloud with a number N_m and N_f of points (3d coordinates), respectively. Therefor, we need to find displacements $D \in \mathbb{R}^{N_m \times 3}$ such that the distance (w.r.t. to some metric, as exact correspondences may not exist) between $P_m + D$ and P_f is minimal. A recently introduced neural network approach called Free Point Transformer (FPT) [5] aims to solve the registration with a model free approach. A shared PointNet [6] is employed to extract a global feature vector from P_f and P_m. Then a multi layer perceptron (MLP) processes the concatenated moving points, moving global feature and fixed global feature and outputs the displacements D. We employ FPT as backbone and baseline architecture and summarize the model as function $D = f(P_m, P_f)$. The prediction of displacements is formulated as a direct regression. In this work we propose to modify the representation of the displacement prediction as follows: For each point $p_i \in P_m$ the k nearest neighbours $p_j \in P_f$ are determined and the set of directed distances $(p_j - p_i)$ are denoted as candidates $C \in \mathbb{R}^{N_m \times k \times 3}$. With the addition of the candidates dimension, an MLP now processes the concatenation of moving points, candidates displacements, moving global feature and fixed global feature. Note, that the model free paradigm remains unaffected as the local MLP introduces no additional communication between points. Output of the modified network g is a scalar field, softmax normalised in the candidates dimension, i.e. $W = g(P_m, P_f)$ with $W \in (0, 1)^{N_m \times k \times 1}$. The softmax operator ensures that the predicted weights sum to one in the candidate dimension and the network remains differentiable. We can now easily determine the displacement field we are looking for by the sum of candidates and weights, i.e.

$$D = \sum_{i=1}^{k} C_{\{i\}} \cdot W_{\{i\}} \tag{1}$$

where $C_{\{i\}} \in \mathbb{R}^{N_m \times 3}$ and $W_{\{i\}} \in (0, 1)^{N_m \times 1}$ denotes the ith candidate subset of C and W, respectively. Similar to the modification of our chosen registration backbone, the proposed displacement representation can be used as drop-in replacement in every point cloud registration network. The number of network parameters stays approximately the same and only marginally increased runtime is observed due to the nearest neighbour search. To further refine the registration results, a second stage network with a reduced number of candidates k can be applied to the warped moving cloud $P_m + D$. Figure 1 illustrates our proposed approach and its direct comparison to prior work.

3 Experiments

3.1 Data

We conduct experiments on MRI scans from the SegThy dataset [8] featuring manually labeled jugular veins, carotid arteries, thyroid, and semi-automatically segmented trachea of 10 subjects. To generate point cloud data, we extract surface points of anatomical segmentations (using an nnUNet [9]) for fixed clouds. Moving clouds (US slices) are created by simulating sweep trajectories with random start and end points projected on the body surface. A spline, with varying control points, guides the US probe along the neck. Pose and image slice are determined by points on the path, their heading, and body surface normals. Trajectories are augmented with random noise and jitter. Each sweep yields 128 slices (approx. 6 seconds at 20 fps), resulting in 1000 sweeps (100 per subject) for training and evaluation, to be registered on 20 fixed clouds (left and right sides considered separately).

3.2 Implementation details

The proposed PyTorch-based registration network is implemented with the moving cloud resampled to 4096 points and the fixed cloud to 16 slices, each with 64 points (1024 in total). The first and second stage networks use 64 and 32 candidates, respectively. Training comprises 50,000 iterations with a batch size of four, utilizing Adam optimizer and on-the-fly random augmentations (translations, rotations). Supervised by known ground displacements, a least square fitting ensures consistent movement. Initially, the moving cloud has all slices stacked in the z-direction (temporal) with a unit distance of 1 (unknown trajectory). Training and evaluation follow a leave-one-out approach, with hyperparameter tuning performed on a single fold for both our method and comparison methods.

3.3 Ablations and baseline methods

To assess the performance of our proposed framework and individual components we conduct several ablation and baseline experiments.

1. 7dof: A baseline that iteratively optimises global rotation, translation and scale based on a label aware Chamfer distance (used as starting point in all other experiments).
2. Single label: Single scale network with only the target anatomy available for training.
3. Single slice: Instead of 16 only a single random slice is sampled from the trajectory. This corresponds to a conventional 2D/3D registration scenario, where the model does not have any information about neighboring slices or global context.
4. B-spline adam: An iterative optimisation method. Point displacements are directly optimised using the label aware Chamfer distance (as in the 7dof baseline) and the displacement field is regularised by a coarse grid of control points describing a B-spline.
5. FPT + multi label: The Free Point Transformer [5] serves as network backbone/baseline for our multi label method. For more details we refer to the methods section.

4   Results

The registration results can be assessed in Figure 2 and Table 1. We employ a number of evaluation metrics, that focus on the accurate alignment of the target anatomy (thyroid) (target registration error (TRE) of predicted points, Haussdorf metric of reconstructed

Tab. 1. Registration results for the SegThy dataset [8]. We report the target registration error (TRE) of predicted points, the (translational and rotational) pose error of the US sweep trajectory, the 95th percentile of the Hausdorff distance (HD95) between the ground truth and reconstructed target anatomy (thyroid) as well as the number of network parameters and runtime.

	TRE [mm]	trans. error [mm]	rot. error [°]	HD95 [mm]	params #	runtime [ms]
7dof	3.26±2.31	7.05±1.82	14.39±3.41	9.38±4.97		45
single label	2.51±1.68	4.80±1.47	12.03±3.72	6.29±4.15	176929	9
single slice	1.85±1.31	4.15±1.54	10.41±3.51	4.63±2.81	176929	9
b-spline adam	1.63±1.40	4.08±2.34	11.51±4.11	4.82±2.71		435
FPT + multi label	1.51±1.23	3.68±1.53	9.13±3.30	3.93±2.05	176419	2
ours (single scale)	1.09±0.84	3.01±1.09	8.02±3.02	2.88±1.27	176929	9
ours	0.97±0.79	2.85±1.19	8.05±2.89	2.77±1.27	353858	14

segmentations) and on the US sweep reconstruction (pose error of the trajectory). Our registration network yields improved results for all metrics w.r.t the conventional optimsation (b-spline adam) and learning based (FPT) baselines. The TRE decreases from 1.63 mm to 0.97 mm (-40%) and 1.51 mm to 0.97 mm (-35%), respectively.

1. Number of labels: Using only a single anatomical label in training and inference drastically worsens the result, even on the available target anatomy. The Hausdorff distance is more than doubled from 2.77 mm to 6.29 mm.

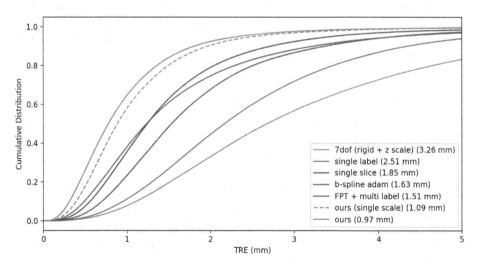

Fig. 2. Cumulative distribution of the target registration error (TRE) in mm of all points corresponding to the anatomical target structure (thyroid) for several baselines, ablation experiments and our method (mean TRE in brackets).

2. Number of slices: When registering the US sweep slice by slice the trajectory pose error for both translation and rotation increases (by 70% and 30%, respectively) while the HD95 metric is still comparable with the results of the optimisation based method (4.63 mm vs. 4.82 mm).

3. Displacement representation: Our main methodological contribution is the proposal of a new representation for displacement prediction. With otherwise identical network architecture (FPT vs. ours (single scale)) the TRE can be improved by about half a centimeter from 1.51 mm to 1.09 mm. Interestingly, employing a second network, that refines the first warping with a reduced candidates space (ours) further reduces the TRE by 12% while a second FPT network does not improve any registration metrics.

5 Conclusion

We have presented a simple yet effective approach to significantly improve registration results of point cloud alignment networks by changing the way displacements are predicted. An extended evaluation with different backbone architectures could give additional insights in the advantages of our method. The results of the 2D/3D US MR registration scenario encourage further steps to be taken for freehand ultrasound in surgical navigation. In ongoing and future work we are curating a clinical dataset to develop and validate our registration framework. In addition to 2D/3D registration, freehand ultrasound reconstruction, in which volumetric ultrasound images are created from one or more untracked sweeps, is of particular clinical interest. In this context, a fast and accurate registration framework can be an important component, e.g. for visual SLAM (simultaneous localization and mapping) approaches. A further promising research direction to improve the registration accuracy is fusion with additional sensors, such as IMUs (inertial measurement units), which are already integrated in the first commercially available ultrasound devices.

References

1. Prevost R, Salehi M, Jagoda S, Kumar N, Sprung J, Ladikos A et al. 3D freehand ultrasound without external tracking using deep learning. MedIA. 2018;48:187–202.
2. Wein W, Lupetti M, Zettinig O, Jagoda S, Salehi M, Markova V et al. Three-dimensional thyroid assessment from untracked 2D ultrasound clips. Proc MICCAI. 2020:514–23.
3. Ferrante E, Paragios N. Non-rigid 2D-3D medical image registration using Markov random fields. Proc MICCAI. 2013:163–70.
4. Markova V, Ronchetti M, Wein W, Zettinig O, Prevost R. Global Multi-modal 2D/3D registration via Local descriptors learning. Proc MICCAI. 2022:269–79.
5. Baum ZM, Hu Y, Barratt DC. Real-time multimodal image registration with partial intraoperative point-set data. MedIA. 2021;74.
6. Qi CR, Su H, Mo K, Guibas LJ. Pointnet: deep learning on point sets for 3d classification and segmentation. Proc CVPR. 2017:652–60.
7. Sun X, Xiao B, Wei F, Liang S, Wei Y. Integral human pose regression. Proc ECCV. 2018:529–45.

8. Krönke M, Eilers C, Dimova D, Köhler M, Buschner G, Schweiger L et al. Tracked 3D ultrasound and deep neural network-based thyroid segmentation reduce interobserver variability in thyroid volumetry. PloS One. 2022;17(7).
9. Isensee F, Jaeger PF, Kohl SA, Petersen J, Maier-Hein KH. nnU-net: a self-configuring method for deep learning-based biomedical image segmentation. Nat Methods. 2021;18(2):203–11.

Joint Learning of Image Registration and Change Detection for Lung CT Images

Temke Kohlbrandt[1], Jan Moltz[1], Stefan Heldmann[1], Alessa Hering[1,3], Jan Lellmann[2]

[1]Fraunhofer Institute for Digital Medicine MEVIS, Bremen/Lübeck, Germany
[2]Institute of Mathematics and Image Computing, University of Lübeck, Germany
[3]Department of Imaging, Radboud University Medical Center, Nijmegen, The Netherlands
temke.kohlbrandt@mevis.fraunhofer.de

Abstract. Intuitive visualization of relevant changes between radiological image pairs in the form of change maps has the potential to not only increase efficiency in diagnostic reading, but also to decrease the number of missed abnormalities. Classically, change maps are created from difference images after an image registration step, which requires a careful balance in order to neither generate artifacts nor disguise relevant changes. We propose jointly learning registration and change map in order to address these limitations. As a proof of concept, the method was tested on NLST lung CT images and synthetically generated data, and shows comparable results to the conventional approach. In a reader study, the use of change maps resulted in a 23% reduction in reading time while maintaining similar recall.

1 Introduction

Medical imaging such as CT and MRI is important in the management of almost all cancer types. Imaging is used from detection, and diagnosis, to treatment planning, and in long-term follow-up. For metastatic cancer, imaging is particularly important because the sites where metastases have grown must be found on the CT scans and followed up during treatment to assess therapeutic success. At the same time, the scan must be examined for other additional abnormalities, so-called incidental findings.

The raising number of cancer cases results in a growing caseload for radiologists. An additional challenge lies in the 'inattentional blindness', when radiologists miss changes or unusual signs because they are concentrating on a specific task [1]. To reduce these problems, methods are being developed to assist radiologists; for example, segmentation and detection of anatomical structures. Image registration can assist radiologists in finding corresponding points in image pairs or in visualizing changes by subtracting the registered images.

Sieren et al. show that the use of difference images generated by a conventional image registration method as an overlay on the original CT images facilitates the evaluation for radiologists by reducing reading time and increasing sensitivity [2]. One problem with creating change maps with a conventional image registration pipeline is overcompensation by the registration, which leads to underestimation of the changes of interest, such as lesion changes. To overcome this limitation, Dufrese et al. [3] jointly estimates deformable registration and lesion change by assigning a weight to the data term in the registration minimization problem based on the changes in brain MR images.

© Der/die Autor(en), exklusiv lizenziert an
Springer Fachmedien Wiesbaden GmbH, ein Teil von Springer Nature 2024
A. Maier et al. (Hrsg.), *Bildverarbeitung für die Medizin 2024*,
Informatik aktuell, https://doi.org/10.1007/978-3-658-44037-4_15

In non-medical contexts, change maps are also of relevance. In [4], binary change maps from previously registered optical aerial images were learned using a siamese neural network. In recent years, an increasing number of methods based on deep learning have been developed for image registration [5]. The advantage of deep-learning-based image registration is the capability to incorporate additional information and tasks, such as joint learning of registration and segmentation [6].

In this work, we introduce a method that jointly learns to establish spatial correspondences and detect diagnostically relevant changes between longitudinal images to create continuous change maps. The aim is to differentiate between natural variations and those of clinical relevance. For comparison, we generate change maps using a conventional approach and test both methods on lung CT images.

2 Materials and methods

2.1 Creating change maps

A straightforward approach to generating change maps involves a sequential method. We use a variational registration approach specialized for lung CT images [7] (Fig. 1 (left)). For each pair of reference and template image $R, T : \mathbb{R}^3 \to \mathbb{R}$ and the associated lung segmentation masks ($M : \mathbb{R}^3 \to \{0, 1\}$) and keypoints ($K \in \mathbb{R}^{n,3}$), the cost function

$$\mathcal{I}(y) := \beta_0 D^{\mathrm{NGF}}(R, T(y)) + \beta_1 D^{\mathrm{key}}(y(K^R), K^T) + \beta_2 D^{\mathrm{mask}}(M^R, M^T(y)) + \beta_3 R^{\mathrm{curv}}(y) \tag{1}$$

is minimized individually to find an optimal deformation $y : \mathbb{R}^3 \to \mathbb{R}^3$. In addition to the normalized gradient field (D^{NGF}) as distance measure, the squared distance of the lung segmentation masks (D^{mask}) and corresponding keypoints, determined by the Förstner operator [7], (D^{key}) are used. The weights β_i were determined empirically using a partial data set. The registration is performed in a coarse-to-fine approach over 3 levels. The conventional change map $\mathrm{CM}_{\mathrm{seq}}$ is obtained by computing the difference image between R and $T(y)$, and normalizing the values to $[0, 1]$.

We propose a joint deep-learning-based method that produces a deformation field and change as its output (Fig. 1 right). We use a U-Net architecture with one head each for the deformation field y (3 channels) and the learned change C (2 channels, 1-hot

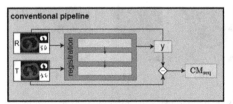 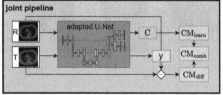

Fig. 1. The conventional sequential registration pipeline *(left)* takes images and their corresponding lung masks and keypoints as input and outputs the deformation y. The joint registration pipeline *(right)* takes only images as input and outputs the change C besides the deformation.

encoded). To ensure that both outputs are well-correlated, the feature map is only split into two separate convolutions in the final layer. Our U-Net is limited to a depth of 2 and an input resolution of $256 \times 256 \times 128$ by the available amount of VRAM (12GB).

To learn the registration with respect to the anatomical conditions of the lung, we employ the same distance measures and regularizers as in Equation 1 using the lung segmentation mask and keypoints. In addition to the curvature regularizer R^{curv}, we use a volume regularizer R^{vol} [8] in the area of the lesions to reduce overcompensation. For this purpose, segmentation masks of the lesions ($L : \mathbb{R}^3 \rightarrow \{0, 1\}$) are used, which are required only for training and not for inference.

For learning the change we use the recall loss L^{recall} from [9]. This loss function reweights the cross-entropy for each epoch, aiming to achieve a balanced precision-recall ratio, particularly in imbalanced datasets. The complete loss function for training is

$$\mathcal{L}(y, C) := \alpha_0 D^{\text{NGF}}(R, T(y)) + \alpha_1 R^{\text{curv}}(y) + \alpha_2 D^{\text{key}}(y(K^R), K^T) + \qquad (2)$$
$$\alpha_3 D^{\text{mask}}(M^R, M^T(y)) + \alpha_4 R^{\text{vol}}(L^R, L^T(y)) + \alpha_5 L^{\text{recall}}(C, |L^R - L^T(y)|)$$

The weights α_i were determined empirically using a partial data set. While training relies on the additional inputs K, M, and L, inference, only requires the R and T.

With the outputs of the network, we create 3 different change maps. The learned change map CM_{learn} is obtained from the change output of the network after a softmax operation. Additionally, we create a change map CM_{diff} from the learned deformation y in the same way as in the conventional sequential approach. To highlight strong changes marked by both change maps, we created a third change map CM_{comb} by pointwise multiplication of the two change maps.

2.2 Data and training

For evaluation, we used the national lung screening trial (NLST) dataset [10] and selected data sets from patients who have imaging data at two time points and at least one lesion. We utilized 250 image pairs for which we also have information regarding the center of gravity and axial diameter to estimate the volume of the lesion. To increase the variability of our data, we generated synthetic images with lesions based on the lung image database consortium (LIDC) dataset [11], which contains images with lesions and associated segmentation masks. Based on the masks, lesions were extracted and

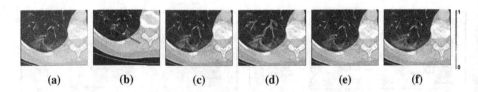

(a)   (b)   (c)   (d)   (e)   (f)

Fig. 2. Exemplary change map visualizations: Sub-images from the reference (a) and template image with an arrow to illustrate the location of the lesion (b). The different change maps are represented as color overlays on the reference image and the color legend: conventional (c), difference (d), combined (e), learned (f).

then inserted into a NLST image, followed by smoothing the boundaries. To model volume changes, we changed the size of the extracted lesions through erosion and inserted them at the corresponding location in the second image of the image pair.

In the conventional image registration pipeline, the images have an average resolution of $512 \times 512 \times 167$ with a voxel size of $0.66 \times 0.66 \times 2$mm. We trained for 50 epochs with a 160/40 pairs split for training and validation; 50 pairs were reserved for evaluation.

2.3 Experiments and evaluation

For evaluation, we binarized the change map using different thresholds on a logarithmic scale, discarded regions with a size of less than 5 voxels, and counted each remaining region as a true positive if it had an overlap with the ground truth region of a lesion. For each threshold, we computed the recall for the synthetic lesions. To determine what size of changes are detected, we created the change maps for each method with the threshold 0.68 and considered the proportion of detected synthetic lesions with respect to the different diameter differences of the lesions. For this purpose, the differences were sorted by magnitude and divided into 10 groups of equal size.

In order to quantify the impact on diagnostic evaluation, we conducted a reader study. Each reader was presented with the same 5 reference images and a rigidly pre-registered template image, and asked to find lung lesions. The study was split into three parts separated by one week. In the first part, no further assistance was given. In the later parts, readers were additionally provided a color-coded overlay of the conventional (second part) and combined learned change map (third part). The reader study was evaluated in terms of reading time as well as precision and recall. The Wilcoxon rank-sum test ($\alpha = 0.05$) was used to examine if there were significant differences between the study parts. We refer to [12] for a more comprehensive discussion of the study.

3 Results

Change maps were created for 50 pairs of images, containing 281 lesions. An example of the colored change maps as an overlay in the reference image is given in Figure 2. In addition, the reference and template image are shown. In CM_{diff} (Fig. 2d), more alterations are delineated due to the less precise registration compared to the conventional approach (Fig. 2c). In this example, a change in lung tissue occurs in addition to a lesion. Both were marked in the difference images as well as in the learned change map CM_{learn} (Fig. 2f). This indicates that other changes besides the known lesions are also learned

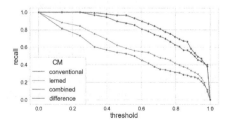

Fig. 3. Recall curves for the change maps (CM) of the different methods across synthetic lesions of all images. The continuous change maps were transformed into binary change maps using various threshold values.

Tab. 1. Mean [minimum; maximum] reading time for the five images in the 3 study parts.

	Reader 1	Reader 2	Reader 3
w/o CM	235.6 s [137.0; 329.5]	348.0 s [298.8; 450.4]	422.5 s [324.3; 617.7]
CM_{seq}	173.6 s [112.6; 267.5]	268.3 s [175.9; 360.5]	331.8 s [226.3; 392.5]
CM_{comb}	258.6 s [221.2; 293.6]	215.3 s [149.5; 279.4]	286.7 s [248.2; 305.8]

by our approach. Figure 3 shows the recall curves across the 141 synthetic lesions for all four change maps. The recall is higher for the change maps created through a difference image (CM_{seq}, CM_{diff}).

When considering the proportion of detected lesions for varying diameter differences, it can be observed that larger changes in lesions can be detected more effectively (Fig 4). For diameter changes smaller than 5.8 mm, the learned methods (CM_{learn}, CM_{diff}) exhibit a higher detection rate of lesions. The average diameter difference for synthetic lesions is 8.99 mm, differing compared to NLST (2.11 mm) and overall lesions (5.71 mm).

For the reader study, overlays were provided of the conventional change map (second part) and the learned change map (third part). Three participants, including a radiologist with 6 years of experience (Reader 1) and two individuals with expertise in medical image processing (Reader 2 and 3), took part in the study. No significant changes in case of mean recall of lesions marked by readers were observed between the study parts (0.29/0.25/0.23). However, a improvement in reading time was observed for Reader 2 and 3 between the first and third parts of the study (each p=0.0079). With each part of the study, Reader 2 and 3 became faster, and the range of reading time decreased across all three readers (Tab. 1). The reading time of all readers decreased by more than 23%.

4 Discussion

In this paper, we introduce an innovative methodology for the generation of change maps, by simultaneous learning deformation fields and change detection. Despite the lower resolution of the images used in the new approach, the results were comparable to the conventional approach. Both methods face challenges in detecting small changes, which could be attributed to the high voxel size and smoothing. However, with our new

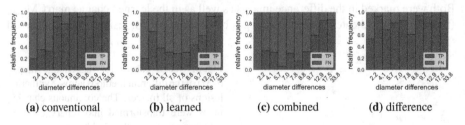

(a) conventional   (b) learned   (c) combined   (d) difference

Fig. 4. The proportion of detected (TP) and undetected (FN) synthetic lesions with respect to the occurring diameter differences. The boundaries for the 10 groups of diameter differences are indicated on the x-axis.

approach, smaller lesions could be detected more effectively. Additionally, it has been demonstrated that our network learns other changes besides the known lesions. Due to the small number of cases in the reader study, no significant changes in recall can be observed. But we observed an improvement in reading time while maintaining the same precision and recall values. Therefore it should be taken into account that getting accustomed to the task can also affect the processing time. Since slight improvements were achieved with our new approach, it can be assumed that, as shown in [2], significant improvements by using a change map can be demonstrated with a larger number of cases.

In the next step, the network will be expanded with a coarse-to-fine strategy in order to improve the registration, and semi-/self-supervised learning methods, such as the contrastive loss, will be applied to learn various changes even without existing segmentation. This study focuses on CT images of the lungs and changes in the lung region and will be extended to other organs. Overall, our proof of concept demonstrated that joint learning of a change map and a deformation field is possible and can provide comparable results to conventional registration in application.

References

1. Drew T, Võ MLH, Wolfe JM. The invisible gorilla strikes again: sustained inattentional blindness in expert observers. Psychol Sci. 2013;24(9):1848–53.
2. Sieren M, Brenne F, Hering A, Kienapfel H, Gebauer N, Oechtering T et al. Rapid study assessment in follow-up whole-body computed tomography in patients with multiple myeloma using a dedicated bone subtraction software. Eur Radiol. 2020;30(6):3198–209.
3. Dufresne E, Fortun D, Kumar B, Kremer S, Noblet V. Joint registration and change detection in longitudinal brain MRI. Proc IEEE ISBI. IEEE. 2020:104–8.
4. Wang Z, Peng C, Zhang Y, Wang N, Luo L. Fully convolutional siamese networks based change detection for optical aerial images with focal contrastive loss. Neurocomputing. 2021;457:155–67.
5. Hering A, Hansen L, Mok TC, Chung AC, Siebert H, Häger S et al. Learn2Reg: comprehensive multi-task medical image registration challenge, dataset and evaluation in the era of deep learning. IEEE Trans Med Imaging. 2022;42(3):697–712.
6. Li B, Niessen WJ, Klein S, Groot Md, Ikram MA, Vernooij MW et al. A hybrid deep learning framework for integrated segmentation and registration: evaluation on longitudinal white matter tract changes. Proc MICCAI. Springer. 2019:645–53.
7. Rühaak J, Polzin T, Heldmann S, Simpson IJ, Handels H, Modersitzki J et al. Estimation of large motion in lung CT by integrating regularized keypoint correspondences into dense deformable registration. IEEE Trans Med Imaging. 2017;36(8):1746–57.
8. Hering A, Häger S, Moltz J, Lessmann N, Heldmann S, Ginneken B van. CNN-based lung CT registration with multiple anatomical constraints. Med Image Anal. 2021;72:102139.
9. Tian J, Mithun NC, Seymour Z, Chiu HP, Kira Z. Striking the right balance: recall loss for semantic segmentation. Proc IEEE ICRA. 2022:5063–9.
10. Team NLSTR. Data from the national lung screening trial (NLST) [Data set]. 2013.
11. Armato III SG, McLennan G, Bidaut L, McNitt-Gray MF. Data From LIDC-IDRI. 2015.
12. Kohlbrandt T. Gemeinsames Lernen von Bildregistrierung und Veränderungskarten für Lungen-CT-Bilder. Masters Thesis, University of Lübeck. 2023.

Abstract: Focused Unsupervised Image Registration for Structure-specific Population Analysis

Jan Ehrhardt[1,2], Hristina Uzunova[2], Paul Kaftan[1], Julia Krüger[3], Roland Opfer[3], Heinz Handels[1,2]

for the Alzheimer's Disease Neuroimaging Initiative
[1]Institute of Medical Informatics, University of Lübeck, Lübeck, Germany
[2]German Research Center for Artificial Intelligence, Lübeck, Germany
[3]jung diagnostics GmbH, Röntgenstraße 24, Hamburg, Germany
jan.ehrhardt@uni-luebeck.de

Population-based analysis of medical images plays an essential role in identification and development of imaging biomarkers. Most commonly the focus lies on a single structure or image region in order to identify variations to discriminate between patient groups. In many applications, existing automatic segmentation tools or trained neural networks are used to identify relevant image structures. However, if new structures are to be analyzed, these approaches have the disadvantage that extensive manually segmented image data are required for development and training. Thus, in our paper [1], we focus on atlas-based segmentation methods for the analysis of image populations. Since, most frequently, high segmentation accuracy is only required in specific image regions while the accuracy in the remaining image area is of less importance, we propose an efficient ROI-based approach for unsupervised learning of deformable atlas-to-image registration to facilitate structure-specific analysis. The proposed approach features a multi-stage registration pipeline using a transformer-based architecture to perform atlas-to-image transfer at high resolution in the specified region of interest and at low resolution in the remaining image space. This reduces computational cost in terms of memory consumption, computation time and energy consumption without significant accuracy loss ind the region of interest. The proposed method was evaluated for predicting cognitive impairment from morphological changes of the hippocampal region in brain MRI images. We compare our approach with models trained on full-resolution and half-resolution images, as well as with a U-net based registration network and iterative optimization-based registration methods. The experiments show that next to the efficient processing of 3D data, our method delivers accurate registration results comparable to state-of-the-art segmentation tools. Furthermore, the proposed method better captures morphological changes in a desired region of interest enabling better distinguishing between different cohorts.

References

1. Ehrhardt J, Uzunova H, Kaftan P, Krüger J, Opfer R, Handels H. Focused unsupervised image registration for structure-specific population analysis. Proc Med Imaging.

Abstract: Combined 3D Dataset for CT- and Point Cloud-based Intra-patient Lung Registration
Lung250M-4B

Fenja Falta[1], Christoph Großbröhmer[1], Alessa Hering[2], Alexander Bigalke[1], Mattias P. Heinrich[1]

[1]Institute of Medical Informatics, University of Lübeck
[2]Departments of Imaging, Radboud University Medical Center, Nijmegen
fenja.falta@student.uni-luebeck.de

Intra-patient lung registration aims to find correspondences between lung images of different respiratory phases, aiding in, e.g., the diagnosis of COPD, estimation of tumour motion in radiotherapy planning or tracking of lung nodules. With recent developments, deep learning-based methods are competing for state-of-the-art in various image registration tasks. Additionally, geometric deep learning on point clouds – in particular learning-based point cloud registration – shows great potential regarding computational efficiency, robustness, and anonymity preservation. Publicly available image datasets for intra-patient lung registration, however, are often not sufficiently large to train deep learning methods properly or include primarily small motions, which transfer poorly to larger deformations. When purely using point cloud data, on the other hand, a fair comparison with state-of-the-art image-based registration methods is not possible and for both expert supervision is desirable. With Lung250M-4B [1], we present a dataset, that aims to tackle these problems. It consists of 248 curated and pre-processed public multi-centric in- and expiratory lung CT scans from 124 patients with large motion between scans. It comprises the DIR-LAB COPDgene [2] data as test data, which is popularly used to evaluate registration methods. Moreover, for each image, corresponding vessel point clouds are provided. For supervision, vein and artery segmentations as well as thousands of image-derived keypoint correspondences are included. Multiple validation scan pairs are annotated with manual landmarks. With all of this, Lung250M-4B is the first dataset to enable a fair comparison between image- and point cloud-based registration methods, while consisting of significantly more image pairs than previous lung CT datasets, and it contains accurate correspondences for supervised learning. The download link for the data, processing scripts and benchmark results are available under https://github.com/multimodallearning/Lung250M-4B.

References

1. Falta F, Großbröhmer C, Hering A, Bigalke A, Heinrich MP. Lung250M-4B: a combined 3D dataset for CT- and point cloud-based intra-patient lung registration. Adv Neural Inf Process Syst. 2023.
2. Castillo R, Castillo E, Fuentes D, Ahmad M, Wood AM, Ludwig MS et al. A reference dataset for deformable image registration spatial accuracy evaluation using the COPDgene study archive. Phys Med Biol. 2013;58(9):2861.

© Der/die Autor(en), exklusiv lizenziert an
Springer Fachmedien Wiesbaden GmbH, ein Teil von Springer Nature 2024
A. Maier et al. (Hrsg.), *Bildverarbeitung für die Medizin 2024*,
Informatik aktuell, https://doi.org/10.1007/978-3-658-44037-4_17

Influence of Prompting Strategies on Segment Anything Model (SAM) for Short-axis Cardiac MRI Segmentation

Josh Stein[1,2], Maxime Di Folco[1], Julia A. Schnabel[1,2,3]

[1]Institute of Machine Learning in Biomedical Imaging, Helmholtz Munich, Neuherberg,
Germany
[2]Technical University of Munich, Munich, Germany
[3]King's College London, London, UK
maxime.difolco@helmholtz-munich.de

Abstract. The segment anything model (SAM) has recently emerged as a significant breakthrough in foundation models, demonstrating remarkable zero-shot
performance in object segmentation tasks. While SAM is designed for generalization, it exhibits limitations in handling specific medical imaging tasks that require
fine-structure segmentation or precise boundaries. In this paper, we focus on the
task of cardiac magnetic resonance imaging (cMRI) short-axis view segmentation
using the SAM foundation model. We conduct a comprehensive investigation of
the impact of different prompting strategies (including bounding boxes, positive
points, negative points, and their combinations) on segmentation performance.
We evaluate on two public datasets using the baseline model and models fine-
tuned with varying amounts of annotated data, ranging from a limited number of
volumes to a fully annotated dataset. Our findings indicate that prompting strategies significantly influence segmentation performance. Combining positive points
with either bounding boxes or negative points shows substantial benefits, but little
to no benefit when combined simultaneously. We further observe that fine-tuning
SAM with a few annotated volumes improves segmentation performance when
properly prompted. Specifically, fine-tuning with bounding boxes has a positive
impact, while fine-tuning without bounding boxes leads to worse results compared
to baseline.

1 Introduction

The segment anything model (SAM) [1] represents a notable and recent breakthrough
in foundation models for computer vision applications. SAM is a model pre-trained on
a dataset containing more than 1 billion masks from 11 million images. It demonstrates
an exceptional zero-shot performance, often rivalling or out-performing prior fully supervised models. This model is specifically engineered for object segmentation with
diverse prompting strategies in the form of points, bounding boxes, and/or textual input.
SAM is designed for a broad generalisation and depth across a variety of segmentation
tasks. Nonetheless, in medical imaging we can encounter more specific tasks such as
segmentation of fine-structure (e.g. lung nodules) or the need of clear boundaries of
segmentation mask (e.g. tumor region), where SAM network is limited [1]. Many recent works have adapted SAM and explored different prompting strategies for medical
segmentation tasks and compared the performance to state-of-the-art segmentation networks on a wide range of datasets, i.e. different imaging modalities and organs [2–5].

© Der/die Autor(en), exklusiv lizenziert an
Springer Fachmedien Wiesbaden GmbH, ein Teil von Springer Nature 2024
A. Maier et al. (Hrsg.), *Bildverarbeitung für die Medizin 2024*,
Informatik aktuell, https://doi.org/10.1007/978-3-658-44037-4_18

Specially, Ma et al. [5] introduced MedSAM which outperforms a baseline U-Net by fine-tuning the image encoder and mask decoder on an extensive medical image dataset composed of more than 1 million images. However, the impact of prompting strategies for specific tasks has not been thoroughly investigated.

In this paper, we aim to investigate the role of the SAM foundation model for the specific task of cMRI short-axis view segmentation. We assess the impact of different prompting strategies (bounding boxes, positive points, negative points and their combinations) on segmentation performance using two publicly available datasets. We further investigate the effect of fine-tuning the model on a varying number of annotated data: from few volumes to a fully annotated dataset.

2 Methods

2.1 Datasets

We experiment with two well-established cardiac imaging datasets, sourced from the the automatic cardiac diagnosis challenge (ACDC) [6] and the multi-centre, multi-vendor, and multi-disease cardiac segmentation challenge (M&Ms) [7]. These datasets exhibit inherent sparsity, as they only provide annotations at end-diastolic and end-systolic phases. The ACDC dataset contains 100 training cases (providing a total of 200 annotated volumes - one for each cardiac phase). 160 volumes were reserved for training and the remaining 40 for validation. The test dataset is composed of 50 cases. Similarly, the M&Ms dataset is composed of 150 training cases (corresponding to 300 training volumes). We split this data into 240 training volumes and 60 validation volumes - the test set contains 136 cases. Notably, the M&Ms dataset encompasses images from diverse vendors and centers. We use the dataset split described in the original work by Campello et al. [7]. We use a variety of pre-processing techniques inspired by nnU-Net [8]. These include random scaling, rotations, Gaussian blurring, brightness, contrast, Gamma correction and mirroring. Images were resized to 224 x 224.

2.2 Segment anything model (SAM):

SAM [1] is the largest foundation model for image segmentation. The model is composed of three parts: an image encoder, a prompt encoder, and a mask decoder. The model can be used without any prompt information, in which case the model segments as many objects as possible. Alternatively, the model can be prompted using text inputs, bounding boxes and positive or negative points. These prompts allow the model to 'focus' on regions of interest. In this paper, we experiment with different prompting strategies using combinations of bounding boxes, positive points and negative points with or without fine-tuning SAM. We fine-tune on a varying number of cases, from 8 to the entire dataset, and learn only the mask decoder (i.e. we freeze the image encoder and prompt encoder, and propagate gradients only through the mask decoder). The default ViT-H model is used for all inference and fine-tuning experiments. We run inference on SAM per class (i.e. we use the left ventricule (LV), the myocardium, and the right ventricle (RV) independently for our tasks) and combine the results into a single output

Tab. 1. Baseline SAM inference results on the **ACDC** dataset. Positive and negative sample counts are per each segmentation class. All Dice standard deviations are less than 0.15. Unless shown, HD standard deviations are less than 5mm and MAD standard deviations are less than 2mm.

Bounding boxes	Pos. samples	Neg. samples	Dice	HD (mm)	MAD(mm)
N	2	0	0.48	38.29 ± 14.14	12.34 ± 5.06
		1	0.66	13.73 ± 8.31	4.67 ± 2.92
N	3	0	0.53	34.09 ± 13.06	10.93 ± 4.36
		1	0.68	13.65 ± 8.10	4.61 ± 2.79
N	5	0	0.60	25.00 ± 12.01	8.24 ± 3.86
		1	**0.69**	13.33 ± 7.51	4.53 ± 2.51
Y	2	0	0.65	14.19	5.31
		1	**0.69**	**12.21**	**4.14**
Y	3	0	0.65	14.21	5.35
		1	0.68	12.79	4.39
Y	5	0	0.66	14.03	5.28
		1	0.68	13.45	4.65

segmentation. We refer to the *baseline* model when referencing experiments without fine-tuning in the experimental section. We evaluate model performance using Dice score, Hausdorff distance (HD) and the mean absolute distance (MAD). Models were fine-tuned for 100 epochs. We use the Adam optimiser ($\beta_1 = 0.9, \beta_2 = 0.999$). An initial learning rate of 1e-4 was empirically determined. We reduce the learning rate on epoch loss plateau with a patience of 5 by a factor of 0.1. A batch size of 1 was used due to GPU memory limitations

3 Experiments and results

3.1 Baseline model

We firstly experimented using the SAM *baseline* model to determine the best prompt setup. We ran inference using combinations of positively sampled points, negatively sampled points and presence/absence of bounding boxes. The Dice score, HD and MAD are reported in Tables 1 and 2 for the ACDC and M&Ms datasets respectively. We observe that in all configurations (with or without bounding boxes and for any number of positive points) using negative samples improves performance for both datasets. The change in improvement reduces when bounding boxes are included in the prompt. For example, on the ACDC dataset (Tab. 1) with 2 positive samples (and a negative sample) the Dice score improves from 0.48 to 0.66 without a bounding box and from 0.65 to 0.69 with a bounding box.

The use of either negative sample points or bounding boxes provide rich spatial information, allowing the network to differentiate between the LV and the myocardium (which envelops the LV). Specifically for the myocarduim, SAM generates poor segmentation masks when prompting with only positive points, as shown in Fig. 1.

Using an increased number of positive sample points tends to have an effect only when prompting with neither bounding boxes nor negative points (the Dice score im-

Tab. 2. Baseline SAM inference results on the **M&Ms** dataset. Positive and negative sample counts are per each segmentation class. All Dice standard deviations are less than 0.15. Unless shown, HD standard deviations are less than 5mm and MAD standard deviations are less than 2mm.

Bounding boxes	Pos. samples	Neg. samples	Dice	HD (mm)	MAD(mm)
N	2	0	0.46	41.30 ± 14.65	13.55 ± 5.36
		1	0.65	14.65 ± 8.75	4.97 ± 3.09
N	3	0	0.48	37.66 ± 13.75	12.29 ± 4.74
		1	0.66	14.24 ± 8.44	4.91 ± 2.96
N	5	0	0.57	27.63 ± 12.20	9.12 ± 3.99
		1	0.67	14.09 ± 8.09	4.83 ± 2.73
Y	2	0	0.66	12.90	4.94
		1	**0.69**	**11.77**	**4.05**
Y	3	0	0.66	12.89	4.95
		1	0.69	11.96	4.17
Y	5	0	0.66	12.80	4.90
		1	0.68	12.39	4.36

proves from 0.48 to 0.60 between 2 and 5 positive points on the ACDC dataset and from 0.46 to 0.57 on the M&Ms dataset).

3.2 Fine-tuned model

We fine-tune using prompts that include two positive points and one negative point, with or without bounding boxes. The results of fine-tuning with bounding boxes are presented in Tabular 3. We observe that fine-tuning improves performance on both datasets, with a larger improvement of 15% achieved on the ACDC dataset. We further observe that training with a greater number of volumes generally increases performance, although the gains are limited. This is especially true for the M&Ms dataset, where fine-tuning with 8 volumes yields a similar Dice score compared to fine-tuning with the fully annotated dataset. Compared to nnU-Net models trained from scratch, we find

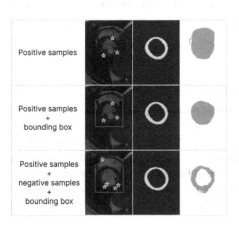

Fig. 1. Effect of different prompting strategies when running inference on the myocardium.

Tab. 3. Inference results for SAM models fine-tuned with limited training data. The models were prompted **with bounding boxes,** two positive sample points and one negative sample per class. Dice standard deviations, HD standard deviations and MAD standard deviations are less than 0.1, 3mm and 1.2mm for all models respectively. Note that the ACDC dataset only has 160 volumes.

Dataset	Metric	0 (baseline)	Number of fine-tuning cases							
			8	24	32	48	80	160	192	240
	Dice	0.69	0.76	0.81	0.82	0.82	0.83	**0.84**	-	-
ACDC	HD (mm)	12.21	9.92	7.42	7.06	7.65	6.33	**5.78**	-	-
	MAD (mm)	4.14	3.50	2.45	2.38	2.48	2.12	**2.02**	-	-
	Dice	0.69	0.76	0.74	0.74	0.75	0.76	0.76	0.76	**0.76**
M&Ms	HD (mm)	11.76	8.12	7.30	7.21	7.07	7.82	6.37	11.77	**6.05**
	MAD (mm)	4.05	2.70	2.66	2.67	2.61	2.68	2.44	2.47	**2.39**

Tab. 4. Inference results of fine-tuned SAM models. The models were prompted **without bounding boxes,** two positive sample points and one negative sample per class. Dice standard deviations are less than 0.1 for all models. Unless shown, MAD standard deviations are less than 2mm.

Dataset	Metric	0 (baseline)	Number of fine-tuning cases			
			8	24	160	240
	Dice	**0.66**	0.61	0.57	0.56	-
ACDC	HD (mm)	**13.73 ± 8.31**	17.11 ± 6.10	20.37 ± 7.64	19.30 ± 6.03	-
	MAD (mm)	**4.67 ± 2.92**	5.99	7.13 ± 2.60	7.02	-
	Dice	**0.65**	0.54	0.62	0.58	0.59
M&Ms	HD (mm)	**14.65 ± 8.75**	23.91 ± 8.49	15.71 ± 5.69	17.89 ± 5.70	16.71 ± 6.04
	MAD (mm)	**4.97 ± 3.09**	8.73 ± 2.81	5.51	6.67 ± 2.08	6.10 ± 2.08

that nnU-Net models are able to out-perform fine-tuned SAM models on both datasets [9]. That said, on the ACDC dataset the SAM models tend to perform better when using less than 32 training volumes. Tabular 4 presents the results when fine-tuning without bounding boxes. We observe that fine-tuning without bounding boxes leads to significantly worse performance on both datasets. From our earlier inference results, we know that not using bounding boxes tends to give very large surface distances. It is possible that the produced segmentations are too large, and the model is not able to learn well-differentiated borders.

4   Discussion and conclusion

In this paper, we experimented with SAM foundation models for cMRI short-axis view segmentation. Specifically, we evaluated different prompting strategies, using bounding boxes, positive and negative points in order to determine their influence on segmentation performance. We initially experiment with the *baseline* model and show that the prompting strategies have a large influence on performance. Our analyses demonstrate that combining positive points either with bounding boxes or negative points has a significant impact, but there is little to no difference when combining bounding boxes and negative points simultaneously. In our experiments, we re-use positive samples for particular classes as negative samples for other classes. Therefore, there is no additional cost of sampling when using negative samples. Models inferred with negative samples yield results very similar to using bounding boxes. For baseline segmentation, we recommend using more positively sampled points (which allows for greater re-use as negative samples), rather than using bounding boxes.

We further fine-tuned SAM using a varying number of annotated volumes. We show that fine-tuning with a limited number of volumes can enhance segmentation performance when appropriately prompted. For this task, we observed that fine-tuning with bounding boxes positively impacts performance, while the absence of bounding boxes resulted in worse results compared to baseline. This is surprising, considering that baseline inference yielded comparable performance between models prompted with and without bounding boxes. We observe that fine-tuned SAM models can be outperformed by specialized nnU-Net models, even with the same amount of training data. Finally, we note that the cost of fine-tuning is relatively small, but can yield significant improvements. When pre-computing image encodings, fine-tuning is fast and efficient.

References

1. Kirillov A, Mintun E, Ravi N, Mao H, Rolland C, Gustafson L et al. Segment anything. 2023;(arXiv:2304.02643).
2. Huang Y, Yang X, Liu L, Zhou H, Chang A, Zhou X et al. Segment anything model for medical images? 2023;(arXiv:2304.14660).
3. Cheng D, Qin Z, Jiang Z, Zhang S, Lao Q, Li K. SAM on medical images: a comprehensive study on three prompt modes. 2023;(arXiv:2305.00035).
4. He S, Bao R, Li J et al. Computer-vision benchmark segment-anything model (SAM) in medical images: accuracy in 12 datasets. 2023.
5. Ma J, He Y, Li F, Han L, You C, Wang B. Segment anything in medical images. 2023;(arXiv:2304.12306).
6. Bernard O, Lalande A, Zotti C et al. Deep learning techniques for automatic MRI cardiac multi-structures segmentation and diagnosis: is the problem solved? IEEE Trans Med Imaging. 2018.
7. Campello VM, Gkontra P, Izquierdo C et al. Multi-centre, multi-vendor and multi-disease cardiac segmentation: the M&Ms challenge. IEEE Trans Med Imaging. 2021;40.
8. Isensee F, Jaeger PF, Kohl SA, Petersen J, Maier-Hein KH. nnU-Net: a self-configuring method for deep learning-based biomedical image segmentation. Nat methods. 2021;18(2):203–11.
9. Stein J, Di Folco M, Schnabel J. Sparse annotation strategies for segmentation of short axis cardiac MRI. 2023;(arXiv:2307.12619).

Abstracting Volumetric Medical Images with Sparse Keypoints for Efficient Geometric Segmentation of Lung Fissures with a Graph CNN

Paul Kaftan[1,2,3], Mattias P. Heinrich[2], Lasse Hansen[4], Volker Rasche[3], Hans A. Kestler[1], Alexander Bigalke[2]

[1] Institute of Medical Systems Biology, Ulm University
[2] Institute of Medical Informatics, University of Lübeck
[3] MoMAN Center for Translational Imaging, Ulm University
[4] EchoScout GmbH, Lübeck
paul.kaftan@uni-ulm.de

Abstract. Volumetric image segmentation often relies on voxel-wise classification using 3D convolutional neural networks (CNNs). However, 3D CNNs are inefficient for detecting thin structures that make up a tiny fraction of the entire image volume. We propose a geometric deep learning framework that leverages the representation of the image as a keypoint (KP) cloud and segments it with a graph convolutional network (GCN). From the sparse point segmentations, 3D meshes of the objects are reconstructed to obtain a dense surface. The method is evaluated for the lung fissure segmentation task on two public data sets of thorax CT images and compared to the nnU-Net as the current state-of-the-art 3D CNN-based method. Our method achieves fast inference times through the sparsity of the point cloud representation while maintaining accuracy. We measure a 34× speed-up at 1.5× the nnU-Net's error with Förstner KPs and a 6× speed-up at 1.3× error with pre-segmentation KPs.

1 Introduction

3D convolutional neural networks (3D CNNs) are common for volumetric image segmentation. However, the 3D image representation is inefficient for small or thin structures as only a tiny fraction of the volume belongs to these objects of interest. Lung fissures are the thin anatomical boundaries between the pulmonary lobes and can restrict the spread of inflammation or neoplasms [1]. They only represent 0.2 % of the volume in a thorax CT. Meanwhile, segmenting the fissures using the state-of-the-art 3D CNN segmentation framework nnU-Net [2] requires 40 s of run time. This is unacceptable in applications like augmented reality, database-scale analyses, and opportunistic screening, where inference time is crucial. In this work, we aim to address the high computational and memory demand of 3D CNNs by sparsifying the image into a point cloud, which can be segmented with point cloud neural networks. Point clouds efficiently encode shape information about anatomical structures and can represent anisotropic data. These properties along with their sparsity make them a desirable abstraction of medical images.

Currently, point cloud segmentation networks are being studied extensively. Especially graph convolutional networks (GCNs) like the dynamic graph CNN (DGCNN)

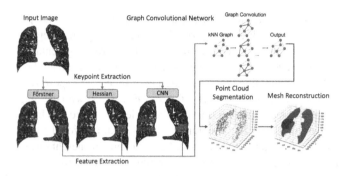

Fig. 1. Overview of the proposed method. We extract a sparse point cloud from the image with one of three different methods. Then, we train a graph convolutional network to segment the points. From the segmented points, a dense object mesh is reconstructed.

[3] provide strong feature extraction capabilities. GCNs are being employed in medical image segmentation. In [4], the nerve segmentation from a 3D CNN is refined by a GCN. In this approach, the GCN post-processing fails if the 3D CNN prediction produces false negatives, which can happen more frequently in segmentation tasks of thin structures. We aim for point cloud extraction with good coverage of the object and focus on the GCN as the primary segmentation model. Other works employ encoder-decoder networks to directly predict a mesh from a volumetric image. For example, Voxel2Mesh [5] is a 3D CNN encoder-decoder with an added GCN for mesh prediction. This approach is inefficient due to the dense image evaluation, which leads to long training and inference times. Instead, we choose to separate the point cloud extraction and the segmentation, yielding a more modular framework that can utilize efficient components.

In this work, we propose a novel framework for keypoint (KP)-based medical image segmentation comprising three major components. First, a point cloud of KPs is extracted from the volumetric image. Then, a GCN segments the point cloud. Finally, 3D meshes are reconstructed from the sparse points of the segmented objects, yielding a dense surface of the target object. An overview of the proposed method is shown in Figure 1. We evaluate the components of our pipeline on lung fissure segmentation in thorax CT images. We show that by focusing on KPs, our pipeline is significantly faster than the nnU-Net and generalizes well to unseen pathological data.

2 Material and methods

2.1 Pipeline for keypoint-based geometric segmentation

We consider three different methods for extracting KPs from input images (Fig. 1, left). Firstly, we employ an established general KP detection method. We compute the Förstner distinctiveness measure followed by non-maximum suppression as described in [6]. The distinctiveness of each voxel is computed from the structure tensor comprising image gradients, yielding high responses on edges and corners. Further, we explore object-specific KP extraction by pre-segmentation. We employ the unsupervised fissure enhancement filter described by [7] and extract its highest $K = 20\,000$ activations as the point cloud. The filter is based on the eigenvalue decomposition of the Hessian matrix and specific fissure gray values. Lastly, we modify MobileNetV3 [8] by replacing 2D convolutions with their 3D counterparts to construct a lightweight 3D CNN for pre-segmentation. We train the network with cross-entropy loss weighted by false negative rate to promote a high recall of fissure points. Since this leads to an over-segmentation, we subsample K of the segmented voxels as KPs. The result of all KP extraction methods is a point cloud $P \in [-1, 1]^{K \times 3}$ containing the normalized coordinates of K points.

We further investigate how including image-based features $F \in \mathbb{R}^{K \times F}$ with the shape information in P improves point segmentation. First, we sample (5^3)-sized patches of normalized image intensity around each KP to obtain an $F = 125$-dimensional feature vector. We compare these patch features to the modality-independent neighborhood descriptor with self-similarity context (SSC) from [9]. An SSC feature vector consists of $F = 12$ image patch differences from the point's neighborhood.

We choose the DGCNN [3] with the EdgeConv graph convolution as our GCN. During training, $N = 2048$ points are sampled randomly from P in each forward pass. Corresponding features in F are concatenated to the coordinates. A k-nearest-Neighbor (kNN) graph G is constructed from P with $k = 40$. We employ the DGCNN without the dynamic graph update and keep G static over all EdgeConv layers. The spatial transformer of the DGCNN is omitted to stabilize the training. Instead, we apply random rigid data augmentation to P. We train with cross-entropy and Dice loss [2]. During testing, we run multiple forward passes with N points until all K points have been segmented.

A sparse point segmentation is not sufficient for most image analysis tasks. Therefore, we fit a dense 3D surface to the segmented points of each object using poisson surface reconstruction (PSR) [10]. PSR finds the surface by solving a Poisson equation for the indicator function of the object described by the points. Points are organized in an octree. We set its maximum depth to 6, balancing the smoothness and resolution of the resulting triangle mesh. Finally, we remove triangles with vertices outside the lung mask and keep only the largest connected component of the mesh.

2.2 Data and experiments

We perform five-fold cross-validation on 380 thorax CT images selected from the TotalSegmentator data set [11]. The provided semi-automatic labels include the pulmonary lobes. We extract fissure label maps by computing the boundaries of the lobes. Labels comprise the left oblique (LOF), right oblique (ROF), and right horizontal fissure (RHF). We compare the different configurations of our pipeline to the state-of-the-art 3D CNN segmentation framework nnU-Net [2]. Since a point-based learning model can focus more on the shape of the objects and less on appearance, we expect our pipeline to generalize better to unseen domains than 3D CNNs. To investigate this, we apply the trained networks to 20 CT images of COPD patients [12] with LOF and ROF annotations from [13]. Target fissure meshes are generated using PSR after label maps have been thinned to one voxel thickness using morphological operations. Between the predicted and the target mesh, we compute the average symmetric surface distance (ASSD), the standard deviation of surface distances (SDSD), and the hausdorff distance (HD). The metrics are averaged over the three fissures. We measure inference times on an NVIDIA RTX 2080Ti GPU (11 GB) and an Intel Xeon Silver 4210R CPU. We implemented all models, KP, and feature extraction methods with GPU acceleration in PyTorch.

Tab. 1. Inference times of our pipeline with different keypoint (KP) extraction methods compared to the nnU-Net (trainable parameters per method in brackets).

Model	KPs	KP extr. [s]	Inference [s]	Mesh rec. [s]	Total [s]
DGCNN	Förstner	0.17 ± 0.05	0.22 ± 0.04	0.96 ± 0.21	1.18 ± 0.22
(0.7M)	Hessian	34.50 ± 11.25	0.26 ± 0.04	2.05 ± 0.55	36.81 ± 11.26
	CNN (3.6M)	0.30 ± 0.14	0.25 ± 0.06	6.23 ± 0.66	6.79 ± 0.67
nnU-Net (31.2M)	–	–	9.44 ± 3.69	34.00 ± 11.28	39.82 ± 11.87

3 Results

Figure 2a shows that CNN KPs led to the lowest surface distances of the three KP methods with an ASSD between 3.07 and 3.56 mm, SDSD between 2.85 and 3.08 mm, and HD between 18.37 and 19.58 mm. In all except Hessian KPs, image patch features gave the best results and SSC was the second best, both clearly outperforming models without image features. Hessian KPs showed an ASSD of 4.81 (SSC) to 5.05 mm (no image features). Förstner KPs had a range of 3.54 (image patch) to 7.36 mm ASSD (no image features). The error of the nnU-Net baseline was lower compared to the variations of our pipeline with ASSD of 2.39 mm, SDSD of 2.59 mm, and HD of 17.90 mm. Figure 3 shows 3D mesh outputs and voxelized label maps.

Table 1 summarizes inference times for KP extraction, point segmentation, and mesh reconstruction. Our pipeline took 1.18 s on average with Förstner KPs, 6.79 s with CNN KPs, and 36.81 s with Hessian. Hessian KP extraction is by far the slowest at 34.5 s. The nnU-Net's 3D CNN inference alone (9.44 s without test-time augmentation and

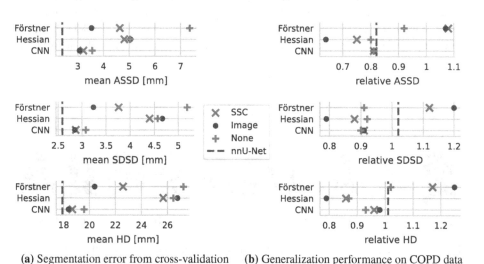

(a) Segmentation error from cross-validation   (b) Generalization performance on COPD data

Fig. 2. Comparison of keypoint and feature extraction methods with the nnU-Net baseline. (a) absolute average symmetric surface distance (ASSD), standard deviation of SD (SDSD), and hausdorff distance (HD) on TotalSegmentator data. (b) SD on COPD data relative to (a).

ensembling) took far longer than the DGCNN (0.22 to 0.25 s). The total nnU-Net run time
with PSR was 39.82 s. PSR computation time is the fastest for Förstner KPs and slowest
for nnU-Net as it depends on the number of segmented points used for reconstruction.
Image patch features were sampled in 0.9 ms, while SSC feature computation took
230 ms on average. The number of trainable parameters of the DGCNN is 0.7 million
compared to the nnU-Net's 31.2 million. The MobileNetV3 for CNN KPs uses 3.6
million parameters.

When applying the trained models to the COPD data set, surface distances were
comparable to or lower than on the source data set (TotalSegmentator), as shown by the
relative metrics depicted in Figure 2b. In this experiment, we excluded the RHF from
the evaluation, as it is not labeled for the COPD data. The nnU-Net baseline showed a
0.82× reduction of the ASSD to 1.95 mm. SDSD and HD did not change significantly.
CNN KPs showed a similar change in ASSD (of 0.81× to 2.33 mm with image features).
Unlike nnU-Net, SDSD and HD are also improved on the COPD data. With Förstner
KPs, only DGCNNs without additional features had a reduced ASSD (of 0.92× to
6.93 mm). Förstner KPs with other features increased all metrics. Hessian KP extraction
yielded the highest decrease in ASSD with image features by 0.64× to 2.67 mm. All
other metrics were also decreased with all features tested.

4 Discussion

In this work, we proposed a pipeline for segmenting thin structures in volumetric images
using a sparse KP cloud representation. We extract KPs, segment them with a DGCNN,
and fit a dense surface mesh to segmented points with PSR. Using sparse inputs and fewer
trainable parameters, our point-based pipeline is much more efficient than the 3D CNN-
based nnU-Net. The pipeline with Förstner KPs produced a 3D mesh 34× faster at 1.5×
error of the nnU-Net or 6× faster at 1.3× error with CNN KPs. Hessian KPs, however,
did not provide a robust pre-segmentation and were slow to compute. We showed that

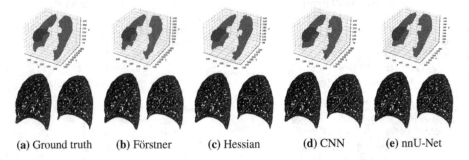

(a) Ground truth   (b) Förstner   (c) Hessian   (d) CNN   (e) nnU-Net

Fig. 3. Qualitative results of our pipeline with different keypoint extraction methods using image
patch features compared to nnU-Net. All variations of our method yield visually convincing
results for this example with well-contrasted fissures. Top row: meshes from Poisson surface
reconstruction. Bottom left: sagittal slices of voxelized label maps of the left oblique fissure (red).
Bottom right: label maps with the right oblique (green) and right horizontal fissure (blue).

the DGCNN can predict fissure points better from sampled image intensities than from the more complex SSC descriptor. Beyond the in-domain evaluation, the method was validated on a data set of COPD patients. Our pipeline and the nnU-Net generalized well to this domain. This means, however, that we could not determine a superior generalization ability of our point-based method compared to the voxel-based network. We aim to further validate our method on other data sets and different thin anatomical structures. Also, PSR mesh reconstruction could be replaced with a faster, learned shape modeling approach.

Acknowledgement. The authors thank the Ulm University Center for Translational Imaging MoMAN (DFG – Projektnummer 447235146) for its support.

References

1. Sofranik RM, Gross BH, Spizarny DL. Radiology of the pleural fissures. Clin Imaging. 1992;16(4):221–229.
2. Isensee F, Jäger PF, Kohl SAA, Petersen J, Maier-Hein KH. Automated design of deep learning methods for biomedical image segmentation. Nat Methods. 2021;18(2):203–211.
3. Fischer M, Neher P, Schüffler P, Xiao S, Ulrich C, Muckenhuber A et al. Enhanced diagnostic fidelity in pathology whole slide image compression via deep learning. Mach Learn Med Imaging. 2023.
4. Balsiger F, Soom Y, Scheidegger O, Reyes M. Learning shape representation on sparse point clouds for volumetric image segmentation. Proc MICCAI. Springer, 2019:273–281.
5. Wickramasinghe U, Remelli E, Knott G, Fua P. Voxel2Mesh: 3D mesh model generation from volumetric data. Proc MICCAI. Springer, 2020:299–308.
6. Heinrich MP, Handels H, Simpson IJA. Estimating large lung motion in COPD patients by symmetric regularised correspondence fields. Proc MICCAI. Springer, 2015:338–345.
7. Wiemker R, Bülow T, Blaffert T. Unsupervised extraction of the pulmonary interlobar fissures from high resolution thoracic CT data. Int Congr Ser. 2005;1281:1121–1126.
8. Howard A, Sandler M, Chu G, Chen LC, Chen B, Tan M et al. Searching for MobileNetV3. 2019;(arXiv:1905.02244).
9. Heinrich MP, Jenkinson M, Papież BW, Brady SM, Schnabel JA. Towards realtime multimodal fusion for image-guided interventions using self-similarities. Proc MICCAI. Springer, 2013:187–194.
10. Kazhdan M, Hoppe H. Screened poisson surface reconstruction. ACM Trans Graph. 2013;32(3):1–13.
11. Wasserthal J, Meyer M, Breit HC, Cyriac J, Yang S, Segeroth M. TotalSegmentator: robust segmentation of 104 anatomical structures in CT images. 2022;(arXiv:2208.05868).
12. Castillo R, Castillo E, Fuentes D, Ahmad M, Wood AM, Ludwig MS et al. A reference dataset for deformable image registration spatial accuracy evaluation using the COPDgene study archive. Phys Med Biol. 2013;58(9):2861–2877.
13. Rühaak J, Polzin T, Heldmann S, Simpson IJA, Handels H, Modersitzki J et al. Estimation of large motion in lung CT by integrating regularized keypoint correspondences into dense deformable registration. IEEE Trans Med Imaging. 2017;36(8):1746–1757.

Advanced Deep Learning for Skin Histoglyphics at Cellular Level

Robert Kreher[1,2], Naveeth Reddy Chitti[1], Georg Hille[1,2], Janine Hürtgen[1,3], Miriam Mengonie[4], Andreas Braun[4], Thomas Tüting[4], Bernhard Preim[1], Sylvia Saalfeld[2,5]

[1]Research Campus *STIMULATE*, Otto-von-Guericke University, Magdeburg, Germany
[2]Department of Simulation and Graphics, Otto-von-Guericke University, Magdeburg, Germany
[3]Institute for Medical Engineering, Otto-von-Guericke-University, Magdeburg, Germany
[4]Laboratory of Experimental Dermatology, Department of Dermatology, University Hospital and Health Campus Immunology Infectiology and Inflammation (GC-I3), Otto-von-Guericke University, Magdeburg, Germany
[5]Computational Medicine, Ilmenau University of Technology, Germany
robert.kreher@ovgu.de

Abstract. In dermatology, the histological examination of skin cross-sections is essential for skin cancer diagnosis and treatment planning. However, the complete coverage of tissue abnormalities is not possible due to time constraints as well as the sheer number of cell groups. We present an automatic segmentation approach of seven tissue classes: vessels, perspiration glands, hair follicles, sebaceous glands, tumor tissue, epidermis and fatty tissue, for a fast processing of the large datasets. Hence, the initial size of the data lends itself to the use of patch-based deep learning models, resulting in good IoU score of 94.2 percent for the cancerous tissue and overall IoU score of 83.6 percent.

1 Introduction

According to the World Cancer Research Fund International (WCRF), skin cancer is one of the most common types of cancer globally [1], with rising incidence rates. Early detection significantly improves the prognosis and reduces the morbidity associated with advanced stages of the disease. Histopathological examination of skin biopsies remains a gold standard for confirming diagnoses, but the increasing volume of cases poses challenges in terms of timely analysis. One notable study by Esteva et al. [2] showcased the effectiveness of a deep learning algorithm in classifying skin cancer images with performance on par with dermatologists.

This study focuses on the examination of skin cross-sections in dermatology, to analyse structures in the vicinity of melanoma. This skin cancer, also called black skin cancer, constitutes to 1.7% of global cancer diagnoses and ranking as the fifth most common cancer in the US [3]. UV exposure is the main risk for melanoma, triggering mutations and fostering an inflammatory environment that supports altered melanocyte survival and spread [4].

Histological imaging provides insight into structure of the cancer tissue and surrounding tissues including vessels. However, evaluation of histology imaging is time-consuming due to the large image data. Here, utilizing deep learning-based image segmentation can speed up the identification of the different tissue types and has therefore great potential in pathology [5]. Kather et al. [6] developed a classifier by training it on images representing eight different tissue types present in human colorectal cancer. The calculation of various features describing the texture within the images resulted in a tissue type classification accuracy of 87.4%.

The aim of our study is to precisely identify and quantify tissue structures in hematoxylin and eosin (H&E) stained histological image data of skin cross-sections for further analysis within clinical research. Employing a patch-based approach, high-resolution images are divided into smaller patches. We adapted a U-Net model by combinations of several loss functions to improve the segmentation results and training speed.

2 Materials and methods

The dataset comprises tissue samples of the upper skin layer, which were H&E-stained and digitized, resulting in 7 color images of 3 patients with a size of approx 3000×9000 pixels. For each image there is a segmentation consisting of 8 different classes (Fig. 1). Here, the important epidermal structures include vessels, perspiration glands, hair follicles, sebaceous glands, tumor tissue, epidermis and fatty tissue, which are important for later evaluations. Other tissue regions contains the remaining tissue structures which are of less importance for the physician's assessment. The segmentation of the ground truth was performed manually by experts and requires a high level of expertise, as both knowledge and experience are necessary to locate all structures in a 2D cross-section.

The number of data samples and the size of the samples tipped the scales in favor of the patch-based approach, which is why the data was subsequently divided into overlapping patches of 256×265. The patch size of 256×256 keeps a balance between the number of patches and the amount of information fed through each patch. To determine this value, both a manual examination of the patches and initial training runs of the networks were carried out. To further reduce the problem, the segmentation labels of irrelevant structures was combined with the background to reduce the number of classes. The scan method itself can be used to separate the foreground from the

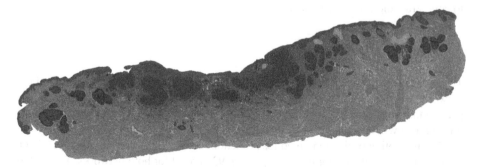

Fig. 1. Tissue sample with segmentation for vessels (violet), perspiration glands (orange), hair follicles (yellow), sebaceous glands (brown), tumor tissue (red), epidermis (blue), adipose tissue (green) and background (white).

background using classic methods (thresholds, flood fill). Furthermore, all patches that do not contain any class information are not fed into the network to reduce the class imbalance.

Subsequently, the data set was divided into 3 folds (2 training, 1 evaluation) for a cross-validation to work out a suitable static evaluation of the following approaches. To obtain the best possible segmentation, two approaches U-Net and PSP Net were compared.

The U-Net [7] was chosen as the basis for the comparison as it is a well-known and widely used network structure for segmentation. A network depth of four levels was used, starting with a number of 32 features, which doubles with each depth level to 256 at the network's bottom. After initial trials, a set of default hyperparameters were established for the training. The network was trained with a batch sizes of four and eight samples. For fast convergence, a learning rate of 0.0005 was chosen, alongside an ADAM optimizer and in total 500 epochs. For the loss function a combination of categorical cross-entropy (CCE), Focal [8] and Jaccard loss was used to counteract the class imbalance.

Since tissue structures consist of groups of cell areas, the idea was to make the local information in the network more usable and to represent it across several pooling layers. The PSP-Net (Pyramid Scene Parsing Network) [9] was selected for this purpose. In the first step, PSP-Net uses a CNN (Convolutional Neural Network) to create a feature map from the input data, then a pyramid parsing module is applied to harvest different sub-region representations, followed by upsampling and concatenation layers to form the final feature representation, which carries both local and global context information. In the last step, the representation is again given into a convolution layer to get the segmentation for each pixel. The pyramid parsing module consists of multiple pooling stages with a deficient pooling kernel size each stage. Pooling with different kernel sizes followed by concatenating the individual representations should ensure that the local information of the pixels benefits the global context information.

The network was trained with a batch sizes of four and eight samples. For fast convergence, a learning rate of 0.0005 was chosen, so was the ADAM optimizer. All tested networks were trained 500 epochs to ensure convergence of all networks. For the loss function a combination of CNN (categorical cross-entropy), Focal and Jaccard loss to counteract the class imbalance.

3 Results

The experiments revealed a notable decrease in mean IoU score during training for both networks when the number of patches was reduced to four compared to using 8 patches per training step. Specifically, the mean IoU score for the U-Net with a patch count of four fell below 70 percent.

The utilization of the combined loss function alongside the patch method yielded a good accuracy for the tumor class, surpassing 93 percent for both networks. The U-Net demonstrated robust segmentation, achieving high accuracies of approximately 82 to 90 percent for the epidermis, sebaceous glands, and hair follicle classes. However, the vessel, perspiration glands, and adipose tissue classes were segmented with slightly

Tab. 1. IoU scores for each Label for U-Net and PSP-Net.

Label	U-Net	PSP-Net
Vessel	0.7089	0.6254
Perspiration glands	0.7433	0.6576
Hair follicle	0.8185	0.6484
Sebaceous glands	0.8451	0.7891
Tumor	0.9419	0.9370
Epidermis	0.9047	0.8697
Adipose tissue	0.7547	0.7172
Background	0.9760	0.9707

lower accuracies, ranging from approximately 70 to 75 percent. In contrast, the PSP-Net exhibited a notable decrease in accuracy, lagging behind by about 10 percent in segmenting these classes, as shown in Table 1.

In summary, the U-Net method was able to achieve a higher mean IoU of 83.6 percent, than the PSP-Net, which had a mean IoU of 77.7 percent.

4 Discussion

The diminished accuracy in labeling vessels and perspiration glands likely stems from class imbalance, limited examples, and their inherent similarity. In the patches, vessels typically manifest individually, whereas perspiration glands tend to appear in groups but exhibit smaller sizes, as depicted in Figure 2. These factors present challenges in effectively distinguishing and accurately labeling these structures.

The decline in the accuracy of adipose tissue identification is likely attributed to the specific cell types present. As illustrated in Figure 3, the depicted regions exhibit minimal tissue presence, predominantly comprising background. This intricacy poses a segmentation challenge for the network, as pooling layers diminish the significance of cell tissue within these areas.

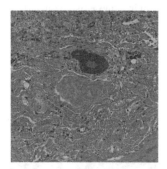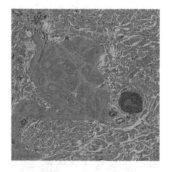

Fig. 2. Examples of the occurrence of vessels (violet) and perspiration glands (orange) in close proximity.

Another challenge impacting accuracy is the network's identification of structures not present in the ground truth but assignable to individual labels (see Figure 4). This underscores the necessity for computer-aided segmentation in scanned histological data, as experts typically face challenges in manually locating all structures in sectional planes. Automated methods play a crucial role in addressing these complexities and enhancing the precision of segmentation tasks.

In comparison with the state of the art, the presented approach achieved competitive results with respect to related deep learning-based segmentation methods of histopathological images, although the specific tissue types and number of classes may vary between most works. For instance, Wang et al. [10] reported an average Dice score for non-melanocytic skin tumors in the range between 87-92 % (vs. our 94 % IoU that roughly corresponds to 96 % Dice) or Liu et al. [11] who achieved a mean IoU of 80 % (vs. our 94 %) on the BCSS challenge regarding breast cancer in histopathological images. Most recently, Li et al. [12] reported a mean classification accuracy of 93 % for various tissues in histopathological image of colorectal cancer patients. However, comparisons between such works must be considered rather indirect, since the database and the clinical objective of those images differ quite vastly and thus, the level of complexity and overall challenge.

The presented study introduces the multilabel segmentation of histological skin cross-sections. With the inclusion of attention modules and careful selection of the loss

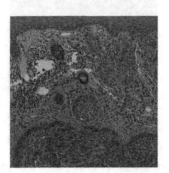 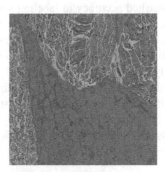

Fig. 3. Example of the background problem in adipose tissue (green).

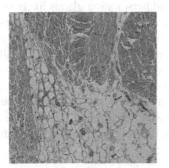 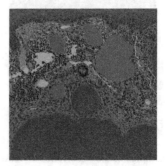

Fig. 4. Example of additional identified tumor areas (cyan).

function, an automatic segmentation of histological data was carried out. The automatic segmentation of the seven classes, i.e., vessels, perspiration glands, hair follicles, sebaceous glands, tumor tissue, epidermis and adipose tissue achieved accuracies between 70 and 94 percent depending on the respective class and can be exploited for further analysis, e.g., morphological analysis, volumetric assessment of tissue classes or a 3D reconstruction aiming at 3D shape analysis of the blood vessels next to the tumor.

References

1. WCRF International: skin cancer statistics. 2022.
2. Esteva A, Kuprel B, Novoa RA, Ko J, Swetter SM, Blau HM et al. Dermatologist-level classification of skin cancer with deep neural networks. Nat. 2017;542(7639):115–8.
3. Saginala K, Barsouk A, Aluru JS, Rawla P, Barsouk A. Epidemiology of melanoma. Med Sci. 2021;9(4):63.
4. Tronnier M, Smolle J, Wolff HH. Ultraviolet irradiation induces acute changes in melanocytic nevi. J Inv Dermatol. 1995;104(4):475–8.
5. Serag A, Ion-Margineanu A, Qureshi H, McMillan R, Saint Martin MJ, Diamond J et al. Translational AI and deep learning in diagnostic pathology. Front Med. 2019;6:185.
6. Kather JN, Weis CA, Bianconi F, Melchers SM, Schad LR, Gaiser T et al. Multi-class texture analysis in colorectal cancer histology. Sci Rep. 2016;6(1):27988.
7. Ronneberger O, Fischer P, Brox T. U-net: convolutional networks for biomedical image segmentation. Proc MICCAI. Springer. 2015:234–41.
8. Lin TY, Goyal P, Girshick R, He K, Dollár P. Focal loss for dense object detection. Proc IEEE. 2017:2980–8.
9. Zhao H, Shi J, Qi X, Wang X, Jia J. Pyramid scene parsing network. Proc IEEE. 2017:2881–90.
10. Wang L, Shao A, Huang F, Liu Z, Wang Y, Huang X et al. Deep learning-based semantic segmentation of non-melanocytic skin tumors in whole-slide histopathological images. Exp Dermatol. 2023.
11. Liu Y, He Q, Duan H, Shi H, Han A, He Y. Using sparse patch annotation for tumor segmentation in histopathological images. Sensors. 2022;22(16):6053.
12. Li YJ, Chou HH, Lin PC, Shen MR, Hsieh SY. A novel deep learning-based algorithm combining histopathological features with tissue areas to predict colorectal cancer survival from whole-slide images. J Transl Med. 2023;21(1):731.

Combining Image- and Geometric-based Deep Learning for Shape Regression

Comparison to Pixel-level Methods for Segmentation in Chest X-ray

Ron Keuth, Mattias P. Heinrich

Institute of Medical Informatics, University of Lübeck
r.keuth@uni-luebeck.de

Abstract. When solving a segmentation task, shaped-base methods can be beneficial compared to pixelwise classification due to geometric understanding of the target object as shape, preventing the generation of anatomical implausible predictions in particular for corrupted data. In this work, we propose a novel hybrid method that combines a lightweight CNN backbone with a geometric neural network (Point Transformer) for shape regression. Using the same CNN encoder, the Point Transformer reaches segmentation quality on per with current state-of-the-art convolutional decoders (4 ± 1.9 vs 3.9 ± 2.9 error in mm and 85 ± 13 vs 88 ± 10 Dice), but crucially, is more stable w.r.t image distortion, starting to outperform them at a corruption level of 30 %.

1 Introduction

Semantic segmentation is a fundamental task of medical image processing. It identifies an image object by classifying each pixel or aligning a shape model comprising anatomical landmarks from a known image to a new one. Recently, deep learning has set a new state-of-the-art in this field, especially the U-Net with its self-adapting nnU-Net framework [1] for the pixel-wise classification approach. However, tackling the shape alignment approach with deep learning is also an active field of research, motivated by the geometric understanding of the object itself, which the pixel-wise classification lacks. This offers several advantages, like addressing limitations such as anatomical implausible predictions of convolutional decoders or opening the possibility of human interaction by propagating local refinements through the whole predicted shape. In [2], ConvLSTM cells are used to predict contour points sequentially on the features of a CNN backbone.Newer work combines such CNN backbones with graph neural networks. In PolyTransform [3], the contour of a predicted segmentation mask is refined by a transformer block, and [4] combines a CNN encoder and a graph convolutional decoder with a new type of image-to-graph skip connections. In this work, we propose a shape-based segmentation pipeline that also utilizes geometric deep learning, yielding promising results using a much smaller CNN encoder (preventing the risk of overfitting) compared to the nnU-Net (factor: 3.7). We formulate the shape-regression in three different approaches and furthermore reveal its higher robustness for corrupted input compared to the pixel-level baselines.

© Der/die Autor(en), exklusiv lizenziert an
Springer Fachmedien Wiesbaden GmbH, ein Teil von Springer Nature 2024
A. Maier et al. (Hrsg.), *Bildverarbeitung für die Medizin 2024*,
Informatik aktuell, https://doi.org/10.1007/978-3-658-44037-4_21

2 Methods

2.1 Pipeline for shape regression

Our proposed pipeline consists of multiple parts (Fig. 1): a convolutional neural network (CNN) backbone extracts features from the input image, followed by a graph neural network (GNN), and finally, a multilayer perceptron (MLP) that maps the generated point features to the desired solution space. To define a 2D point cloud for shape regression, we start from an initial shape (randomly picked from another training sample) and add four additional points for each landmark's local neighbourhood, which were obtained by sampling its offsets from a normal distribution with a small standard derivation. We then sample (bilinear interpolation) image features from the respective positions.

As a CNN-backbone, we adopt an ImageNet-pretrained ResNet18 [5] by cropping it to the first 12 layers and replacing the last two convolutions with dilated convolution to obtain a higher resolution feature map of 32×32 pixels with 64 channels.

We explore two GNN architectures in our pipeline. As a baseline, we chose the well-established PointNet [6] and the Point Transformer [7], which applies the transformer's self-attention mechanism to the local neighbourhood for each point in the point cloud. This enables us to compare the PointNet's performance to the new state-of-the-art. In our pipeline, the GNN takes the $L \cdot 5 = 830$ landmarks, including their additional four sampling points, and projects each in a $K = 128$ feature space. We then select only those point features that correspond to the L landmarks of the initial shape and feed the $L \times K$ feature matrix to the MLP head, which generates the final prediction. This MLP head is shared for all L points and consists of three layers doubling K and projecting them to the desired dimensionality M, where M differs depending on the employed type of shape regression.

All our models are trained with the same hyperparameters: We use the Adam optimiser and reduce its learning rate $1e - 3$ with factor 0.1, if the validation loss has not decreased in the last 30 epochs. We train our models in a supervised manner, reducing the $L2$ distance (first term of Eq. 1) between the predicted and ground truth shape for 500 epochs. As evaluation metrics, we chose the dice similarity coefficient (DSC) and the average surface distance (ASD) in mm and average over five random initial shapes.

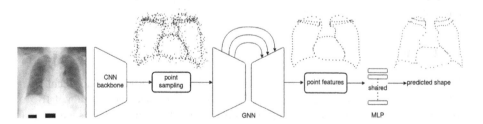

Fig. 1. A schematic overview of our pipeline for shape regression: A pretrained CNN backbone extracts image features, which are sampled in a point cloud for the geometric neural network (GNN) using a random initial shape of the training data. A shared MLP head finally predicts the shape directly or via relative displacement for each landmark.

2.1.1 Formulation of shape regression. In the following, we describe our three different formulations of shape regression.

With the first method, $M = 2$ holds the *relative displacements* in x and y direction for the current landmark. We limit the possible value space to a local neighbourhood of 45×45 pixels (in the image space), and we require a smooth displacement field, which is added to the $L2$ distance loss as regularisation

$$\mathcal{L}_{\text{disp}} = (1 - \lambda_{\mathcal{R}})||S^* - S_{\text{init}} + U||_2^2 + \lambda_{\mathcal{R}}||\nabla U||^2 \tag{1}$$

with $S^*, S_{\text{init}} \in \mathbb{R}^{L \times 2}$ describing the ground truth and randomly picked initial shape with its relative displacement field $U \in \mathbb{R}^{L \times 2}$. We use finite differences to calculate ∇U. $\lambda_{\mathcal{R}} \in [0, 1]$ weights the impact of the regularisation term. In our experiments, we obtain the best results with $\lambda_{\mathcal{R}} = 0.2$.

Secondly, we formulate the shape regression as a *heatmap regression* [8]. For this, we define the range of potential displacements as the same local neighbourhood as in the previous approach. We cover this neighbourhood with an $11 \times 11 = 121 = M$ regular grid G and let the model predict the likelihood of each grid point being the new position of the landmark. To obtain the likelihood, we normalize the logits with a softmax and calculate the relative displacement via the weighted sum over all grid points' coordinates in G.

As a last approach, we formulate the problem as a *direct shape regression*. Therefore, the final MLP head predicts the likelihood ($M = 160$) for each of the 160 training shapes given the image and initial shape. We use these likelihoods as weights in a linear combination of all training shapes to generate the predicted shape.

2.2 Pixel-level baselines

For a comparison to segmentation using a pixel-wise classification, we chose two well-established deep learning architectures. As upper baseline, we use the nnU-Net framework [1] to train two U-Nets on our training split (with the all fold option) to avoid overlapping of lungs and clavicles. However, to make a direct comparison using the same feature input, we additionally train an LR-ASPP head [9] on the same pretrained CNN backbone, but omit the skip connection from the intermediate encoder layer to make the comparison fair. We train it using the same hyperparameters as our pipeline but replace the $L2$ loss with a weighted binary cross entropy loss.

3   Results

We train and test our methods on the Japanese Society of Radiological Technology (JSRT) Dataset [10]. The JSRT consists of 247 chest X-rays with a resolution of 1024×1024 pixels and an isotropic pixel spacing of 0.175 mm. Each image comes with human expert landmark annotations ($L = 166$) for the four anatomical structures of the right lung (44), left lung (50), heart (26), right clavicle (23), and left clavicle (23) (Fig. 2a). For our experiments, we downsample the dataset to 256×256 pixels and divide it into a custom split of 160 training and 87 test images. We use the mean shape of the training split as lower baseline in our experiments.

Tab. 1. The average surface distance (ASD) in mm and the dice similarity score (DSC) in percent for the 87 test images (using five initial shapes). Point Transformer and PointNet are used as GNN in our pipeline (Fig. 1) with the three regression approaches: displacement, heatmap, and shape (Sec. 2.1.1). The best result for shape-based and pixel-level approaches is highlighted in bold.

Structure	Metric	Point Transformer			PointNet	Mean Shape	Pixel-Level Baseline	
		Disp.	Heatmap	Shape	Disp.		LR-ASPP	nnU-Net
Lungs	ASD	3.5±1.5	3.6±1.7	6.7±3.1	3.8±1.7	11.4±5.1	2.9±2.1	1.4±0.6
	DSC	94.5±2.7	94.2±2.9	89.2±5.5	93.9±3.0	82.1±7.4	96.2±0.9	98.1±0.8
Heart	ASD	5.3±2.3	5.3±2.7	9.0±3.7	5.8±3.0	13.2±7.0	4.5±3.3	3.0±1.2
	DSC	91.8±3.9	91.7±4.3	84.8±6.7	91.1±5.0	77.2±12.0	93.6±2.2	95.2±2.1
Clavicles	ASD	3.8±1.7	3.9±1.7	5.0±2.2	4.6±2.1	7.8±3.8	4.5±3.2	1.1±0.3
	DSC	73.0±11.6	71.8±11.2	58.5±22.1	61.3±16.1	37.8±27.0	76.8±5.4	93.4±2.7
Average	ASD	4.0±1.9	4.1±2.0	6.5±3.3	4.5±2.3	10.3±5.5	3.9±2.9	1.6±1.0
	DSC	85.3±12.7	84.8±13.0	76.0±20.6	80.3±18.8	63.4±28.0	87.9±9.8	95.6±2.9

In general, the quantitative results in Tab. 1 show that the pixel-level baselines outperform the graph-based models, with the nnU-Net as the overall best performance,

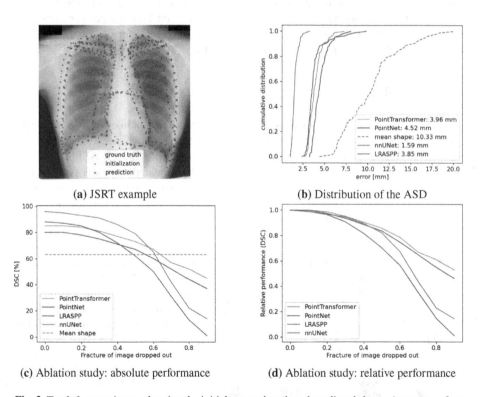

(a) JSRT example

(b) Distribution of the ASD

(c) Ablation study: absolute performance

(d) Ablation study: relative performance

Fig. 2. Top left, a test image showing the initial, ground truth and predicted shape. Average surface distance (ASD) for the test split (top right) and results of our ablation study (bottom).

with an ASD of 1.6 ± 1 mm and a DSC of $96 \pm 3\,\%$. Comparing the three different shape regression approaches of the Point Transformer (Sec. 2.1.1), the performance of the direct displacement and heatmap regression are nearly identical (4 mm error and 85 % DSC), with a minor superiority for the direct displacement formulation for smaller structures like the clavicles (3.8 ± 1.7 mm vs 3.9 ± 1.7 mm). The direct shape regression performs significantly worse, with a gap of nearly 3.5 mm in error and 9 % DSC. We find the Point Transformer outperforms the PointNet in all three approaches (exemplified by the displacement approach with a gap of 5 % DSC). Taking the ASD distribution (Fig. 2b) into consideration, it can be seen that the LR-ASPP has the lowest consistency in its predictions and drops below the performance of the Point Transformer in 10.34 % of all test images.

As an ablation study, we compare the robustness of all models by masking out an area in the input image like in [4]. The position of the mask is chosen randomly, and its size is defined as a fracture of the image size increasing linearly from 0 to 1 with a step size of 0.1. For each sampling point, we mask the test images and evaluate the models. Our experiment shows higher robustness of our proposed pipeline to corrupted input than the pixel-level baselines, with the Point Transformer surpassing the PointNet. Considering the decline in relative DSC performance (Fig. 2d), the pixel-level baselines drop faster and being outperformed by the shape-based approaches at an image masking of 50%. However, for the absolute performance (Fig. 2c), the Point Transformer performs only best in the case of 60 % corruption. Below this mark, it is outperformed by the nnU-Net and above it, the mean shape scores the highest DSC.

4   Discussion

According to the quantitative results in Tab. 1, our proposed pipeline is surpassed by the nnU-Net. However, when using the same lightweight CNN backbone, we can show that its performance is comparable to pixel-level approaches like the LR-ASPP. Note that for shape-based methods, the DSC tends to be underestimated, as some performance is lost due to the conversion from (subpixel) landmark position to mask. Likewise, for pixel-level baselines, the ASD tends underestimated, as it is calculated on the overall segmentation contour instead of L landmarks.

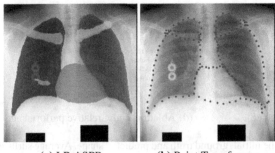

(a) LR-ASPP   (b) Point Transformer

Fig. 3. Predictions of a test image showing an advantage of shape-based segmentation. The two ports in the left lung cause a domain shift and result in a false positive error by the pixelwise classification. In contrast, such anatomical implausibilities cannot be generated with a shape-based approach.

Our ablation study shows an advantage of our method in terms of higher robustness regarding input corruption. In particular, our shape-based Point Transformer outperforms the LR-ASPP at an early stage of 30 % input corruption (Fig. 2c). Fig. 3 demonstrates another superiority of our method, where two ports for injecting medication caused a little domain shift, resulting in a false positive in the LR-ASPP's prediction. Our shape-based method, however, cannot produce such errors due to their anatomical implausibility.

In conclusion, we propose a combination of a CNN backbone and a geometric neural network for shape-based segmentation. We can show that our approach is in reach of the performance of pixel-level methods like the LR-ASPP when the same CNN backbone is used. Furthermore, we demonstrate the benefit of a shape-based approach being less sensitive to image corruption.

In our future work, we will investigate stronger CNN backbones and further optimization of hyperparameters, as well as a possible refinement with a cascade approach [11] to narrow the performance gap to the nnU-Net. Besides that, we plan to take advantage of the geometric understanding of the shape by our model to use it in a human in the loop situation, where it accelerates the annotations process of segmentation mask by allowing to automatically propagate a manual refinement of one single landmark to the whole predicted shape.

References

1. Isensee F, Jaeger PF, Kohl SAA, Petersen J, Maier-Hein KH. nnU-Net: a self-configuring method for deep learning-based biomedical image segmentation. Nat Methods. 2021;18:203–11.
2. Castrejon L, Kundu K, Urtasun R, Fidler S. Annotating object instances with a polygon-RNN. Proc IEEE CVPR. 2017.
3. Liang J, Homayounfar N, Ma WC, Xiong Y, Hu R, Urtasun R. PolyTransform: deep polygon transformer for instance segmentation. Proc IEEE CVPR. 2020.
4. Gaggion N, Mansilla L, Mosquera C, Milone DH, Ferrante E. Improving anatomical plausibility in medical image segmentation via hybrid graph neural networks: applications to chest X-ray analysis. IEEE Trans Med Imaging. 2023;42(2):546–56.
5. He K, Zhang X, Ren S, Sun J. Deep residual learning for image recognition. Proc IEEE CVPR. 2016.
6. Qi CR, Su H, Mo K, Guibas LJ. PointNet: deep learning on point sets for 3D classification and segmentation. Proc IEEE CVPR. 2017.
7. Zhao H, Jiang L, Jia J, Torr PH, Koltun V. Point transformer. Proc IEEE ICCV. 2021:16259–68.
8. Bulat A, Tzimiropoulos G. Human pose estimation via convolutional part heatmap regression. Proc ECCV. 2016:717–32.
9. Howard A, Sandler M, Chu G, Chen LC, Chen B, Tan M et al. Searching for MobileNetV3. Proc IEEE CVPR. 2019.
10. Shiraishi J, Katsuragawa S, Ikezoe J, Matsumoto T, Kobayashi T, Komatsu Ki et al. Development of a digital image database for chest radiographs with and without a lung nodule: Receiver operating characteristic analysis of radiologists' detection of pulmonary nodules. Am J Roentgenol. 2000;174(1):71–4.
11. Ha IY, Wilms M, Heinrich MP. Multi-object segmentation in chest X-ray using cascaded regression ferns. Proc BVM. 2017:254–9.

Abstract: Multi-dataset Approach to Medical Image Segmentation
MultiTalent

Constantin Ulrich[1,4,5], Fabian Isensee[1,2], Tassilo Wald[1,2], Maximilian Zenk[1,5], Michael Baumgartner[1,2,6], Klaus H. Maier-Hein[1,3]

[1]Division of Medical Image Computing, German Cancer Research Center (DKFZ), Heidelberg, Germany
[2]Helmholtz Imaging, DKFZ, Heidelberg, Germany
[3]Pattern Analysis and Learning Group, Department of Radiation Oncology, Heidelberg University Hospital, Heidelberg, Germany
[4]National Center for Tumor Diseases (NCT), NCT Heidelberg, A partnership between DKFZ and University Medical Center Heidelberg
[5]Medical Faculty Heidelberg, University of Heidelberg, Heidelberg, Germany
[6]Faculty of Mathematics and Computer Science, Heidelberg University, Germany
constantin.ulrich@dkfz-heidelberg.de

The medical imaging community generates a wealth of data-sets, many of which are openly accessible and annotated for specific diseases and tasks such as multi-organ or lesion segmentation. Current practices continue to limit model training and supervised pre-training to one or a few similar datasets, neglecting the synergistic potential of other available annotated data. We propose MultiTalent, a method that leverages multiple CT datasets with diverse and conflicting class definitions to train a single model for a comprehensive structure segmentation [1]. Our results demonstrate improved segmentation performance compared to previous related approaches, systematically, also compared to single-dataset training using state-of-the-art methods, especially for lesion segmentation and other challenging structures. We show that MultiTalent also represents a powerful foundation model that offers a superior pre-training for various segmentation tasks compared to commonly used supervised or unsupervised pre-training baselines. Our findings offer a new direction for the medical imaging community to effectively utilize the wealth of available data for improved segmentation performance. The code and model weights are publicly available: https://github.com/MIC-DKFZ/MultiTalent.

References

1. Ulrich C, Isensee F, Wald T, Zenk M, Baumgartner M, Maier-Hein KH. MultiTalent: a multi-dataset approach to medical image segmentation. Proc MICCAI. 2023.

© Der/die Autor(en), exklusiv lizenziert an
Springer Fachmedien Wiesbaden GmbH, ein Teil von Springer Nature 2024
A. Maier et al. (Hrsg.), *Bildverarbeitung für die Medizin 2024*,
Informatik aktuell, https://doi.org/10.1007/978-3-658-44037-4_22

Abstract: 3D Medical Image Segmentation with Transformer-based Scaling of ConvNets
MedNeXt

Saikat Roy[1,3], Gregor Koehler[1,3], Michael Baumgartner[1,3,4], Constantin Ulrich[1,5], Fabian Isensee[1,4], Paul F. Jaeger[4,6], Klaus Maier-Hein[1,2]

[1]Division of Medical Image Computing (MIC), German Cancer Research Center (DKFZ), Heidelberg, Germany
[2]Pattern Analysis and Learning Group, Department of Radiation Oncology, Heidelberg University Hospital, Germany
[3]Faculty of Mathematics and Computer Science, Heidelberg University, Germany
[4]Helmholtz Imaging, German Cancer Research Center, Heidelberg, Germany
[5]National Center for Tumor Diseases (NCT), NCT Heidelberg, A partnership between DKFZ and University Medical Center Heidelberg
[6]Interactive Machine Learning Group, German Cancer Research Center, Heidelberg, Germany
saikat.roy@dkfz-heidelberg.de

Transformer-based architectures have seen widespread adoption recently for medical image segmentation. However, achieving performances equivalent to those in natural images are challenging due to the absence of large-scale annotated datasets. In contrast, convolutional networks have higher inductive biases and consequently, are easier to train to high performance. Recently, the ConvNeXt architecture attempted to improve the standard ConvNet by upgrading the popular ResNet blocks to mirror Transformer blocks. In this work, we extend upon this to design a modernized and scalable convolutional architecture customized to challenges of dense segmentation tasks in data-scarce medical settings. In this work, we introduce the MedNeXt architecture which is a *Transformer-inspired*, scalable large-kernel network for medical image segmentation with 4 key features – 1) *Fully* ConvNeXt 3D Encoder-Decoder architecture to leverage network-wide benefits of the block design, 2) Residual ConvNeXt blocks for *up and downsampling* to preserve semantic richness across scales, 3) *Upkern*, an algorithm to iteratively increase kernel size by upsampling small kernel networks, thus preventing performance saturation on limited data, 4) *Compound scaling* of depth, width and kernel size to leverage the benefits of large-scale variants of the MedNeXt architecture. With state-of-the-art performance on 4 popular segmentation tasks, across variations in imaging modalities (CT, MRI) and dataset sizes, MedNeXt represents a *modernized* deep architecture for medical image segmentation. This work was originally published in [1]. Our code is made publicly available at: https://github.com/MIC-DKFZ/MedNeXt.

References

1. Roy S, Koehler G, Ulrich C, Baumgartner M, Petersen J, Isensee F et al. Mednext: transformer-driven scaling of convnets for medical image segmentation. Int Conf Med Image Comput Assist Interv. Springer. 2023:405–15.

© Der/die Autor(en), exklusiv lizenziert an
Springer Fachmedien Wiesbaden GmbH, ein Teil von Springer Nature 2024
A. Maier et al. (Hrsg.), *Bildverarbeitung für die Medizin 2024*,
Informatik aktuell, https://doi.org/10.1007/978-3-658-44037-4_23

Abstract: Baseline Pipeline for Automated Eye Redness Extraction with Relation to Clinical Grading

Philipp Ostheimer[1], Arno Lins[4], Bernhard Steger[2], Vito Romano[3], Marco Augustin[4], Daniel Baumgarten[1]

[1]Institute of Electrical and Biomedical Engineering, UMIT TIROL, Austria
[2]Department of Ophthalmology and Optometry, Medical University of Innsbruck, Austria
[3]Department of Medical and Surgical Specialties, Radiological Sciences and Public Health, University of Brescia, Italy
[4]Occyo GmbH, Innsbruck, Austria
philipp.ostheimer@umit-tirol.at

An essential bio-marker to detect ocular surface diseases like dry eye disease is ocular redness. In clinical routine, this marker is graded by visual comparison to reference image scales. We aim at supporting clinicians in this time-consuming and subjective task by determining a redness score from images, obtained with a novel device for standardized ocular surface photography (Cornea Dome Lens, Occyo GmbH, Innsbruck, Austria). Therefore, in a previous work [1], we presented a baseline pipeline to automatically determine eye redness. Regions of interest were cropped from the recordings based on the iris center and split up into smaller squared sub-regions called tiles. Each of these tiles was classified by a machine learning model and the redness is extracted for the relevant regions. Using the pipeline, images from 36 healthy and 37 pathological eyes were divided into 5840 tiles (80 per eye). A typical split of 80/10/10 % was used as training, validation and test set, respectively, to train the machine learning model. Hereby, the Random Forest model employed in the baseline was replaced by a deep learning model (ResNet50) to improve the performance. This model showed an accuracy of 0.920 and an F1-score of 0.919 on the test data set compared to an accuracy of 0.856 and an F1-score of 0.855 for the Random Forest [2]. In a follow-up work, we were able to relate the resulting redness scores with gradings from clinicians [3]. A positive relation between the scores and the gradings was observed. In the future, we will expand our data set and include more features (e.g., vessel density) to define a meaningful indicator for eye redness grading, which can be used as support in the clinical routine.

References

1. Ostheimer P, Lins A, Massow B, Steger B, Baumgarten D, Augustin M. Extraction of eye redness for standardized ocular surface photography. Ophthalmic Med Image Anal. Springer. 2022:193–202.
2. Ostheimer P, Steger B, Romano V, Augustin M, Baumgarten D. Automated ocular surface classification for redness extraction of standardized ocular surface photographs. Biomed Eng. 2023;68(s2):12.
3. Ostheimer P, Lins A, Steger B, Romano V, Augustin M, Baumgarten D. Ocular surface redness determination using a novel photography system with reference to clinical gradings. Ophthalmology Vis Sci. 2023;64(8):2379–9.

Abstract: Reducing Domain Shift in Deep Learning for OCT Segmentation using Image Manipulations

Marc S. Seibel[1], Joshua Niemeijer[2], Marc Rowedder[1], Helge Sudkamp[4], Timo Kepp[1,3], Gereon Hüttmann[5], Heinz Handels[1,3]

[1] Institute of Medical Informatics, University of Lübeck, Lübeck, Germany
[2] German Aerospace Center (DLR), Braunschweig, Germany
[3] German Research Center for Artificial Intelligence, Lübeck, Germany
[4] Visotec GmbH, Lübeck, Germany
[5] Institute of Biomedical Optics, University of Lübeck, Lübeck, Germany
marc.seibel@uni-luebeck.de

Medical segmentation of optical coherence tomography (OCT) images using deep neural networks (DNNs) has been intensively studied in recent years, but generalization across datasets from different OCT devices is still a considerable challenge. In this work, we focus on the novel self-examination low-cost full-field (SELFF)-OCT, a handheld imaging device for home-monitoring of retinopathies, and the clinically used Spectralis-OCT. Images from both devices exhibit different characteristics, leading to different representations within DNNs and consequently to a reduced segmentation quality when switching between devices. To robustly segment OCT images from an OCT-scanner unseen during training, we alter the appearance of the images using manipulation methods ranging from traditional data augmentation to noise-based methods to learning-based style transfer methods. We evaluate the effect of the manipulation methods with respect to segmentation quality and changes in the feature space of the DNN. Reducing the domain shift with style transfer methods results in a significantly better segmentation of pigment epithelial detachment (PED). We evaluate the obtained segmentation networks qualitatively using t-SNE and quantitatively by measuring the univariate Wasserstein distance between feature representations across domains. We find that the segmentation quality of PED is negatively correlated with the distance between training and test distributions.f To obtain the best segmentation performance, we find that style transfer should be applied either at train or test time (but not at both), depending on which domain is used for training. Our methods and results help researchers to choose and evaluate image manipulation methods for developing OCT segmentation models which are robust against domain shifts. This paper was accepted and will be presented at the SPIE for Computer-Aided Diagnosis 2024 [1].

References

1. Seibel MS, Niemeijer J, Rowedder M, Kepp T, Hüttmann G, Handels H. Reducing the impact of domain shift in deep learning for OCT segmentation using image manipulations. Proc BVM. 2024.

© Der/die Autor(en), exklusiv lizenziert an
Springer Fachmedien Wiesbaden GmbH, ein Teil von Springer Nature 2024
A. Maier et al. (Hrsg.), *Bildverarbeitung für die Medizin 2024*,
Informatik aktuell, https://doi.org/10.1007/978-3-658-44037-4_25

Neural Implicit k-space with Trainable Periodic Activation Functions for Cardiac MR Imaging

Patrick T. Haft[1], Wenqi Huang[1], Gastao Cruz[2], Daniel Rueckert[1,3], Veronika A. Zimmer[1], Kerstin Hammernik[1]

[1]Technical University of Munich, Munich, Germany
[2]University of Michigan, Michigan, United States
[3]Imperial College London, London, United Kingdom
patrick.haft@tum.de

Abstract. In MRI reconstruction, neural implicit k-space (NIK) representation maps spatial frequencies to k-space intensity values using an MLP with periodic activation functions. However, the choice of hyperparameters for periodic activation functions is challenging and influences training stability. In this work, we introduce and study the effectiveness of trainable (non-)periodic activation functions for NIK in the context of non-Cartesian Cardiac MRI. Evaluated on 42 radially sampled datasets from 6 subjects, NIKs with the proposed trainable activation functions outperform qualitatively and quantitatively other state-of-the-art reconstruction methods, including NIK with fixed periodic activation functions.

1 Introduction

Implicit neural representation (INR) continuously parametrizes an arbitrary signal implicitly by a trained neural network. Input values, e.g., pixel coordinates in an image, are mapped by the trained neural network to attribute values, e.g., RGB values. INR can be applied to various types of signals, such as sound, images, videos, or 3D shapes [1]. In [2], a novel framework for ECG-triggered non-Cartesian Cardiac Magnetic Resonance (MR) Imaging was developed. The method learned an INR in k-space (NIK), resulting in improved artifact removal and spatio-temporal resolution for cardiac MRI, which is the leading modality to assess cardiac function and morphology. Beyond MRI, INRs have also been used for deformable image registration of 4D chest computed tomography (CT) images [3, 4]. These works underpin that periodic activation functions are crucial for reconstructing high-frequency information.

Initially, INRs used multi-layer perceptrons (MLP) with rectified linear unit (ReLU) activations [5]. In follow-up work, MLPs with the periodic sine activation function outperformed ReLU-MLPs in capturing fine details [6]. Detailed representations were successfully created for various signal types by using dubbed sinusoidal networks (SIRENs). Further advancements in INR have been made by incorporating complex Gabor wavelets as activation functions, leading to the development of wavelet implicit neural representation (WIRE) [7]. WIRE's use of complex Gabor wavelets as activation functions results in increased robustness to signal noise, improved accuracy, and reduced training time compared to previous INR methods. These works show that more complex activation functions than ReLU are required to capture fine details. However, the choice of hyper-parameters and training stability is challenging.

© Der/die Autor(en), exklusiv lizenziert an
Springer Fachmedien Wiesbaden GmbH, ein Teil von Springer Nature 2024
A. Maier et al. (Hrsg.), *Bildverarbeitung für die Medizin 2024*,
Informatik aktuell, https://doi.org/10.1007/978-3-658-44037-4_26

To overcome these challenges, we propose trainable periodic and non-periodic activation functions for NIK. The effectiveness of using a trainable activation function instead of choosing a predefined one has been successfully shown for other deep learning applications [8–11]. We expand the framework for ECG-triggered non-Cartesian Cardiac MR Imaging [2] by adding support for trainable (non-)periodic activation functions. The evaluation shows the superior performance of the implemented models compared to several state-of-the-art reconstruction methods, including the original NIK with sine activation functions for Cardiac MRI.

2 Materials and methods

2.1 Neural implicit k-space representation

In this work, we used a slightly modified version of NIK [2] illustrated in Figure 1 (a). The model learns a mapping $f : V \rightarrow K$, with $V \subseteq \mathbb{R}^3$ representing k-space coordinates and $K \subseteq \mathbb{C}^j$ representing the j-dimensional complex signal vector space. Whereby j is defined as the number of coils. A k-space coordinate $v = [t, k_x, k_y]^\top \in V$ consists of three elements: measured time point t and spatial frequencies k_x and k_y. During training, the k-space coordinate $v_m = [t_m, k_{xm}, k_{ym}]^\top \in V$ of a sample $m = 1, 2, ..., M$ is fed through the network, where M is the total number of samples. The optimizer minimizes the error between the predicted vector and the corresponding k-space signal vector $y_m \in K$. During inference, signal values of k-space points on a Cartesian grid

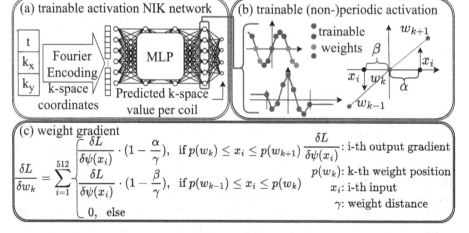

Fig. 1. Schematic illustration of the NIK with trainable periodic activation functions. (a) the MLP predicts the complex k-space intensity per coil from the input feature t, k_x, and k_y, which represent time point and k-space coordinates. (b) the input of the (non-)periodic activation is interpolated between two weights. The first plot (purple, blue, green) shows a trainable periodic activation function with sine initialization. The second plot illustrates an already trained non-periodic activation function with Gabor wavelet initialization. (c) The final gradient of one weight is the sum of all gradients of this weight over all features.

are predicted by the model. The inverse fast Fourier transform and coil combination are applied to the complete k-space to obtain the final reconstruction.

NIK [2] uses a multi-layer perception (MLP) with 8 hidden layers and 512 features. A random Gaussian matrix B, with entries independently drawn from a normal distribution $\mathcal{N}(0, 1)$, is generated for each element in the k-space coordinate $v = [t, k_x, k_y]$. The matrix B is used for positional encoding of v with Fourier features [12] defined as $\gamma(v) = [\cos(2\pi Bv), \sin(2\pi Bv)]$. While the original NIK uses sine activation functions, which is inspired by [6], we introduce trainable activation functions in Sec. 2.2.

2.2 Trainable activation functions

We define trainable non-periodic activation functions $\psi(x)$ applied to the input x as linear weighted combination of two neighboring trainable weights w_{k-1} and w_k. Outside the interval $[v_{min}, v_{max}]$ the weights are extrapolated. Hence, $\psi(x)$ reads as

$$\psi(x) = \begin{cases} w_n, & \text{if } x \geq v_{max} \\ w_1, & \text{if } x \leq v_{min} \\ w_k \dfrac{p(w_{k+1}) - x}{p(w_{k+1}) - p(w_k)} + w_{k+1} \dfrac{x - p(w_k)}{p(w_{k+1}) - p(w_k)}, & \text{if } p(w_k) \leq x \leq p(w_{k+1}) \end{cases}$$

where $p(w_k)$ defines the position on the natural number line. The trainable weights allow us to learn an activation function that does not require frequency-tuning of fixed periodic activations, and also allows us to capture high frequency details.

In the periodic case, the input x is mapped into the interval $[v_{min}, v_{max}]$. Hence, the function repeats with a period of $v_{max} - v_{min}$. Before training, the weights are initialized by a pre-defined function. The sine function was used for the periodic version, inspired by [6]. In the non-periodic case, the Gabor wavelet function was used, inspired by [7].

2.3 Experimental setup

2.3.1 Dataset. We evaluated our method on the cardiac MR dataset used in [2]. The dataset consists of 6 healthy subjects with 7 short-axis slices each and 20 measured heartbeats, acquired on an 1.5 T scanner (Ingenia, Philips, Best, The Netherlands). To evaluate the performance of accelerated data acquisition, only 4 heartbeats were used. IRB approval and informed consent were obtained for all in vivo experiments. Following sequence parameters were used for acquisition: short axis slice; 28 receiver coils; FOV = 256×256 mm^2; 8 mm slice thickness; resolution = 2×2 mm^2; TE/TR = 1.16/2.3 ms; b-SSFP readout; radial tiny golden angle of ~23.6°; flip angle 60°; 8960 radial spokes acquired; nominal scan time ~20 s; ECG-triggered breath-hold acquisition.

2.3.2 Training settings. The training was performed on an Nvidia Quadro RTX 6000 (24 GB). To optimize the model, the Adam optimizer was used with a learning rate of $3 \cdot 10^{-5}$ for the linear layer parameters and $3 \cdot 10^{-3}$ for the parameters of the trainable activation functions. The trainable (non-)periodic activation function were implemented in

Tab. 1. Mean and standard deviation of all reconstruction methods for NRMSE, PSNR, SSIM.

Model	NRMSE	PSNR (dB)	SSIM
Trainable sine NIK (proposed)	*0.181 ± 0.036*	*33.795 ± 1.936*	*0.861 ± 0.040*
Trainable Gabor wavelet NIK (proposed)	0.186 ± 0.035	33.534 ± 2.049	0.854 ± 0.040
NIK [2]	0.193 ± 0.059	33.359 ± 2.210	0.850 ± 0.037
CG-SENSE [14]	0.217 ± 0.036	32.185 ± 1.725	0.768 ± 0.048
L+S [15]	0.214 ± 0.032	32.301 ± 1.645	0.772 ± 0.043
INUFFT	0.334 ± 0.057	28.471 ± 1.702	0.620 ± 0.063

Optox (https://github.com/midas-tum/optox), PyTorch, and CUDA. The number of trainable weights was set to 31 similar to [10]. The interval $[v_{min}, v_{max}]$ was set empirically to $[-\frac{\pi}{5}, \frac{\pi}{5}]$ for sine and to $[-0.3, 0.3]$ for Gabor initialization. As in the NIK framework [2], the high dynamic range loss was used during training, which was inspired by [13]. The models were trained for 1500 epochs, which resulted in a training time ranging from 34 to 59 minutes, depending on the slice. All other hyperparameters were consistent with [2].

2.3.3 Evaluation. The proposed NIK with trainable (non-)periodic activation functions and the original NIK [2] with sine activation were compared to inverse NUFFT (INUFFT), conjugate gradient sENSE (CG-SENSE) [14], and low rank plus sparse (L+S) [15]. The evaluation is based on the average and standard deviation of three metrics: the normalized root mean squared error (NRMSE), peak signal-to-noise ratio (PSNR), and structural-similarity index (SSIM). To calculate the metrics, the CG-SENSE reconstruction [14] with the data of 20 heartbeats was used as reference.

3 Results

Table 1 shows that the proposed trainable periodic sine NIK and trainable non-periodic Gabor wavelet NIK outperform all other methods for every metric. This indicates that the proposed models produce improved reconstruction results. Trainable periodic sine NIK performs superior to the trainable non-periodic Gabor wavelet NIK in all cases.

Qualitative results comparing the different methods are shown in Figure 2. The error maps (bottom row) indicate that the proposed trainable periodic sine NIK, trainable non-periodic Gabor wavelet NIK, and the original NIK implementation outperform the other methods. Especially at edges, it is evident that the other models struggle to generate accurate reconstructions, whereas the proposed and original NIK implementations demonstrate superior results. Furthermore, the error maps in Figure 2 confirm the improved reconstruction result of the proposed version compared to the original implementation. The visual comparison verifies that trainable periodic sine NIK is superior to the trainable non-periodic Gabor wavelet NIK on this dataset.

Figure 3 shows the trainable periodic activation functions of all layers, which were initialized with $\sin(x \cdot 30)$ before training. Figure 3 demonstrates that the shapes of the activation functions changed during training.

4   Discussion

In this work, we explored the effectiveness of trainable activation functions for INRs. We proposed periodic and non-periodic activation functions and incorporated them into the framework for ECG-triggered non-Cartesian Cardiac MR Imaging [2]. The quantitative and visual evaluation demonstrated that NIKs [2] with trainable activation functions outperform all other reconstructions methods, including the original version, and produce finer details in the reconstruction results.

Further research is needed to find optimal model parameters for the trainable NIK version. The parameters used in the performance evaluation for the trainable NIK were consistent with those in [2], which were optimized for the original NIK version. Furthermore, other types of interpolation could be tested. For example, the linear interpolation could be replaced with b-spline interpolation. Trainable (non-)periodic activation functions could be applied to other INR tasks or, more generally, to other deep learning

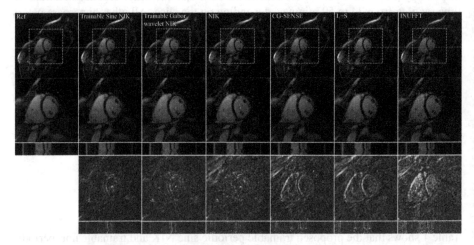

Fig. 2. Reconstructed images from four heartbeats data. The second row shows the zoomed view visualized by the yellow box in the first row, with the corresponding error map in row four. Row three shows the x-t profile, with the corresponding error map in row five.

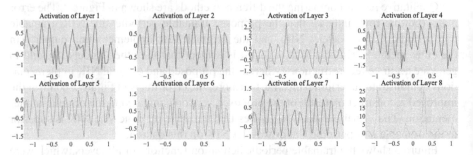

Fig. 3. Example of a trainable periodic activation functions after training.

models where activation functions play a crucial role, e.g., for image registration as in [3, 4].

References

1. Chen Z, Zhang H. Learning implicit fields for generative shape modeling. Proc IEEE CVPR. 2019:5939–48.
2. Huang W, Li HB, Pan J, Cruz G, Rueckert D, Hammernik K. Neural implicit k-space for binning-free non-aartesian cardiac MR imaging. Proc MICCAI. Springer. 2023:548–60.
3. Wolterink JM, Zwienenberg JC, Brune C. Implicit neural representations for deformable image registration. Int Conf Med Imag Deep Learn. 2022:1349–59.
4. Zimmer V, Hammernik K, et al. Towards generalised neural implicit representations for image registration. DGM4MICCAI@MICCAI. 2023, in print.
5. Mildenhall B, Srinivasan PP, Tancik M, Barron JT, Ramamoorthi R, Ng R. NeRF: representing scenes as neural radiance fields for view synthesis. Commun ACM. 2021;65(1):99–106.
6. Sitzmann V, Martel J, Bergman A, Lindell D, Wetzstein G. Implicit neural representations with periodic activation functions. Adv Neural Inf Process Syst. 2020;33:7462–73.
7. Saragadam V, LeJeune D, Tan J, Balakrishnan G, Veeraraghavan A, Baraniuk RG. WIRE: wavelet implicit neural representations. Proc IEEE CVPR. 2023:18507–16.
8. Agostinelli F, Hoffman M, Sadowski P, Baldi P. Learning activation functions to improve deep neural networks. arXiv preprint arXiv:1412.6830. 2014.
9. Chen Y, Pock T. Trainable nonlinear reaction diffusion: a flexible framework for fast and effective image restoration. IEEE Trans Pattern Anal Mach Intell. 2016;39(6):1256–72.
10. Kobler E, Klatzer T, Hammernik K, Pock T. Variational networks: connecting variational methods and deep learning. Proc GCPR. Springer. 2017:281–93.
11. Hammernik K, Klatzer T, Kobler E, Recht MP, Sodickson DK, Pock T et al. Learning a variational network for reconstruction of accelerated MRI data. Magn Reson Med. 2018;79(6):3055–71.
12. Tancik M, Srinivasan P, Mildenhall B, Fridovich-Keil S, Raghavan N, Singhal U et al. Fourier features let networks learn high frequency functions in low dimensional domains. Adv Neural Inf Process Syst. 2020;33:7537–47.
13. Mildenhall B, Hedman P, Martin-Brualla R, Srinivasan PP, Barron JT. NeRF in the dark: high dynamic range view synthesis from noisy raw images. Proc IEEE CVPR. 2022:16190–9.
14. Pruessmann KP, Weiger M, Börnert P, Boesiger P. Advances in sensitivity encoding with arbitrary k-Space trajectories. Magn Reson Med. 2001;46(4):638–51.
15. Otazo R, Candes E, Sodickson DK. Low-rank plus sparse matrix decomposition for accelerated dynamic MRI with separation of background and dynamic components. Magn Reson Med. 2015;73(3):1125–36.

Effect of Training Epoch Number on Patient Data Memorization in Unconditional Latent Diffusion Models

Salman U. Hassan Dar[1,2,3], Isabelle Ayx[4], Marie Kapusta[1], Theano Papavassiliu[2,3,5], Stefan O. Schoenberg[2,4], Sandy Engelhardt[1,2,3]

[1]Department of Internal Medicine III, Heidelberg University Hospital, Heidelberg, Germany
[2]AI Health Innovation Cluster, Heidelberg, Germany
[3]DZHK (German Centre for Cardiovascular Research), Heidelberg, Germany
[4]Department of Radiology and Nuclear Medicine, University Medical Centre Mannheim, Mannheim, Germany
[5]First Department of Medicine-Cardiology, University Medical Centre Mannheim, Mannheim, Germany
salmanulhassan.dar@med.uni-heidelberg.de

Abstract. Deep diffusion models hold great promise for open data sharing while preserving patient privacy by utilizing synthetic high quality data as surrogates for real patient data. Despite the promise, such models are also prone to patient data memorization, where generative models synthesize patient data copies instead of novel samples. This can compromise patient privacy and further lead to patient re-identification. Given the risks, it is of considerable importance to investigate the reasons underlying memorization in such models. One aspect that is typically ignored is number of epochs while training, and over-training a model can lead to memorization. Here, we evaluate the effect of over-training on memorization. We train diffusion models on a publicly available chest X-ray dataset for varying number of epochs and detect patient data copies among synthesized samples using self-supervised models. Our results suggest that over-training can result in enhanced data memorization and it is an important aspect that should be considered while training generative models.

1 Introduction

Recent advances in deep generative modeling models have enabled the possibility of open data sharing without compromising patient privacy. Generative models learn data distribution and generate novel synthetic samples, and since these samples do not belong to a patient, they can be used as surrogates for the real data [1]. In fact, few synthetic datasets or trained generative models have already been made publicly available [1–3].

Currently latent diffusion models (LDMs) hold the position as state-of-the-art in medical image synthesis [1, 4]. Regardless of their capability to generate high quality and diverse images, an aspect that is typically ignored is the capacity of these networks to memorize patient images. A few recent studies suggest that these models are prone to memorization and generate patient copies [5–7]. This brings the whole notion regarding generative models for open data sharing into question, given that one of the main objective is to share data while preserving patient privacy. Therefore, understanding the underlying reasons leading to memorization and mitigating them is essential for safe open data sharing.

Here, we investigate the effect of training epoch number on memorization in 2D unconditional latent diffusion models. Currently, there is no standard criterion to choose optimum training epoch number for generative models in medical imaging, and typically studies just report a number without performing thorough evaluation. Moreover, the metrics typically reported to compare generative models in terms of quality and diversity can have desirable values even when the models memorize training patient data. To this end, we train LDMs on a publicly available chest X-ray dataset, and assess memorization as a function of training epochs. We detect patient data replicas generated by trained LDM via self-supervised models trained through a contrastive learning approach. Our results suggest that over-training the models enhances memorization, and it is an important aspect that should be considered while utilizing generative models for open data sharing.

2 Materials and methods

2.1 Generative modeling via latent diffusion models

Latent diffusion models (LDMs) belong to a family of generative models that learn data distribution through sequential denoising in a lower dimensional latent space (Fig. 1). The lower dimensional latent space is learned using an auto-encoder, which is trained to first project an image x onto its latent space representation z_0 using an encoder $\mathcal{E}$. While training the auto-encoder, the projection onto the latent space is followed by reconstruction via a decoder $\mathcal{D}$ that enforces the latent space to retain meaningful information while performing compression.

Afterwards, a denoising diffusion probabilistic model is trained in the latent space. First, noise modeled as normal distribution is gradually added to the latent representation (z_0) in small increments (Δt) with a variance schedule β_t. Consequently, at any time (t), the conditional distribution of z_t given z_{t-1} $(q(z_t|z_{t-1}))$ also follows a normal distribution with mean $\sqrt{1 - \beta_t} z_{t-1}$ and variance $\beta_t I$. The diffusion model is then trained to approximate $q(z_{t-1}|z_t)$ via a neural network $\hat{q}_\theta (z_{t-1}|z_t)$. Upon training, the network can be used to generate new samples by starting with normal distribution $z_T \sim \mathcal{N}(0, I)$, and obtaining z_0 through progressive denoising. The decoder $\mathcal{D}$ can then be used to obtain novel sample from image distribution.

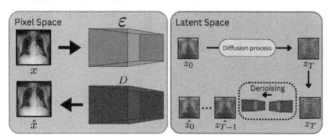

Fig. 1. Latent diffusion model.

2.2 Memorization assessment

Despite the ability of such models to generate high-quality and diverse images, such models are also prone to data memorization [5, 6]. Data memorization is a phenomenon where the models can generate copies of training data samples instead of novel realistic samples. An important question arises as to what constitutes a copy. Here, a copy is defined as a synthesized sample that shares the same anatomical structure with a training sample with minor variations such as rotation, flipping or slight changes in contrast [5].

2.2.1 Self-supervised training.

To detect patient data copies/replicas we trained a model via contrastive learning (Fig. 2a). The model projects each sample onto a lower dimensional embedding space with the aim to bring each sample closer to its variation, and push each sample away from other samples. One naive approach is to have one positive pair $(y_j, y_{j'})$ and one negative pair (y_j, y_k) for each sample, where y_j is the jth training sample, $y_{j'}$ is its variation and y_k is kth sample with $j \neq k$. However, we observed that such approach was unable to push samples within negative pairs away from each other. For this purpose, we increased the number of negative pairs per sample [8]. In each batch B of size K, first, variation or each sample was obtained via rotation or flipping, making $2K$ samples in total. In vectorized form these $2K$ samples can be presented as $B' = [y_1, y_{1'}, ..., y_K, y_{K'}]$. Afterwards, positive and negative pairs were created. Each sample consisted of 1 positive and $2(K - 1)$ negative pairs. The network was trained to minimize the normalized temperature-scaled cross entropy (NT-Xent) loss [8]. All samples within B' are fed to a model f_θ to obtain corresponding their embeddings $B'_E = [e_1, e_{1'}, ..., e_K, e_{K'}]$. For each jth sample (y_j) within B, NT-Xent loss can then be expressed as

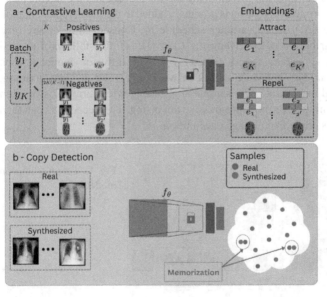

Fig. 2. a) A self-supervised model is trained to project images onto a lower dimensional embedding space, where a sample is attracted to its variations and repelled from all other samples in a batch. b) Synthetic samples lying very close to training samples are categorized as copies.

$$\mathcal{L}_j = -\log \frac{\exp\left(s_{e_j,e_j'}/\tau\right)}{\sum_{k=1}^{2K} \mathbf{1}_{[k \neq j]} \exp\left(s_{e_j,e_k}/\tau\right)} - \log \frac{\exp\left(s_{e_j',e_j}/\tau\right)}{\sum_{k=1}^{2K} \mathbf{1}_{[k \neq j']} \exp\left(s_{e_{j'},e_k}/\tau\right)} \quad (1)$$

where s_{e_j,e_k} denotes similarity between embeddings e_j and e_k, $\mathbf{1}_{[k \neq j]}$ is an indicator function that is 1 if $k \neq j'$ and 0 otherwise, and τ is a constant set to 0.07.

2.2.2 Copy detection. To detect patient data copies, the trained self-supervised model f_θ was utilized (Fig. 2b). First, all training, validation and synthetic samples were passed through the network to obtain their corresponding embeddings. Next, Pearson's correlation coefficient was computed between all pairs of training and validation sample embeddings, and for each training sample closest validation sample was selected. Afterwards, a threshold value (ρ) was defined as 95th percentile of the correlation values between training and corresponding closest validation sample embeddings. Finally, for each training sample, the closest synthetic sample was selected as a copy candidate based on correlations between training and synthetic sample embeddings. All copy candidates having correlation values greater than ρ were categorized as copies.

2.3 Dataset and network training

We used publicly available NIH chest X-ray dataset consisting of patients with common thorax diseases [9]. Originally the dataset consists of 112,120 X-ray images of 30,805 unique patients. For proof of concept demonstration and reduced computational complexity, we utilized 20,000 images where 10,000 were reserved for training and 10,000 for validation. All images were resized to have a resolution of 512x512, and pixel intensity was normalized in the range [-1,1].

For the training of LDM, network architecture, training procedures, hyperparameters and loss functions were adopted from https://github.com/Warvito/generative_chestxray, which is based on the MONAI framework [3]. For memorization detection, the architecture was adopted from Packhäuser et al [10]. The input layer was modified to have 1-channel input layer and the output classification dense layer was replaced by a dense layer mapping features to a 128 dimensional vector. Model was trained for 200 epochs with Adam optimizer having learning rate η reducing from 10^{-4} to half with the cosine annealing learning rate schedule.

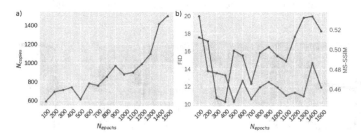

Fig. 3. a) No. of copies detected (N_{copies}) and b) FID/MS-SSIM in models trained for epochs (N_{epochs}) in range [100-1500].

3 Results

We first assess memorization in 2D unconditional LDMs by training LDMs for no. of epochs (N_{epochs}) in range [100-1500]. For each epoch, the trained models were used to generate 10,000 synthetic samples. All training, validation and synthetic samples (10,000 each) were then passed through the self-supervised network to obtain corresponding embeddings. Patient data copies were then detected based on the threshold value (ρ) as described in Section 2.2.2. Figure 3a shows no. of copies (N_{copies}) as a function of N_{epochs}. N_{copies} increases with N_{epochs}, implying that over-training can lead to enhanced memorization. Figure 4 shows a few detected copies with their closest training samples as detected by the self-supervised model for N_{epochs} = 1500. It can be seen that the detected copies show strong resemblance to the training samples.

An important point worth noting is that models with very high memorization can also have desirable quantitative metrics typically used to assess the generative models. Two widely used metrics include Fréchet inception distance (FID) for image quality assessment, and multi-scale structural similarity index measure (MS-SSIM) for data diversity. Figure 3b shows FID calculated using a model pre-trained on the NIH dataset adopted from Cohen et al. [11], and MS-SSIM as a function of N_{epochs}. After an initial decrease, FID starts oscillating around similar values as opposed to N_{copies} which keeps on increasing with N_{epochs}. MS-SSIM seems to show an initial decreasing and later an increasing trend, compared to MS-SSIM value of 0.46 in the real validation data. However, it only quantifies data diversity and gives no information regarding the quality of the synthesized images and data memorization. Taken together, these results suggest that LDMs trained without a proper stopping criterion can lead to enhanced memorization, and multiple aspects must be taken into consideration while training.

4 Discussion

Here, we assess the effect of training epoch number on memorization in LDMs. To our knowledge, this is the first study focusing on effect of training length on memorization. Our results show that increasing epoch number leads to enhanced memorization. It is an important aspect that is typically ignored while training. While evaluating generative models, the focus is primarily on improving quantitative measures reflecting quality and diversity of images. These metrics can have desirable values even when models memorize almost all data points. The performed study calls for an urgent need for devising new metrics that can enable high-quality, diverse and safe image synthesis.

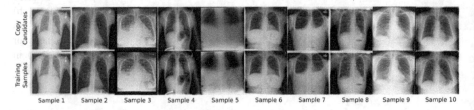

Fig. 4. Representative copy candidates with their closest training samples.

Acknowledgement. This work was supported through state funds approved by the State Parliament of Baden-Württemberg for the Innovation Campus Health + Life Science Alliance Heidelberg Mannheim, BMBF-SWAG Project 01KD2215D, and Informatics for life project through Klaus Tschira Foundation. The authors also gratefully acknowledge the data storage service SDS@hd supported by the Ministry of Science, Research and the Arts Baden-Württemberg (MWK) and the German Research Foundation (DFG) through grant INST 35/1314-1 FUGG and INST 35/1503-1 FUGG.

References

1. Pinaya WHL, Tudosiu PD, Dafflon J, Da Costa PF, Fernandez V, Nachev P et al. Brain imaging generation with latent diffusion models. Deep Generative Models. Cham: Springer Nature Switzerland, 2022:117–26.
2. Hamamci IE, Er S, Simsar E, Tezcan A, Simsek AG, Almas F et al. GenerateCT: text-guided 3D chest CT generation. arXiv preprint arXiv:2305.16037. 2023.
3. Pinaya WH, Graham MS, Kerfoot E, Tudosiu PD, Dafflon J, Fernandez V et al. Generative ai for medical imaging: extending the monai framework. arXiv preprint arXiv:2307.15208. 2023.
4. Khader F, Müller-Franzes G, Tayebi Arasteh S, Han T, Haarburger C, Schulze-Hagen M et al. Denoising diffusion probabilistic models for 3D medical image generation. Sci Rep. 2023;13(1):7303.
5. Dar SUH, Ghanaat A, Kahmann J, Ayx I, Papavassiliou T, Schoenberg SO et al. Investigating data memorization in 3d latent diffusion models for medical image synthesis. arXiv preprint arXiv:2307.01148. 2023.
6. Akbar MU, Wang W, Eklund A. Beware of diffusion models for synthesizing medical images: a comparison with GANs in terms of memorizing brain tumor images. arXiv preprint arXiv:2305.07644. 2023.
7. Fernandez V, Sanchez P, Pinaya WHL, Jacenków G, Tsaftaris SA, Cardoso J. Privacy distillation: reducing re-identification risk of multimodal diffusion models. arXiv preprint arXiv:2306.01322. 2023.
8. Chen T, Kornblith S, Norouzi M, Hinton G. A simple framework for contrastive learning of visual representations. Proceedings of the 37th International Conference on Machine Learning. Ed. by III HD, Singh A. Vol. 119. (Proc Mach Learn Research). PMLR, 2020:1597–607.
9. Wang X, Peng Y, Lu L, Lu Z, Bagheri M, Summers RM. ChestX-ray8: hospital-scale chest X-ray database and benchmarks on weakly-supervised classification and localization of common thorax diseases. Proc IEEE. 2017.
10. Packhäuser K, Gündel S, Münster N, Syben C, Christlein V, Maier A. Deep learning-based patient re-identification is able to exploit the biometric nature of medical chest X-ray data. Sci Rep. 2022;12(1):14851.
11. Cohen JP, Viviano JD, Bertin P, Morrison P, Torabian P, Guarrera M et al. TorchXRayVision: a library of chest X-ray datasets and models. Proc IEEE. 2022.

Exploring GPT-4 as MR Sequence and Reconstruction Programming Assistant
GPT4MR

Moritz Zaiss[1,2,3], Junaid R. Rajput[1,6], Hoai N. Dang[1], Vladimir Golkov[4,5],
Daniel Cremers[4,5], Florian Knoll[2], Andreas Maier[6]

[1]Institute of Neuroradiology, University Hospital Erlangen, Friedrich-Alexander-Universität Erlangen-Nürnberg (FAU), Erlangen, Germany
[2]Department Artificial Intelligence in Biomedical Engineering, Friedrich-Alexander-Universität Erlangen-Nürnberg (FAU), Erlangen, Germany
[3]Magnetic Resonance Center, Max-Planck-Institute for Biological Cybernetics, Tübingen, Germany
[4]Technical University of Munich, Munich, Germany
[5]Munich Center for Machine Learning, Munich, Germany
[6]Pattern Recognition Lab Friedrich-Alexander-University Erlangen-Nürnberg
moritz.zaiss@uk-erlangen.de

Abstract. In this study, we explore the potential of generative pre-trained transformer (GPT), as a coding assistant for MRI sequence programming using the Pulseq framework. The programming of MRI sequences is traditionally a complex and time-consuming task, and the Pulseq standard has recently simplified this process. It allows researchers to define and generate complex pulse sequences used in MRI experiments. Leveraging GPT-4's capabilities in natural language generation, we adapted it for MRI sequence programming, creating a specialized assistant named GPT4MR. Our tests involved generating various MRI sequences, revealing that GPT-4, guided by a tailored prompt, outperformed GPT-3.5, producing fewer errors and demonstrating improved reasoning. Despite limitations in handling complex sequences, GPT4MR corrected its own errors and successfully generated code with step-by-step instructions. The study showcases GPT4MR's ability to accelerate MRI sequence development, even for novel ideas absent in its training set. While further research and improvement are needed to address complexity limitations, a well-designed prompt enhances performance. The findings propose GPT4MR as a valuable MRI sequence programming assistant, streamlining prototyping and development. The future prospect involves integrating a PyPulseq plugin into lightweight, open-source LLMs, potentially revolutionizing MRI sequence development and prototyping.

1 Introduction

Magnetic resonance (MR) imaging, a non-invasive technique that uses static and dynamic magnetic fields and radiofrequency pulses, has become clinically efficient with the discovery of optimized MR sequences [1]. These sequences, which efficiently utilize radiofrequency pulses and spatial magnetic field gradients, enable rapid image acquisition. The strategic placement of these components is critical in the development of

© Der/die Autor(en), exklusiv lizenziert an
Springer Fachmedien Wiesbaden GmbH, ein Teil von Springer Nature 2024
A. Maier et al. (Hrsg.), *Bildverarbeitung für die Medizin 2024*,
Informatik aktuell, https://doi.org/10.1007/978-3-658-44037-4_28

MR sequences, especially in medicine where the generation of tissue contrast is of paramount importance. MR exhibits exceptional properties in soft tissues, leading to diverse applications in routine medical imaging. The direct correlation between the MR image contrast and the actual MR sequence with its numerous free parameters leads to the question of whether both image and contrast generation can be fully automated. This complicated task can be solved with the help of the Pulseq [2] and MR-zero [3] tools. However, programming MRI sequences remains a challenging and time-consuming task for researchers, technicians, and students alike. This study explores the potential of generative pre-trained transformer (GPT-4) [4], an advanced large language model (LLM) proficient in programming and natural language generation, as an MRI sequence programming assistant within the Pulseq framework. This exploration aims to accelerate MR prototyping in development and education.

2 Materials and methods

2.1 PyPulseq

Pulse sequence design is a crucial aspect of MRI research, yet multi-vendor studies demand familiarity with diverse hardware programming environments. PyPulseq addresses this challenge by facilitating vendor-neutral pulse sequence design in Python [2]. The generated pulse sequences can be exported as .seq files, compatible with Siemens, GE, and Bruker hardware, using their respective Pulseq interpreters. This tool caters to MRI pulse sequence designers, researchers, students, and other users interested in a versatile and accessible platform. It serves as a Python adaptation of the Pulseq framework, originally scripted in Matlab.

2.2 MR-zero

MR-zero [3] is a comprehensive framework that replicates the entire MRI pipeline, encompassing sequence and phantom definition, signal simulation, and image reconstruction. MR-zero uses a state-of-the-art Bloch simulation that enables accurate ADC signal calculation with less time and noise compared to isochromatic Monte Carlo simulations. MR-zero was developed with PyTorch and runs on CUDA-enabled GPUs. It supports automatic differentiation by backpropagation to optimize sequence parameters or phantom values based on loss functions considering the reconstructed image of the simulated signal.

2.3 GPT4MR

GPT is a type of LLM known for its advanced natural language understanding and generation capabilities. ChatGPT [5] is just a variant of GPT that was developed specifically for conversational AI applications. It is trained to predict words based on context from large text databases. Through this training, they are able to generate human-like speech, making them valuable for a wide range of natural language understanding and generation tasks.

We used ChatGPT with the models GPT-3.5 and GPT-4. We adapted it for MRI sequence programming by adding a custom prompt to turn it into an MRI and Py-Pulseq coding assistant abbreviated here by GPT4MR. The prompt contained general instructions as well as PyPulseq function definitions and examples, principles known as in-context few-shot learning [6, 7] and Chain-of-Thought Prompting [8]. Chain of thought prompting guides the LLM through a step-by-step thinking process. This involves presenting the prompt with a few-shot exemplar that outlines the logical reasoning steps. On the other hand, in-context learning empowers the prompt to generate responses or predictions by leveraging the specific context provided to it.

We tested the AI model's ability to generate simple pulse sequences, composite binomial pulses, a spin echo EPI sequence with reconstruction, and a Lissajous-EPI. The spin echo EPI and Lissajous-EPI sequences are simulated for a synthetic brain phantom by using the MR-zero [3] pipeline. Instructions to reconstruct the simulated signals were also given to GPT4MR with the additional task to use the torchkbnufft [9] package for a non-uniform FFT. we have provided an open Colab notebook [10] that contains the GPT4MR prompt, comprehensive examples, instructions and a platform for testing GPT-4 as an MR coding assistant.

3   Results

In our initial attempts, native GPT models often generated erroneous code, mainly using non-existing PyPulseq subfunctions. The performance is considerably improved using our tailored GPT4MR prompt, allowing it to generate MRI sequences with fewer or no errors (Fig. 1). GPT-4 outperformed GPT-3.5 in terms of number of bugs and reasoning/explaining. However, our study also revealed GPT-4's limitations in handling more complex sequence ideas or fully replicating existing sequence concepts. Prompts like "Code a spin echo EPI" lead to running code, but conceptual sequence errors (Fig. 2). Interestingly, GPT4MR was able to correct its own errors when problems were pointed out. When instructed with step-by-step instructions of the sequence implementation as

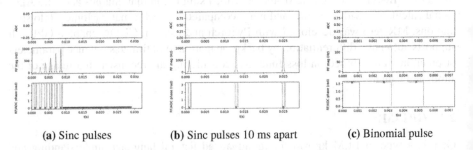

(a) Sinc pulses   (b) Sinc pulses 10 ms apart   (c) Binomial pulse

Fig. 1. Sequence plots of prompts for generating pulse trains. Prompt a: "Can you generate a pypulseq file containing 6 sinc pulses, with increasing flipangle from 1 to 90 degree and after the last pulse we have an ADC event of 20 ms". Promt b: "Can you play out 3 sinc pulses. The distance between the pulses should be 10 ms each. The rf flipangle are 90, 180, 180". Prompt c: "What is a binomial rf pulse in MRI? Can you create one using pypulseq?".

plain text, GPT4MR was able to generate correct and running code in a single try for a spin echo EPI (Fig. 3), and a Lissajous EPI (Fig. 4). While timings, gradient moments etc. were not always 100% correct or optimal, running codes were produced and an easy-to-alter base sequence as well as a correct EPI FFT reconstruction (Fig. 3), as well as a non-uniform FFT reconstruction using the advanced torchkbnufft package, which yields a better outcome compared to linear re-gridding, were generated (Fig. 4).

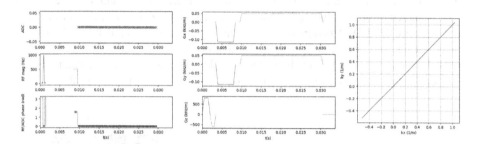

Fig. 2. Sequence plot of prompt for generating spin echo EPI sequence. Prompt: "Code a spin echo EPI". Here our assistant GPT4MR fails, this resembles a gradient echo sequence, but only a single too short diagonal k-space line is acquired.

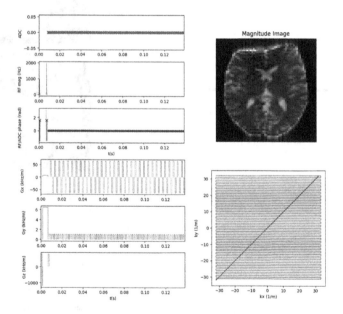

Fig. 3. Spin-Echo EPI coded by GPT4MR in the first attempt using a step-by-step detailed prompt. This is a correct implementation, just the spin echo TE does not match the time of k-space center acquisition. The reconstruction shows the typical EPI distortion artifact, but line flips and shifts were implemented correctly by GPT4MR.

4   Discussion

Our findings indicate that LLMs have the potential to serve as a valuable MRI sequence programming assistant, enabling faster development of novel MRI sequences,
reconstruction, or building blocks. Our last two chosen examples cannot be found on
the internet (i.e. in the training set of GPT-4), demonstrating GPT4MR's capacity to
accelerate the realization of new MRI sequence ideas. However, its limitations in dealing with complex ideas and sequences necessitate further research and improvement. A
well-designed prompt including PyPulseq documentation can improve the performance
considerably. GPT4MR understood programming hints and altered the code accordingly, forming a sparring partner for fast MR prototyping. We have first evidence that
GPT-4-vision can also directly interpret uploaded images of sequence diagrams and
deliver the correct code implementation. We propose a versatile prompt that enables

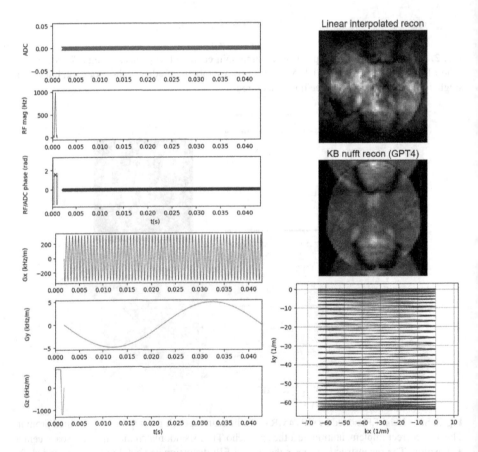

Fig. 4. Lissajous EPI coded by GPT4MR in the first attempt. This is a correct implementation, only
the k-space coverage is not yet ideal. The torchkbnufft package was used via GPT for non-uniform
FFT reconstruction.

GPT-4 to act as a Pulseq coding assistant for MRI sequence/reconstruction development and prototyping, streamlining the process. As a future outlook, integrating a PyPulseq plugin into (free, leightweight, open source) [11] LLMs could create a powerful tool for MRI sequence development and prototyping.

References

1. Carr HY. Steady-state free precession in nuclear magnetic resonance. Phys Rev. 1958;112:1693–701.
2. Ravi KS, Geethanath S, Vaughan JT. PyPulseq: a Python package for MRI pulse sequence design. J Open Source Softw. 2019;4:1725.
3. Loktyushin A, Herz K, Dang N, Glang F, Deshmane A, Weinmuller S et al. MRzero: automated discovery of MRI sequences using supervised learning. Magn Reson Med. 2020;86:709–24.
4. OpenAI. GPT-4 Technical Report. ArXiv. 2023;abs/2303.08774.
5. OpenAI. OpenAI: introducing ChatGPT. 2022.
6. Brown TB, Mann B, Ryder N, Subbiah M, Kaplan J, Dhariwal P et al. Language models are few-shot learners. ArXiv. 2020;abs/2005.14165.
7. Dai D, Sun Y, Dong L, Hao Y, Sui Z, Wei F. Why can GPT learn in-context? Language models secretly perform gradient descent as meta-optimizers. ArXiv. 2023;abs/2212.10559.
8. Wei J, Wang X, Schuurmans D, Bosma M, Chi EHh, Xia F et al. Chain of thought prompting elicits reasoning in large language models. ArXiv. 2022;abs/2201.11903.
9. https://github.com/mmuckley/torchkbnufft.
10. https://colab.research.google.com/drive/1RoubncbIAOBmX7IFy_OXeJFKI3DQK_F1.
11. Touvron H, Lavril T, Izacard G, Martinet X, Lachaux MA, Lacroix T et al. LLaMA: open and efficient foundation language models. ArXiv. 2023;abs/2302.13971.

Abstract: Understanding Silent Failures in Medical Image Classification

Till J. Bungert[1,2], Levin Kobelke[1,2], Paul F. Jaeger[1,2]

[1]Interactive Machine Learning Group, German Cancer Research Center (DKFZ), Heidelberg, Germany
[2]Helmholtz Imaging, DKFZ, Heidelberg, Germany
till.bungert@dkfz-heidelberg.de

To ensure the reliable use of classification systems in medical applications, it is crucial to prevent silent failures. This can be achieved by either designing classifiers that are robust enough to avoid failures in the first place, or by detecting remaining failures using confidence scoring functions (CSFs). A predominant source of failures in image classification is distribution shifts between training data and deployment data. To understand the current state of silent failure prevention in medical imaging, we conduct the first comprehensive analysis comparing various CSFs in four biomedical tasks and a diverse range of distribution shifts. Based on the result that none of the benchmarked CSFs can reliably prevent silent failures, we conclude that a deeper understanding of the root causes of failures in the data is required. To facilitate this, we introduce SF-Visuals, an interactive analysis tool that uses latent space clustering to visualize shifts and failures. On the basis of various examples, we demonstrate how this tool can help researchers gain insight into the requirements for safe application of classification systems in the medical domain. The open-source benchmark and tool are at: https://github.com/IML-DKFZ/sf-visuals. [1]

References

1. Bungert TJ, Kobelke L, Jäger PF. Understanding silent failures in medical image classification. Proc MICCAI. 2023:400–10.

© Der/die Autor(en), exklusiv lizenziert an
Springer Fachmedien Wiesbaden GmbH, ein Teil von Springer Nature 2024
A. Maier et al. (Hrsg.), *Bildverarbeitung für die Medizin 2024*,
Informatik aktuell, https://doi.org/10.1007/978-3-658-44037-4_29

Abstract: Advancing Large-scale Deformable 3D Registration with Differentiable Volumetric Rasterisation of Point Clouds

Chasing Clouds

Mattias P. Heinrich[1], Alexander Bigalke[1], Christoph Großbröhmer[1], Lasse Hansen[2]

[1]Institute of Medical Informatics, University of Lübeck, Germany
[2]EchoScout GmbH, Lübeck, Germany
mattias.heinrich@uni-luebeck.de

3D point clouds are an efficient and privacy-preserving representation of medical scans highly suitable for complex segmentation and registration tasks. Yet, current loss functions for training self-supervised geometric networks are insufficient to handle large-scale clouds and provide robust derivatives. Here, we present Differentiable Volumetric Rasterisation of Point Clouds (DiVRoC) that overcomes those limitations and provides highly accurate learning- or optimisation-based deformable 3D registration [1]. The key contribution is the derivation of a reverse grid-sampling operation with gradients for the motion vectors that can rapidly transform between grid-based volumetric and sparse point representations. It enables scalable regularisation and loss computation on 3D point clouds with >100k points being orders of magnitude faster than a Chamfer loss. The concept includes geometric registration networks that can be robustly trained in an unsupervised fashion and act on sparser point clouds. This is followed by a regularisation model that enables extrapolation for high-resolution distance metrics. Our experiments on the challenging PVT1010 lung dataset [2] that includes large motion of COPD patients between inspiration and expiration demonstrate state-of-the-art accuracies for training a PointPWC-Net and/or alignment based on Adam instance optimisation. The model reduces registration errors to approx. 2.4 mm and runs on very large point clouds in one second. The DiVRoC module can also be used to learn shape models for 3D surfaces [3]. Implementation details to use DiVRoC as drop-in replacement for point distances, a new out-of-domain dataset for evaluation and demos for realtime inference can be found at https://github.com/mattiaspaul/ChasingClouds.

References

1. Heinrich MP, Bigalke A, Großbröhmer C, Hansen L. Chasing clouds: differentiable volumetric rasterisation of point clouds as a highly efficient and accurate loss for large-scale deformable 3D registration. Proc. IEEE CVF. 2023:8026–36.
2. Shen Z, Feydy J, Liu P, Curiale AH, San Jose Estepar R, San Jose Estepar R et al. Accurate point cloud registration with robust optimal transport. NeurIPS. 2021:5373–89.
3. Hempe H, Bigalke A, Heinrich MP. Shape matters: detecting vertebral fractures using differentiable point-based shape decoding. Proc CVPR. 2023.

© Der/die Autor(en), exklusiv lizenziert an
Springer Fachmedien Wiesbaden GmbH, ein Teil von Springer Nature 2024
A. Maier et al. (Hrsg.), *Bildverarbeitung für die Medizin 2024*,
Informatik aktuell, https://doi.org/10.1007/978-3-658-44037-4_30

Harmonized Import of Clinical Research Data for the Open Source Image Analysis Platform Kaapana

Lucas Kulla[1], Philipp Schader[1,2], Klaus Maier-Hein[1,3], Marco Nolden[1,3]

[1]Division of Medical Computing, Deutsches Krebsforschungszentrum (DKFZ) Heidelberg
German Cancer Research Center (DKFZ) Heidelberg, Division of Medical Image Computing,
Germany
[2]Faculty of Mathematics and Computer Science, Heidelberg University, Heidelberg, Germany
[3]Pattern Analysis and Learning Group, Department of Radiation Oncology, Heidelberg
University Hospital, Heidelberg, Germany
lucas.kulla@dkfz-heidelberg.de

Abstract. While the DICOM standard facilitates a consistent approach to image data, integrating clinical and patient data from unstructured formats into medical image analysis platforms remains a complex challenge. To address this problem, we propose a web-based tool for interactive harmonization of semi-structured data tables and facilitating their integration into image analysis platforms such as Kaapana. Harmonization is performed with respect to a given schema. The approach supports researchers throughout the data lifecycle by enabling the interactive creation of migration scripts to extend the life of data in changing environments. The proposed tool helps researchers enhance data utilization in the medical field by making unharmonized data available. Despite its potential, the proposed solution has limitations when handling large data sets and faces potential security issues due to the use of JavaScript. Nevertheless, it offers considerable benefits by assisting in data harmonization, enabling the use of data from various sources, and therefore reducing costs by eliminating the need for redundant data collection.

1 Introduction

For image-based medical data, the DICOM standard is broadly adopted. However, for non-imaging medical data, a similar standardization is less established, and research data often exists in disparate tabular data formats such as CSV and XLSX. This data fragmentation and lack of standardization complicates the comprehensive analysis of collected data and, consequently, the gain of new insights that are crucial to advancing medical research. While image analysis platforms, like Kaapana, can handle imaging data or incorporate structured data sets into the analysis, they cannot deal with clinical data from semi-structured datasets. The lack of a mechanism to harmonize and import different data sources prevents comprehensive data analytics with imaging and clinical data combined. Therefore, additional tooling enabling researchers to efficiently harmonize semi-structured data is needed to allow the integration of such data into analysis pipelines and make them available for computational research in medicine.

Data harmonization plays a pivotal role in ensuring the quality and usability of clinical research data. Tools such as AutoMed, developed by Boyd et al. [1], focus on local-to-global schema mappings to integrate semi-structured datasets, but the tool itself

© Der/die Autor(en), exklusiv lizenziert an
Springer Fachmedien Wiesbaden GmbH, ein Teil von Springer Nature 2024
A. Maier et al. (Hrsg.), *Bildverarbeitung für die Medizin 2024*,
Informatik aktuell, https://doi.org/10.1007/978-3-658-44037-4_31

is now unavailable. Teoman and Sinaci's data-curation-tool[1] harmonizes data but only aligns to the HL7 FHIR profile[2], lacking the flexibility of a general schema mapping. The Darwin framework by Hillenbrand et al. [2] offers data migration and schema evolution strategies, emphasizing decisions on migrating legacy entities. However, it's not fully implemented. Jia et al. present a method for transforming relational databases to MongoDB [3], focusing on database-specific issues like performance. Uniquely, our tool provides a user-focused harmonization approach, directly compatible with formats such as XSLX, and employs use-case tailored schemas, going beyond the limitations of database-only solutions.

The main objective was to develop a tool that allows the import of semi-structured data into the Kaapana platform. It is intended to promote a uniform data standard that simplifies data integration and enables efficient and uniform data processing within the platform. The problem was approached by conducting a structured analysis of scenarios and selecting an appropriate open-source tool as a baseline for the specified requirements using a weight sum model. This tool was then tailored to meet specific requirements through an iterative adaptation and testing process. The finalized tool was integrated into the kaapana-persistence layer extension within the Kaapana platform. As a result, a web-based application was developed to improve data interoperability and migration The application allows users to import tabular data and convert it into a harmonized structure. It offers two functionalities: users without a predefined schema can generate a JSON schema that reflects the input data structure, while users with an existing reference schema can ensure data consistency. The application also includes a mechanism for schema evolution, allowing users to adapt and modify schemas and migrate the data to meet changing data requirements. Additionally, the tool enables advanced data manipulation using JavaScript, allowing users to perform complex transformations directly in their browser. Overall, this application provides a first solution for managing data interoperability, migration, and manipulation.

2 Materials and methods

The requirements engineering process was split into two phases. Initially, scenarios were defined that the application should or must fulfill (2.1). A technology selection was conducted using a weighted sum model (WSM). Existing tools were identified, and evaluated against predefined criteria, and the most suitable one was selected for our specific requirements.

2.1 Data integration and transformation scenarios

In the beginning, 4 scenarios were defined in which the application should support the user. The main focus is on the import of tables with and without schema, as well as the use of Java-Script (JS) transformations and the ability to change a schema.

---

[1] https://github.com/fair4health/data-curation-tool
[2] https://www.hl7.org/fhir

- Scenario 1: Import tabular data without a schema - Import data from CSV, XLS, or XLSX files without a preexisting schema. This provides flexibility and allows the user to create an initial schema based on the first data set. The derived schema can later be used to import similar data.
- Scenario 2: Import tabular data with reference schema - Import data from CSV, XLS, or XLSX files into an existing schema. This scenario is integral for ensuring data consistency and harmonization. The reference schema prescribes a clear structure and format. On import, the user maps the data columns to the schema properties, ensuring that the data aligns with the pre-established format.
- Scenario 3: Apply complex Java-Script transformation on tabular data - To enable more complex harmonization not covered by the first two scenarios, the user may apply arbitrary transformations to the input dataset. These transformations can be expressed in Java-Script so that they can be directly executed within the browser and do not require a backend service to run.
- Scenario 4: Create a new version of a schema - Update an existing schema to a new version. This makes it easier to evolve schemas when data requirements change, which in turn makes the tool more versatile and ensures data longevity.

In addition to the scenarios, the tool is designed to provide an interactive, easy-to-use interface compatible with popular web browsers. It should enable internationalization for user accessibility and support the import of files up to 1 GB in size.

2.2 Score based selection of technologies

The issue of data harmonization has led to the development of numerous tools. Our search on GitHub for open-source projects meeting our criteria included terms such as csv import, xls import, data harmonization and data mapping in TypeScript and JavaScript languages. Results were filtered for relevance and license. Promising projects were tested against predefined criteria derived from 2.1 as well as the requirement of compatibility with the Kaapana platform using a WSM. They consisted of nine factors, each with distinct weights. The most important criteria included the CSV file import capability and the use of React or Vue for easy integration. Six projects were evaluated based on the WSM. The tools achieved a score ranging from 300 to 568 out of a possible 1000 points. react-spreadsheet-import [4] achieved the highest score with 568 points, followed by react-admin-import-csv [5] with 484 points, and react-csv-importer [6] with 397 points. There are two groups of tools in the ranking, the first group scored between 300 and 400 points, whereas the second group scored between 484 and 568 points. To validate the robustness of the ranking, a sensitivity analysis was conducted, reaffirming the position of the tool in the ranking.

After evaluating various tools, the open-source project react-spreadsheet-import, version 2.0.8 [4] was chosen as the foundation for the tool. Built on React 17, the chosen application splits the import process into four steps: Upload, Header Selection, Column Matching and Data Validation, facilitated via a dialog form. It supports importing CSV, XLS, and XLSX files, offers post-import column mapping to a single predefined schema, validates data based on these fields, and finally presents the data as a JSON Object. Despite its strengths, some aspects from 2.1 weren't met. These centered around dynamic schema creation enhancements, necessitating algorithms for real-time schema generation, column alignment, and anomaly handling. Additional features were integrated, like tools for direct schema editing, CSV data download, and modules facilitating data and schema API upload. Complex data transformations were enabled via JS. For optimal integration with the kaapana-persistence API, React was updated to version 18.2.0, aligning all related dependencies.

2.3 Kaapana

To integrate the harmonized clinical data into a comprehensive analysis pipeline, the application was integrated into the Kaapana Platform. Kaapana is a Kubernetes-based[3], open-source medical data analysis framework tailored for AI workflows and federated learning in radiology and radiotherapy. The extension component of Kaapana works like an app store, facilitating component management and standardizing workflows. The platform provides the kaapana-persistence extension (version 0.2.0), offering a RESTful API for schema storage and data import. With this extension, stored data is available in different areas of the platform, e.g., in a different analysis pipeline.[7]

3 Results

3.1 Implementation

Based on the scenarios from 2.1 the react-spreadsheet-import was extended to allow data harmonization in the following way: The user initiates the procedure by selecting the Start Harmonization option and uploading their data file, which may be in CSV, XLS, or XLSX format (step 1, 1). File sizes up to 80MB can be imported in around 30 seconds. The user has the option to choose a predefined schema that can be selected at the start of the upload process (step 2). Otherwise, the system automatically generates a schema reflecting the data's inherent structure. In the case of XLS, XLSX files, the user must then specify the worksheet of interest (step 3). Following this, the header row must be selected to finalize the import (step 4). Afterward, in the mapping phase, the user aligns the data columns with corresponding fields from the schema (see 5, 2). In the case that no schema is selected, the newly generated schema is used, and the mapping is automatically done. In both cases, a user has the option to add validation rules, like flagging any discrepancies, such as non-unique identifiers. After this step, the data is validated against the rules. If errors occur, they are highlighted, and the option to validate the data is given (step 6). For users in need of advanced data manipulation, they

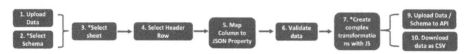

Fig. 1. Visualization of the workflow to harmonize clinical research data. * means mandatory.

---

[3]https://kubernetes.io

can opt for the migration editor, which enables the creation and execution of JavaScript-based transformations on the dataset (see 7). After transformation, if needed, users can enhance the schema by adding new properties or adjusting it through the Edit schema tool. The result of this process enables users to either upload the unified data and its corresponding schema to the kaapana persistence API or opt for a local download in CSV format (step 9,10). The project's transparency is guaranteed by making the web interface's source code publicly available on GitHub[4] under the MIT License.

3.1.1   Evaluation. The tool's functionality was assessed against the scenarios from 2.1 which it supported. Certain non-functional requirements, such as handling files over 1 GB, have not been met. For further evaluation, two medical datasets with overlapping attributes were harmonized into a single schema. The QIN-HeadNeck [8] collection comprises PET/CT 18F-FDG scans of head and neck cancer patients, along with augmented segmentations and clinical data. In contrast, the RADCURE dataset offers CT images and segmentations of the same patient category, clinical, demographic, and treatment details [9]. Initially, QIN-HeadNeck was imported without a schema, setting its first header as a guide and later uploaded to the API using the identifier urn:kaapana:HeadNeck. The RADCURE dataset leveraged the earlier-created schema, requiring mapping tweaks such as alignment of PatientID to id and Sex to Gender, while also introducing new fields (Fig. 2). More complex harmonization was executed on the TNM classification between the datasets. While QIN-HeadNeck used labels like Final T and values like 4b, RAD-CURE employed labels T with values formatted T4b. Using the JS editor, RADCURE's values were altered from T4b to match 4b. Post-transformation, the schema was updated, validated, and, along with the datasets, uploaded to the kaapana-persistence API, optimizing its utility on the Kaapana platform.

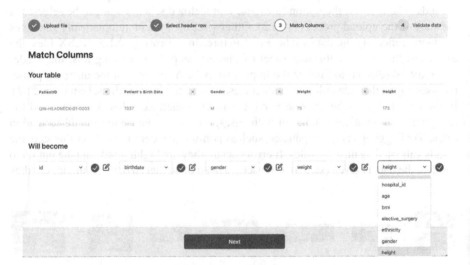

Fig. 2. Column mapping to schema attributes using a dropdown menu.

---

[4]https://github.com/lucaskulla/SpreadSheetImporter

4 Discussion

This work presents a web-based tool for importing and harmonizing semi-structured clinical research data into the Kaapana platform. Based on a preexisting application (see 2.2) that provides basic functionality like importing tabular data in an interactive manner, a tool fulfilling extended scenarios was created. The functionality for mapping tabular data to any JSON-Schema was introduced and evaluated on real-world data by harmonizing two datasets. Capabilities for developing, testing, and executing complex JS transformations on the data were added, allowing for arbitrary transformations.

While the resulting tool meets most requirements, it struggles to handle large files as all processes run within the browser. On a 2022 MacBook Pro, the import of an 80 MB XLSX table took about 30 seconds on average. Limitations in the current approach that need to be addressed in an upcoming version include usability improvements like allowing users to save their progress, user guidance in the creation of complex transformations as well as improving the overall performance.

The resulting web-based tool supports researchers routinely interacting with inhomogeneous clinical research data. By providing a simple interactive interface for data import and harmonization, the tool directly addresses the challenges associated with incorporating inhomogeneous clinical data into image analysis pipelines. While there are still hurdles to overcome, the tool supports data-driven research by facilitating clean, harmonized datasets.

Acknowledgement. Part of this project was supported by the Helmholtz Metadata Collaboration (HMC).

References

1. Boyd M, Kittivoravitkul S, Lazanitis C, McBrien P, Rizopoulos N. AutoMed: a BAV data integration system for heterogeneous data sources. 2004. Ed. by Persson A, Stirna J:82–97.
2. Hillenbrand A, Störl U, Nabiyev S, Klettke M. Self-adapting data migration in the context of schema evolution in NoSQL databases. Distrib Parallel Databases. 2022;40(1):5–25.
3. Jia T, Zhao X, Wang Z, Gong D, Ding G. Model transformation and data migration from relational database to MongoDB. Proc IEEE. 2016:60–7.
4. Masiulis K, JulitorK, Karlsson H, Tordgeman J, Fiddler J, Butola A et al. UgnisSoftware. Computer Program. 2023.
5. Winding B, songkeith, Kowalski M, Flavien, Akker Kvd, Cramer S et al. benwinding/react-admin-import-csv. Computer Program. 2023.
6. Matantsev N, Stehr T, Arney T, Bismut D, Dahl TKK, Multani PS et al. beamworks/react-csv-importer. Computer Program. 2023.
7. Scherer J, Kades K, Gao H, Schader P, Parekh K, Parampottupadam S et al. kaapana/kaapana: v0.2.0. Computer Program. Version 0.2.0. 2022.
8. Agarwal M. Patient survival prediction. 2021.
9. Welch ML, Kim S, Hope A, Huang SH, Lu Z, Marsilla J et al. Computed tomography images from large head and neck cohort (RADCURE). Version 1. [Data set]. 2023.

Interactive Exploration of Conditional Statistical Shape Models in the Web-browser

exploreCOSMOS

Maximilian Hahn, Bernhard Egger

Friedrich-Alexander-Universtitat Erlangen-Nürnberg
bernhard.egger@fau.de

Abstract. Statistical Shape Models of faces and various body parts are heavily used in medical image analysis, computer vision and visualization. Whilst the field is well explored with many existing tools, all of them aim at experts, which limits their applicability. We demonstrate the first tool that enables the convenient exploration of statistical shape models in the browser, with the capability to manipulate the faces in a targeted manner. This manipulation is performed via a posterior model given partial observations. We release our code and application on GitHub https://github.com/maximilian-hahn/exploreCOSMOS.

1 Introduction

Statistical shape models (SSMs) serve as a powerful tool for analyzing and interpreting complex shapes in various fields, such as medical imaging, computer graphics and computer vision [1]. One key motivation for utilizing SSMs is their ability to overcome the limitations of individual shape analysis. Traditional methods often struggle to effectively capture the variations found within a shape dataset, making it challenging to accurately represent and compare shapes. SSMs address this issue by aligning the set of shapes to a reference shape and thus being able to create a mean shape and generate a comprehensive representation of shape variation. We propose an interactive web-based application that allows the user to visualize and modify instances of their SSM via a 3D mesh. Shape variations of the model can be explored and the user can add constraints such that a posterior model can be computed that alters the appearance of the model by satisfying those user-given constraints. These constraints could be the movement of selected vertices of the 3D mesh representing the model or marking them with either predefined or user-created landmarks, ensuring that these vertices remain in place. With these constraints, the posterior mesh has vertices at the defined positions, and the statistically most probable positions for the rest of the vertices are computed so that the whole shape fits as well as possible into the statistical model. This enables the user to explore a SSM, aid in avatar creation or 3D modeling tasks, and realize visualizations by generating faces with desired features [1–3].

While these things are possible by, for example, utilizing the Scala library Scalismo[1] [1], that approach requires more understanding of the topic, programming effort, and time to set up the development environment. In contrast to that, we concentrated on

---

[1]https://github.com/unibas-gravis/scalismo

© Der/die Autor(en), exklusiv lizenziert an
Springer Fachmedien Wiesbaden GmbH, ein Teil von Springer Nature 2024
A. Maier et al. (Hrsg.), *Bildverarbeitung für die Medizin 2024*,
Informatik aktuell, https://doi.org/10.1007/978-3-658-44037-4_32

making this application as easily accessible for everyone as possible and only requiring minimal prior knowledge on the topic in order to be able to use it. The result is a web application that can be accessed by any modern browser without the need to install anything. Our user interface is compatible with the Statismo file format [4] and can handle any shape model in that format. For a quick start, we provide a simple face model that has a free license. To the best of our knowledge, this is the first interactive graphical user interface that allows shape model exploration and posterior model creation in the web browser.

2 Methods

Statistical shape models are mathematical representations used to capture and analyze the variability of shapes within a given dataset. SSMs represent this data in a compact way by incorporating a mean shape as well as their variations to that mean shape.

A SSM is built from shapes in dense correspondence to a common reference shape allowing to compute the difference in position of each vertex, consisting of an x, y, and z coordinate. Each shape is then represented as a shape vector s containing this difference to the reference shape, the so-called deformation. For this section, we follow the formulation of SSMs as done in [2]. With this, the mean shape is just the arithmetic mean over all given shape vectors: $\mu = \frac{1}{n} \sum_{i=1}^{n} s_i$. To model the class of shapes as a multivariate normal distribution $\mathcal{N}(\mu, \Sigma)$, the covariance matrix can be computed with $\Sigma = \frac{1}{n} \sum_{i=1}^{n} (s_i - \mu) \cdot (s_i - \mu)^T$. Principal component analysis can then be used to decompose the covariance matrix Σ into its eigenvectors and eigenvalues: $\Sigma = U \cdot D^2 \cdot U^T$. U is a matrix whose i-th column is the eigenvector, or principal component, q_i of Σ,

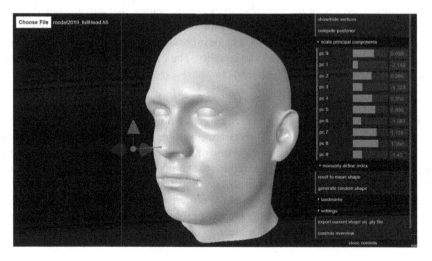

Fig. 1. Screenshot of the proposed user interface after generating a random face from the Basel Face Model 2019 [5] and its corresponding principal components on the right. We can now modify the face by adding observations, e.g., here we move the tip of the nose forward and then compute and display the mean face shape of the posterior; size of controls adjusted for readability.

ordered from largest to smallest, and D^2 is a diagonal matrix with the corresponding eigenvalues $D_{ii}^2 = \lambda_i$ as diagonal entries. Each principal component now represents an independent characteristic shape variation of the shape class and the eigenvalues quantify the variance σ^2, meaning that D holds the standard deviation σ. To generate new shape vectors based on the model, the following equation can be used

$$s = \mu + Q \cdot \alpha \tag{1}$$

μ represents the mean shape, Q is defined as $Q = U \cdot D$, holding n columns with principal components, where each entry of the n principal components is multiplied with the corresponding standard deviation. α is then a vector with n values that follows a standard multivariate normal distribution $p(\alpha) \sim \mathcal{N}(0, I_n)$, thus scaling the corresponding principal components after matrix-vector-multiplication. Generating a new normally distributed α and recalculating the Eq. 1 provides a new shape vector s, that represents a new shape variation of the given shape class.

A particular strength of SSMs is that they are capable of reconstructing a full shape from only partial information. This reconstruction is performed via a posterior shape model, which is a SSM that has been updated by incorporating given observations to calculate a new mean and covariance, the posterior mean and posterior covariance. These observations are the given partial information. They can consist of positional changes of certain vertices specified by the user or of user-created or predefined landmarks of the shape class at hand.

To get to the posterior mean and covariance from the given observations, the approach is to repurpose Eq. 1 in the sense that the shape vector s is now given as a partial shape vector s_p, where only those vertices occur that correspond to the observations [2]. Because now s_p has fewer entries than s, it is essential to also reduce the size of the complete model's μ and Q that appear in Eq. 1 for it to be consistent with the dimensions again. Thus, a sub-vector μ_p and sub-matrix Q_p are defined that only include the entries and rows of μ and Q, that correspond to the observations in s_p [2]. This leads to the adjusted equation: $s_p = \mu_p + Q_p \cdot \alpha$. The next consideration is what values the α vector has to consist of in order to fulfill the equality. The easiest way to get this α is to solve the previous equation for it, which leads to

$$\alpha = Q_p^{-1} \cdot (s_p - \mu_p) \tag{2}$$

Calculating the inverse of Q_p can be pretty computation-intensive, especially when many observations and principal components are given, as the size of the matrix increases with them. Since Q_p is also not a quadratic matrix, one has to resort to the generalized or pseudo inverse. There are ways to reduce the complexity and optimize this part of the process [2] but for simplicity reasons this work just relies on the pseudo inverse of Q_p. The new α can then be used to compute the posterior mean by just applying it to Eq. 1. The result is a vector that represents the most probable shape in the model factoring in the given observations, the posterior mean.

3 Implementation

Our application is implemented as a web-based application. We choose JavaScript, HTML and CSS at the core of our implementation, this has the additional benefit that everything runs locally, and no data has to be sent to the server, which is particularly useful when working in a privacy-constrained setting. To realize the 3D component, three.js[2] is used, which is the most popular JavaScript library for displaying 3D content on the web and based on WebGL. With the help of the integrated raycaster and event listeners, we select the nearest vertex of the mesh to the clicked position and mark it with a helper object that represents the 3D coordinate system axes, as can be seen in Figure 1. With that, the user can move the selected vertex in the desired direction and thus modify the shape. For most of the other controls, dat.GUI[3] is used as a lightweight controller library that organizes buttons and sliders in a folder-like manner and internally generates the needed HTML and CSS code to display them in the window. It enables interaction with the given 3D scene by changing variables and executing functions.

The user can also load in their own SSM if it follows the Statismo file format [4]. We extend the implementation using jsfive[4] to parse the hdf5 files. With the help of the PLYExporter add-on in three.js, the modified face mesh can be exported and downloaded as a .ply file. Additionally, we use the library Toastify.js[5] for notifications. In order to compute the posterior mean mentioned in section 2, the hardware-accelerated library Tensorflow.js[6] is used. It provides good performance for matrix operations, which is necessary for large models. Since Tensorflow.js doesn't include a function for the pseudo inverse of a matrix needed for the computation, we had to resort to the worse-performing ml-matrix library[7] and convert the data types between them to implement Eq. 2.

4 Results

We tested our user interface with the Basel Face Model [5] since it can nicely visualize the features of this application. What the user interface looks like in use can be seen in

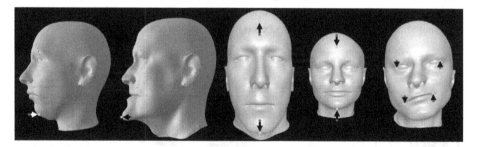

Fig. 2. Examples of face manipulations by moving specific points (original position in red, new position in green). The statistical model enables these manipulations and the resulting faces appear natural (from left to right): receding and protruding chin, long face, short face and asymmetric face.

---

[2] https://github.com/mrdoob/three.js
[3] https://github.com/dataarts/dat.gui
[4] https://github.com/usnistgov/jsfive
[5] https://github.com/apvarun/toastify-js
[6] https://github.com/tensorflow/tfjs
[7] https://github.com/mljs/matrix

Figure 1. Our application allows the user to take all existing principal components of the model into account and generate new shapes by scaling them. They can be defined individually or generated randomly all at once by using the "generate random shape" option and reset to zero by the "reset to mean shape" option.

In addition, our implementation offers an easy way to generate characteristic shapes. Figure 2 shows such possible shapes for faces. All these examples were realized by just moving two to four vertices, and were done in less than a minute. How the interactive design process looks like to generate these results can be seen in Figure 3.

To demonstrate a potential clinical use case, we present the application of nose reconstruction [3] in Figure 4. We show how different kinds of noses could look like on a given patient's face, with potential application in surgery planning.

In order to determine the usability of our tool, a small user study was performed based on four experts with experience in the field of SSMs. The participants had to complete three tasks with the help of this application: First, modify the displayed shape by scaling the principal components. Second, modify the shape in a way that it has a very long nose, and third, modify the shape until it looks alien-like to oneself. These tasks were performed on a model based on a single face [6]. It is a highly flexible model, which is especially helpful when the goal shape doesn't directly relate to a possible human face anymore, such as the face of an alien. Figure 5 shows examples of what the resulting shapes could look like. After completing the tasks, the participants took a small survey. Regarding the difficulty of completing the tasks, the results show a 2.5 on a scale from 1 to 5, the overall experience using the application was a 4 out of 5, and the intuitiveness of the user interface a 3.25. These results are fairly balanced but have a slight tendency toward the desired end of the spectrum. The participants spent 2 to 10 minutes to solve the tasks, being 5 minutes on average, which speaks for how fast one is able to modify shapes in a desired manner using the application. Furthermore, the participants were asked for feedback. One response described the expectation that after deleting all landmarks and recomputing the posterior, the model should reset to its original shape, which it didn't. This behavior was implemented afterward.

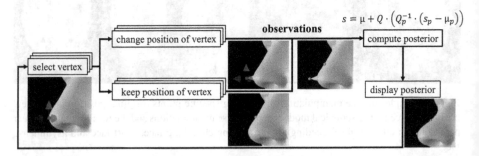

Fig. 3. Our interactive design process is structured as follows: we select vertex points on the face surface and decide if they should stay at the current position or if their position should be modified. The posterior is then calculated based on those observations and displayed to the user. The user can then refine the designed face by readjusting existing observations or adding new observations.

Fig. 4. Potential application: We guide different versions for a nose reconstruction for a given face (many observations) and few guiding landmarks on the nose (additional observations) (from left to right): initial shape with missing nose and landmarks, slim, wide, big, small and hooked.

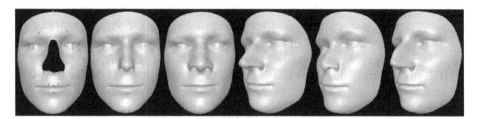

Fig. 5. Possible solutions for the tasks in our user study (from left to right): initial shape, shape with long nose, shape with adjusted principal components and two alien-like shapes.

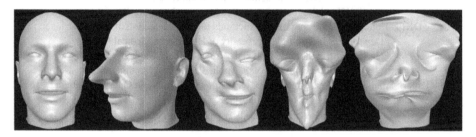

5 Conclusion

We presented the first web-based GUI to visualize 3D SSMs and explore reconstructions given partial observations. The tool enables fast exploration of basic features of SSMs and can be applied in a teaching setting, to design particular shapes or potentially even in clinical guidance. The tool is shared as open-source and can be run in the browser.

References

1. Lüthi M, Gerig T, Jud C, Vetter T. Gaussian process morphable models. IEEE Trans Pattern Anal Mach Intell. 2017;40(8):1860–73.
2. Albrecht T, Lüthi M, Gerig T, Vetter T. Posterior shape models. Med Image Anal. 2013;17(8):959–73.
3. Basso C, Vetter T. Statistically motivated 3D faces reconstruction. Procs 2nd Int Conf Reconstruct Soft Facial Parts. Vol. 31. (2). Citeseer. 2005.
4. Lüthi M, Blanc R, Albrecht T, Gass T, Goksel O, Büchler P et al. Statismo-a framework for PCA based statistical models. Insight J. 2012;2012:1–18.
5. Gerig T, Morel-Forster A, Blumer C, Egger B, Luthi M, Schoenborn S et al. Morphable Face Models : an open framework. Proc IEEE Int COnf Autom Face Gesture Recogn. 2018:75–82.
6. Sutherland S, Egger B, Tenenbaum J. Building 3D generative models from minimal data. Int J Comput Vis. 2023:1–26.

Abstract: Anatomy-informed Data Augmentation for Enhanced Prostate Cancer Detection

Balint Kovacs[1,2,3], Nils Netzer[2,3], Michael Baumgartner[1,4,5], Carolin Eith[2,3], Dimitrios Bounias[1,3], Clara Meinzer[2], Paul F. Jäger[5,6], Kevin S. Zhang[2], Ralf Floca[1], Adrian Schrader[2,3], Fabian Isensee[1,5], Regula Gnirs[2], Magdalena Görtz[7,8], Viktoria Schütz[8], Albrecht Stenzinger[9], Markus Hohenfellner[8], Heinz-Peter Schlemmer[2], Ivo Wolf[10], David Bonekamp[2], Klaus H. Maier-Hein[1,11]

[1]German Cancer Research Center (DKFZ) Heidelberg, Division of Medical Image Computing
[2]DKFZ Heidelberg, Division of Radiology
[3]Medical Faculty Heidelberg, Heidelberg University, Heidelberg
[4]Faculty of Mathematics and Computer Science, Heidelberg University
[5]DKFZ Heidelberg, Helmholtz Imaging
[6]DKFZ Heidelberg, Interactive Machine Learning Group
[7]DKFZ Heidelberg, Multiparametric methods for early detection of prostate cancer
[8]Department of Urology, University of Heidelberg Medical Center
[9]Institute of Pathology, University of Heidelberg Medical Center
[10]Mannheim University of Applied Sciences, Mannheim
[11]Pattern Analysis and Learning Group, Department of Radiation Oncology, Heidelberg University Hospital, Heidelberg
balint.kovacs@dkfz-heidelberg.de

Data augmentation (DA) is a key factor in medical image analysis, such as in prostate cancer (PCa) detection on magnetic resonance images. State-of-the-art computer-aided diagnosis systems still rely on simplistic spatial transformations to preserve the pathological label post transformation. However, such augmentations do not substantially increase the organ and tumor shape variability in the training set, limiting the model's generalization ability. We propose a new anatomy-informed transformation that leverages information from adjacent organs to simulate typical physiological deformations of the prostate and generates unique lesion shapes without altering their label. Due to its lightweight computational requirements, it can be easily integrated into common DA frameworks. We demonstrate the effectiveness of our augmentation on a dataset of 774 biopsy-confirmed examinations, by evaluating a state-of-the-art method for PCa detection with different augmentation settings [1].

References

1. Kovacs B et al. Anatomy-informed data augmentation for enhanced prostate cancer detection. Int Conf Med Image Comput Assist Interv. Springer. 2023:531–40.

Abstract: Reformulating COPD Classification on Chest CT Scans as Anomaly Detection using Contrastive Representations

cOOpD

Silvia D. Almeida[1,2,3], Carsten T. Lüth[4,5], Tobias Norajitra[1,3], Tassilo Wald[1,5], Marco Nolden[1], Paul F. Jäger[4,5], Claus P. Heussel[3,6], Jürgen Biederer[3,7], Oliver Weinheimer[3,7], Klaus H. Maier-Hein[1,3,5]

[1]Division of Medical Image Computing, German Cancer Research Center, Heidelberg, Germany
[2]Medical Faculty, Heidelberg University, Heidelberg, Germany
[3]Translational Lung Research Center Heidelberg (TLRC), Member of the German Center for Lung Research (DZL), Heidelberg, Germany
[4]Interactive Machine Learning Group, German Cancer Research Center, Heidelberg, Germany
[5]Helmholtz Imaging, German Cancer Research Center, Heidelberg, Germany
[6]Diagnostic and Interventional Radiology with Nuclear Medicine, Thoraxklinik at University Hospital, Heidelberg, Germany
[7]Diagnostic and Interventional Radiology, University Hospital, Heidelberg, Germany
silvia.diasalmeida@dkfz-heidelberg.de

Classification of heterogeneous diseases is challenging due to their complexity, variability of symptoms and imaging findings. Chronic obstructive pulmonary disease (COPD) is a prime example, being underdiagnosed despite being the third leading cause of death. Its sparse, diffuse and heterogeneous appearance on computed tomography challenges supervised binary classification. We reformulate COPD binary classification as an anomaly detection task, proposing cOOpD: heterogeneous pathological regions are detected as out-of-distribution (OOD) from normal homogeneous lung regions. To this end, we learn representations of unlabeled lung regions employing a self-supervised contrastive pretext model, potentially capturing specific characteristics of diseased and healthy unlabeled regions. A generative model then learns the distribution of healthy representations and identifies abnormalities (stemming from COPD) as deviations. Patient-level scores are obtained by aggregating region OOD scores. We show that cOOpD achieves the best performance on two public datasets, with an increase of 8.2% and 7.7% in terms of AUROC compared to the previous supervised state-of-the-art. Additionally, cOOpD yields well-interpretable spatial anomaly maps and patient-level scores which we show to be of additional value in identifying individuals in the early stage of progression. Experiments in artificially designed real-world prevalence settings further support that anomaly detection is a powerful way of tackling COPD classification [1].

References

1. Almeida SD, Lüth CT, et al. cOOpD: reformulating COPD classification on chest CT scans as anomaly detection using contrastive representations. Proc MICCAI. 2023.

© Der/die Autor(en), exklusiv lizenziert an
Springer Fachmedien Wiesbaden GmbH, ein Teil von Springer Nature 2024
A. Maier et al. (Hrsg.), *Bildverarbeitung für die Medizin 2024*,
Informatik aktuell, https://doi.org/10.1007/978-3-658-44037-4_34

Abstract: Handling Label Uncertainty on the Example of Automatic Detection of Shepherd's Crook RCA in Coronary CT Angiography

Felix Denzinger[1,2], Michael Wels[2], Oliver Taubmann[2], Florian Kordon[1],
Fabian Wagner[2], Stephanie Mehltretter[1], Mehmet A. Gülsün[2], Max Schöbinger[2],
Florian André[3], Sebastian Buß[3], Johannes Görich[3], Michael Sühling[2],
Andreas Maier[1], Katharina Breininger[4]

[1]Pattern Recognition Lab, FAU Erlangen-Nürnberg, Erlangen, Germany
[2]Siemens Healthineers AG, Computed Tomography, Forchheim, Germany
[3]Das Radiologische Zentrum, Sinsheim-Eberbach-Erbach-Walldorf-Heidelberg, Germany
[4]Department Artificial Intelligence in Biomedical Engineering, FAU Erlangen-Nürnberg
felix.denzinger@fau.de

Coronary artery disease (CAD) is often treated minimally invasively with a catheter being inserted into the diseased coronary vessel. If a patient exhibits a shepherd's crook (SC) right coronary artery (RCA) – an anatomical norm variant of the coronary vasculature – the complexity of this procedure is increased. Automated reporting of this variant from coronary CT angiography screening would ease prior risk assessment. We propose a 1D convolutional neural network which leverages a sequence of residual dilated convolutions to automatically determine this norm variant from a prior extracted vessel centerline. As the SC RCA is not clearly defined with respect to concrete measurements, labeling also includes qualitative aspects. Therefore, 4.23 % samples in our dataset of 519 RCA centerlines were labeled as unsure SC RCAs, with 5.97 % being labeled as sure SC RCAs. We explore measures to handle this label uncertainty, namely global/model-wise random assignment, exclusion, and soft label assignment. Furthermore, we evaluate how this uncertainty can be leveraged for the determination of a rejection class. With our best configuration, we reach an area under the receiver operating characteristic curve (AUC) of 0.938 on confident labels. Moreover, we observe an increase of up to 0.020 AUC when rejecting 10 % of the data and leveraging the labeling uncertainty information in the exclusion process [1].

References

1. Denzinger F, Wels M, Taubmann O, Kordon F, Wagner F, Mehltretter S et al. Handling label uncertainty on the example of automatic detection of shepherd's crook RCA in coronary CT angiography. Proc IEEE ISBI. 2023:1–5.

© Der/die Autor(en), exklusiv lizenziert an
Springer Fachmedien Wiesbaden GmbH, ein Teil von Springer Nature 2024
A. Maier et al. (Hrsg.), *Bildverarbeitung für die Medizin 2024*,
Informatik aktuell, https://doi.org/10.1007/978-3-658-44037-4_35

Segment-wise Evaluation in X-ray Angiography Stenosis Detection

Antonia Popp[1,2,3], Alaa Abd El Al[1,3], Marie Hoffmann[1,3], Ann Laube[2,3,5],
Peter McGranaghan[1,3,6,7], Volkmar Falk[1,3,5], Anja Hennemuth[2,3,4,5],
Alexander Meyer[1,3]

[1]Department of Cardiothoracic and Vascular Surgery, DHZC Berlin, Germany
[2]Institute of Computer-Assisted Cardiovascular Medicine, DHZC Berlin, Germany
[3]Charité – Universitätsmedizin Berlin, corporate member of Freie Universität Berlin,
Humboldt-Universität zu Berlin, and Berlin Institute of Health, Germany
[4]Fraunhofer Institute for Digital Medicine MEVIS, Berlin, Germany
[5]DZHK (German Centre for Cardiovascular Research), partner site Berlin
[6]Baptist Health South Florida, Miami, Florida, USA
[7]Semmelweis University, Budapest, Hungary
antonia.popp@dhzc-charite.de

Abstract. X-ray coronary angiography is the gold standard imaging modality for the assessment of coronary artery disease (CAD). The SYNTAX score is a recommended instrument for therapy decision-making and predicts the postprocedural risk associated with the two revascularization strategies: percutaneous coronary intervention (PCI) and coronary artery bypass graft (CABG). The score requires expert assessment and manual measurements of coronary angiograms for stenosis characterization. In this work we propose a deep learning workflow for automated stenosis detection to facilitate the calculation of the SYNTAX score. We use a region-based convolutional neural network for object detection, fine-tuned on a public dataset consisting of angiography frames with annotated stenotic regions. The model is evaluated on angiographic video sequences of complex CAD patients from the German Heart Center of the Charité University Hospital (DHZC), Berlin. We provide a customized graphical tool for cardiac experts that allows correction and segment annotation of the detected stenotic regions. The model reached a precision of 78.39% in the frame-wise object detection task on the clinical dataset. For the task of predicting the presence of coronary stenoses at the patient level, the model achieved a sensitivity of 49.55% for stenoses of all degrees and 59.18% for stenoses of relevant degrees (>75%). The results suggest that our stenosis detection tool can facilitate visual assessment of CAD in angiography data and encourage to investigate further development towards fully automated calculation of the SYNTAX score.

1 Introduction

Coronary artery disease (CAD) is the leading cause of death worldwide [1]. CAD is caused by pathological narrowing of the coronary arteries due to atherosclerotic plaque. This leads to reduced blood flow followed by insufficient supply of the heart muscles and increases the risk of ischaemia [2]. In clinical environments, treatment options for

© Der/die Autor(en), exklusiv lizenziert an
Springer Fachmedien Wiesbaden GmbH, ein Teil von Springer Nature 2024
A. Maier et al. (Hrsg.), *Bildverarbeitung für die Medizin 2024*,
Informatik aktuell, https://doi.org/10.1007/978-3-658-44037-4_36

patients with (complex) CAD are discussed in meetings of cardiac experts, known as heart teams, with the aim of identifying the optimal disease management strategy [3].

X-ray coronary angiography (XA) is the primary imaging modality for CAD assessment [4]. During cardiac catheterization, contrast agent is injected into the coronary arteries which enables vessel lumen visualization in x-ray video sequences. The heart team uses these XA sequences along with clinical patient data as basis for discussions about appropriate treatment and intervention planning. The latest Guidelines on Myocardial Revascularization advocate the SYNTAX score as an instrument for transparent and objective therapy decision-making [5]. The SYNTAX score quantifies the complexity of CAD to estimate the postprocedural risk associated with the two common revascularization strategies: percutaneous coronary intervention (PCI) and coronary artery bypass graft (CABG) [6]. The score depends on the location of the stenosis, with high scores for proximal vessel segments and low scores for distal segments. However, due to the time-consuming parameterization process, the score is barely used in clinical practice and many clinicians make decisions based on individual knowledge and experience. Since analyzing angiograms is also complicated by complex patient-specific vessel anatomy, low image quality, heart movement and insufficient spatial representation in 2D, decisions are accompanied by high uncertainty and inconsistency. Automating the CAD assessment process could enable guideline-compliant decision making, reduce inappropriate use of therapy methods and improve overall clinical outcomes.

Recent approaches on automated CAD assessment mainly use convolutional neural networks (CNNs) for (semantic) artery segmentation [7–9] and subsequent stenosis classification [10, 11]. Some studies investigate direct stenosis detection using CNN-based object detection models and achieve reliable results in angiographic images [12, 13]. Including temporal information enables stenosis detection and tracking on entire video sequences [14]. However, the evaluation of these methods is limited to single XA frames. In clinical practice multiple videos of different projection angles are considered for visual detection of stenoses. None of the studies above use data with segmental information about the stenoses, which is mandatory to calculate the SYNTAX score.

In this work we present an automated stenosis detection model which we evaluate on a clinical dataset of complex CAD patients from the German Heart Center of the Charité University Hospital (DHZC), Berlin. The data includes all XA video sequences recorded during the catheter examination. We provide a customized annotation tool for cardiac experts which displays the automatically detected regions of interest (ROIs) and allows the user to review and edit detected stenoses and annotate corresponding segments. The additional segment annotations allow us to evaluate the detection performance segment by segment.

2 Materials and methods

Our workflow for automated stenosis detection and evaluation includes two steps. First, a trained stenosis detection model is applied to all XA video frames in the clinical test dataset and predicts regions likely to show a stenosis. Subsequently, the marked stenotic regions are reviewed by a cardiac expert and visually annotated with the corresponding segment using a customized annotation tool.

2.1 Data

The stenosis detection model was trained on the public dataset by Danilov et al. [12], which includes 8325 XA frames (images) from 100 CAD patients. Each image is annotated with one or more stenotic regions.

We evaluated the model on a clinical dataset assembled from XA sequences from two DHZC cohorts. The first cohort consisted of 126 CAD patients with complex triple vessel disease and high SYNTAX scores who were being prepared to receive CABG surgery. The second cohort included 16 CAD patients with complex LAD segment stenoses who were eligible for hybrid PCI and CABG surgery.

During an XA examination several video sequences are recorded from different projection angles, showing the coronary arteries filled with contrast medium. The number of XA videos recorded per patient in the clinical dataset ranges from 3 to 79 with a mean of 18.7, resulting in a total of 2, 590 sequences that consist of 130, 620 frames. The XA videos were exported directly from a clinical system without pre-selection and show the right coronary arteries, left coronary arteries, the aorta or the catheter track. In total, there are 553 stenoses in the test dataset. Of these, 316 have a stenotic degree of $> 75\%$ and require treatment, thus, are considered as relevant stenoses.

2.2 Stenosis detection model

As a baseline, we used the pre-trained Faster R-CNN ResNet-101 V2, as it achieves the highest accuracy in detecting stenotic regions among multiple object detection networks [12]. Faster R-CNN is a CNN for object detection, including a region proposal network (RPN) that shares full-image convolutional features with the detection network [15]. It predicts the coordinates of a bounding box and the corresponding confidence score at each predicted position. The model was initialized with pre-trained weights [16] and fine-tuned over 10^5 iterations using the weighted smooth L1 loss for localization, the weighted focal loss for classification and a gradually decreasing learning rate.

2.3 Customized annotation tool

The trained model predicts stenotic regions on each frame of the clinical test dataset, but only regions with a confidence score of $> 90\%$ were considered as ROIs for evaluation. To allow verification and segment annotation of the ROIs by cardiac experts, we developed a customized software which shows the ROIs on the XA images and allows graphical interaction such as removal of false detections and boundary annotation of missed stenotic regions. For each ROI containing a stenosis the user can assign the stenotic degree and the coronary artery segment. The detected ROIs were verified and assessed by one cardiac expert.

3 Results

The stenosis detection model was evaluated using the local clinical dataset of complex CAD patients as test set (Sec. 2.1). It contains information about stenotic segments in the patient, the predicted stenotic regions and corresponding segment annotations by the cardiac expert. The analysis of one patient included simultaneous identification of present stenoses by visual inspection of all XA recordings, review of the predicted ROIs and assignment of stenosis degree and vessel segment of correctly depicted stenoses. The annotation process was time-consuming with a mean time of 17.5 minutes per patient and required a high level of experience in analyzing XA data. Due to the large number of frames in the dataset, missed stenoses in frames were not marked by the expert and only detected stenoses were considered for evaluation on image level.

The presence of a stenosis in a patient is confirmed by visual inspection of the XA recordings. A stenosis is considered to be detected by the model if it is shown correctly on at least one frame of the patient's XA recordings. 274 out of 553 stenoses in the clinical dataset were successfully detected by the model, resulting in a sensitivity of 49.55%. 187 out of the 316 relevant stenoses with a stenotic degree of > 75% were detected by the model, resulting in a sensitivity of 59.18%. Figure 1 shows for each coronary segment the number of patients in which a present stenosis was successfully detected.

Looking at the performance at the frame level, the model predicted 13, 381 regions, of which 10, 490 show a stenosis, giving a precision of 78.39%.

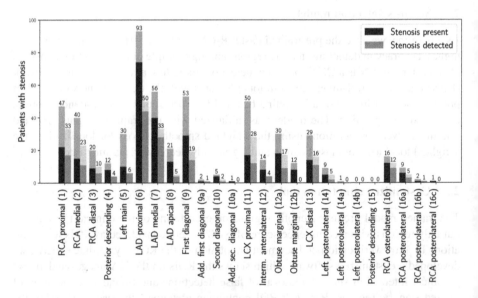

Fig. 1. Number of patients who actually have a stenosis in the segment (blue bar) and who have a relevant stenosis (>75%) in the segment (dark blue). Number of patients for whom the stenosis in the respective segment was successfully detected by the model (orange bar) and for whom a relevant stenosis was successfully detected (dark orange).

4 Discussion

We evaluated the detection performance of a fine-tuned Faster R-CNN [12, 15] on a clinical dataset of complex CAD patients. For segment-wise evaluation we provide a customized tool for a user-friendly review of predicted stenoses and segment annotation.

Regarding the detection performance on XA frame level, the model predicted stenotic regions with a fair level of precision. Investigating the same model architecture, Danilov et al. [12] achieved a higher precision (95%), which can be explained by the selection of high-contrast frames containing at least one stenosis. Ling et al. [13] achieved a comparable precision (82%), but used a smaller dataset of selected frames. Similar to clinical practice, analyzing the frames of full XA sequences complicates automated image processing, especially when faced with varying image quality, insufficient contrast agent and complex patient anatomy. Our test dataset incorporates these challenges, resulting in missed stenotic regions (Fig. 2b) and false detections (Fig. 2c).

Considering the stenoses present in the clinical dataset, most stenoses occurred in the main branches or proximal segments (1, 2, 6, 7, 9, 11) (Fig. 1). Descending arteries contained less stenoses (4, 9a-10a, 14a-15, 16a-c). Considering the detection performance, stenoses occurring in smaller vessels (4, 8, 9, 12) were detected less often, which can be explained by insufficient pixel representation. Stenoses in the right coronary arteries (RCA) were detected more frequently compared to the left coronary arteries (LAD and LCX). Similar to visual inspection, stenoses in the RCA segments are easier to identify due to increased contrast and vessel diameter. The model is more successful in detecting relevant stenoses compared to stenoses of all degrees, as higher changes in the vessel diameter increase detection confidence. The clinical usefulness of the current model is limited as the detection accuracy is not excellent. Lowering the confidence scores for ROI selection (Sec. 2.3) would increase detection sensitivity on the patient level but simultaneously increases the number of false detections on the frame level.

Future work includes model improvement by using a larger clinical dataset with higher variety in CAD complexity for training and evaluation. The constructed stenosis detection dataset enhanced by the annotation of the segments allows further investigation of advanced CAD evaluation such as automated prediction of the stenotic segment.

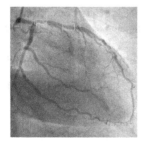 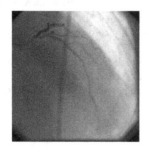 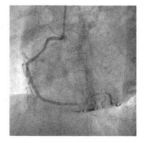

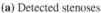

(a) Detected stenoses   (b) Missed stenosis   (c) False detection

Fig. 2. Cases of successful (a) and unsuccessful (b,c) stenosis detection.

The assessment and quantification of CAD through a fully automated calculation of the SYNTAX score can facilitate and improve clinical decision-making in heart team discussions.

References

1. Wang H, Naghavi M, Allen C, Barber RM. Global, regional, and national life expectancy, all-cause mortality, and cause-specific mortality for 249 causes of death, 1980-2015: a systematic analysis for the Global Burden of Disease Study 2015. Lancet. 2016;388(10053):1459–544.
2. Libby P, Theroux P. Pathophysiology of coronary artery disease. Circulation. 2005;(25):3481–8.
3. Holmes DR, Rich JB, Zoghbi WA, Mack MJ. The heart team of cardiovascular care. J Am Coll Cardiol. 2013;61(9):903–7.
4. Rigatelli G, Gianese F, Zuin M. Modern atlas of invasive coronary angiography views: a practical approach for fellows and young interventionalists. Int J Cardiovasc Imaging. 2021.
5. Neumann FJ, Sousa-Uva M, Ahlsson A, Alfonso F, Banning AP, Benedetto U et al. ESC/EACTS Guidelines on myocardial revascularization. Eur Heart J. 2019;40(2):87–165.
6. Sianos G, Morel MA, Kappetein AP, Morice MC. The SYNTAX score: an angiographic tool grading the complexity of coronary artery disease. Eurointervention. 2005.
7. Zhu X, Cheng Z, Wang S, Chen X, Lu G. Coronary angiography image segmentation based on PSPNet. Comput Methods Programs Biomed. 2021;200:105897.
8. Iyer K, Najarian CP, Fattah AA, Arthurs CJ, Soroushmehr SMR, Subban V et al. AngioNet: a convolutional neural network for vessel segmentation in X-ray angiography. Sci Rep. 2021;11(1):18066.
9. Zhao C, Bober R, Tang H, Tang J, Dong M, Zhang C et al. Semantic segmentation to extract coronary arteries in invasive coronary angiograms. J Adv Comput Math. 2022;9:76–85.
10. Zhao C, Vij A, Malhotra S, Tang J, Tang H, Pienta D et al. Automatic extraction and stenosis evaluation of coronary arteries in invasive coronary angiograms. Comput Biol Med. 2021;136:104667.
11. Zhou Y, Guo H, Song J, Chen Y, Wang J. Review of vessel segmentation and stenosis classification in X-ray coronary angiography. Processing WCSP. 2021:1–5.
12. Danilov VV, Klyshnikov KY, Gerget OM, Kutikhin AG, Ganyukov VI, Frangi AF et al. Real-time coronary artery stenosis detection based on modern neural networks. Sci Rep. 2021;11(1):7582.
13. Ling H, Chen B, Guan R, Xiao Y, Yan H, Chen Q et al. Deep learning model for coronary angiography. J Cardiovasc Transl Res. 2023;16(4):896–904.
14. Pang K, Ai D, Fang H, Fan J, Song H, Yang J. Stenosis-DetNet: Sequence consistency-based stenosis detection for X-ray coronary angiography. Computerized Medical Imaging and Graphics. 2021;89:101900.
15. Ren S, He K, Girshick R, Sun J. Faster R-CNN: towards real-time object detection with region proposal networks. Adv Neural Inf Process Syst. 2015;28.
16. Lin TY, Maire M, Belongie S, Bourdev L, Garshick R, Hays J et al. Microsoft COCO: common objects in context. Proc ECCV. 2014:740–55.

Automated Mitotic Index Calculation via Deep Learning and Immunohistochemistry

Jonas Ammeling[1], Moritz Hecker[1], Jonathan Ganz[1], Taryn A. Donovan[2],
Robert Klopfleisch[3], Christof A. Bertram[4], Katharina Breininger[5], Marc Aubreville[1]

[1]Technische Hochschule Ingolstadt, Ingolstadt, Germany
[2]The Schwarzman Animal Medical Center, New York, USA
[3]Institute of Veterinary Pathology, Freie Universität Berlin, Germany
[4]Institute of Pathology, University of Veterinary Medicine Vienna, Vienna, Austria
[5]Department Artificial Intelligence in Biomedical Engineering, Friedrich-Alexander-Universität
Erlangen-Nürnberg, Erlangen, Germany
jonas.ammeling@thi.de

Abstract. The volume-corrected mitotic index (M/V-Index) has demonstrated prognostic value in invasive breast carcinomas. However, despite its prognostic significance, it is not established as the standard method for assessing aggressive biological behaviour, due to the high additional workload associated with determining the epithelial proportion. In this work, we show that the use of a deep learning pipeline solely trained with an annotation-free, immunohistochemistry-based approach, provides accurate estimates of epithelial segmentation in canine mammary carcinomas. We compare our automatic framework with the manually annotated M/V-Index in a study with three board-certified pathologists. Our results indicate that the deep learning-based pipeline shows expert-level performance, while providing time efficiency and reproducibility.

1 Introduction

The accurate assessment of mitotic activity in histopathology plays an essential role in cancer diagnosis, prognosis, and treatment decisions. The mitotic count (MC), which represents the number of mitotic figures in a given area of tissue is a key parameter in many grading schemes used to assess the proliferation rate and aggressiveness of various malignancies. The prognostic significance of the MC is limited due to high inter-observer variability, poor reproducibility and the labor-intensive nature of this microscopic task. Additionally, varying cellular densities of different tumors can limit the interpretability of the MC across cases. Haapasalo & Collan [1] introduced the volume corrected mitotic index (M/V-Index) in an effort to standardize the counting of mitotic figures. The M/V-Index standardizes the MC by dividing it by the area fraction of the epithelial tissue estimated subjectively or by using a point grid and adjusting it for the size of a high power field, resulting in an estimate of the number of mitotic figures per square millimeter. Jannink et al. [2] demonstrated that the M/V-Index, along with tumor size and lymph node status, offered better prognostic information for human breast cancer than the uncorrected MC. Despite its significance, the M/V-Index is not widely adopted due to the additional effort required in estimating the epithelial tissue fraction, leading to higher inter-observer variability. Hence, the faster and simpler uncorrected

© Der/die Autor(en), exklusiv lizenziert an
Springer Fachmedien Wiesbaden GmbH, ein Teil von Springer Nature 2024
A. Maier et al. (Hrsg.), *Bildverarbeitung für die Medizin 2024*,
Informatik aktuell, https://doi.org/10.1007/978-3-658-44037-4_37

MC remains the preferred method for assessing tumor proliferation. In this study, we provide an automated framework for the calculation of the M/V-Index on hematoxilin and eosin (H&E)-stained images. The framework is developed in an annotation-free fashion (i.e. not requiring any human labelling effort for estimating the area fraction of the epithelial tissue) by using immunohistochemistry (IHC) as a reference standard [3] and leveraging an existing model for MC estimation [4]. This framework provides the first proof of concept that the M/V-Index can be estimated with accuracy, efficiency and reproducibility, offering a more objective method to assess tumor proliferation.

2 Materials

The dataset consisted of 50 canine mammary carcinoma samples collected at the University of Veterinary Medicine, Vienna. The samples were first stained with standard H&E and scanned with a 3DHistech Panoramic Scann II at 40× magnification (0.25 µm/px). After scanning, the slides were destained and then restained with the pan-cytokeratin AE1/AE3 primary antibody, which is specific for cytokeratin proteins commonly found in epithelial tissues. The IHC slides were rescanned using the same scanner and magnification. The process of restaining the slides resulted in 50 H&E and IHC whole slide image (WSI) pairs which were co-registered using a robust quad-tree based WSI registration method [5]. Due to some staining artefacts and alignment errors, 9 samples were removed from the dataset. Of the remaining 41 samples, 12 were kept as a hold-out test set. The remaining 29 samples were used in a 5-fold Monte Carlo cross-validation where the samples were randomly divided into 20 training and 9 validation cases. For each slide in the hold-out test set, a region of interest (ROI) with an area of 2.37 mm^2 equivalent to 10 high power fields (HPFs) in a microscope with an ocular Field Number (FN) of 22 mm was selected and annotated for epithelial tissue by a board-certified pathologist.

3 Methods

To reduce the overall amount of manual labelling for our automated M/V-Index system, we automatically generated the training data for tumor epithelium segmentation from the IHC slides, which were then transferred by the registration method to the H&E slides on which we trained our segmentation network.

3.1 Automatic tumor epithelium segmentation on H&E

For tumor epithelium mask generation, we created an IHC map from downsampled WSIs, excluding irrelevant areas. The IHC map was created by applying color deconvolution and then using the cytokeratin channel to generate a binary mask by first applying a Gaussian blur filter and then Otsu's adaptive thresholding method, followed by a closing operation to remove small interruptions. Patches with at least 5% non-zero values in the IHC map were then processed at full resolution, first using color deconvolution, followed by binary thresholding and an opening operation to remove small noise from staining artefacts and intensity variations. Finally, a closing operation with a large circular kernel resulted in a coarse segmentation mask (Fig. 1) that was helpful in mitigating small alignment errors from the registration process. Bulten et al. [3] used a similar pipeline on prostate samples, however they used additional human labelling to further optimize the masks. The tumor epithelium segmentation network was based on a U-Net architecture, consisting of an EfficientNet-b0 encoder and a classical encoder composed of up-sampling and convolutional layer. The network was trained on patches of size 1024×1024 at a resolution of 0.5 µm/px and a batch size of 4. We used the Adam optimizer with an initial learning rate of 0.001 and an exponentially decaying learning rate schedule with a factor of 0.99. The loss function consisted of a weighted combination with factor 0.5 of dice loss and binary cross-entropy loss. To make the model more robust to the noisy training masks, we used label smoothing with a factor of 0.1 for the targets in the cross-entropy loss function. The model was trained with standard online augmentation including random flipping, rotation, Gaussian blurring, and changes in brightness, contrast, saturation and hue.

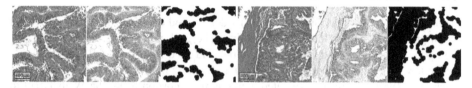

Fig. 1. Two example patches from the mask generation process. (left) H&E patch, (middle) IHC patch, (right) automatically generated mask (white: epithelial tissue, black: background).

3.2 Mitotic count estimation

The mitotic count estimation network was based on DA-RetinaNet [4], a one-stage RetinaNet object detector with a ResNet-18 backbone, trained with domain adversarial training on the MIDOG 21 [6] training dataset, which consists of 200 human breast cancer images from four different scanners. No further annotations or fine tuning were considered necessary due to the morphological similarity between the two species. For further details on the implementation of the network, the reader is referred to Wilm et al. [4].

3.3 Volume corrected mitotic index

The volume corrected mitotic index (M/V-Index) was originally proposed by Haapasalo & Collan [1] in order to standardize the MC based on the cellular density of the tumor. The formula for calculating the M/V-Index is

$$\text{M/V-Index} = k \sum_{i=1}^{n} \frac{\text{MC}_i}{\text{Vv}_i} \tag{1}$$

where n is the number of microscope fields studied, MC is the number of mitotic figures in a selected field, Vv is the volume fraction (in per cent) of the neoplastic tissue in the same field, either estimated subjectively or with point-counting, and k is a coefficient characterizing the microscope: $k = 100/\pi r^2$ where r in (in mm) is the radius of the circular microscope field. To adapt the formula for a digital evaluation we defined $k = 100/A$, where A is the area (in mm^2) of the evaluated ROI. Here we set $k = 100/2.37$ mm^2, where 2.37 mm^2 is the area of 10 HPFs at 40$\times$ magnification (0.25 µm/px). The MC was estimated by first dividing the image into overlapping patches of size 512$\times$512 at 40$\times$ magnification (0.25 µm/px). The predictions of the MC estimation model are then fused and transformed into the original coordinate space. Similarly, Vv is estimated using the segmentation model on overlapping patches of size 1024$\times$1024 at 20$\times$ magnification (0.5 µm/px). The concatenated result of the epithelium segmentation is then used as a mask to filter mitotic figures that are within the epithelial tissue region. Finally, the M/V-Index is calculated as $k \times$ MC/Vv over the entire ROI.

3.4 Manual vs. automatic M/V-index

Three board-certified pathologists manually determined the M/V-Index using a Weibel point grid [2] to reduce interrater variability. The grid, adjusted to the ROI size, had 432 points, equivalent to the 42-point Weibel grid used for a single HPF. Pathologists separately annotated epithelium proportion and mitotic figures, measuring the time for each task. We compare the estimated epithelium proportion using the Weibel grid to the ground truth calculated from the epithelium masks of our pathologist. The ground truth for the M/V-Index is calculated by first filtering all mitotic figure annotations from our pathologists through the ground truth epithelium mask and then averaging the M/V-Index of the individual pathologists.

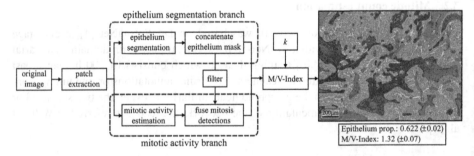

Fig. 2. Automated volume corrected mitotic index (M/V-Index) framework. The image on the right shows the epithelium segmentation in orange. Green boxes represent mitotic figures detected within the epithelium mask. Red boxes represent mitotic figures filtered out by the epithelium mask. The results below the image present algorithm-derived mean and standard deviation for both epithelium proportion and the M/V-Index.

Tab. 1. Results from the comparison between the manual and automatic M/V-Index to the ground truth. Displayed are the mean absolute error (MAE), and Pearson's correlation coefficient.

Metric	Agent	MAE	Pearson's r
Epithelium Proportion	Pathologists	0.06 ± 0.02	0.95 ± 0.04
	Algorithm	0.06 ± 0.01	0.83 ± 0.11
MV-Index	Pathologists	7.39 ± 1.37	0.87 ± 0.06
	Algorithm	4.51 ± 0.25	0.78 ± 0.02

4 Results

The epithelium segmentation algorithm achieved an average intersection-over-union (IOU) of 0.71 (±0.01) and F1 score of 0.83 (±0.01) on the hold-out test set. Qualitative results are in Figure 3. A comparison of results between manual and automatic M/V-Index is in Table 1. The mean absolute error (MAE) for epithelium proportion was consistent among pathologists and the algorithm, shown in Figure 4 (left). For the M/V-Index, the average MAE was 7.39 (±1.37) for pathologists and 4.51 (±0.25) for the algorithm, displayed in Figure 4 (right). In our study, pathologists took an average of 12 minutes, while the algorithm only took 20 seconds to calculate the M/V-Index on a ROI. Using the Weibel grid, pathologists spent an average of 6 minutes assessing only the epithelium proportion per ROI.

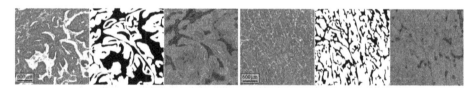

Fig. 3. Tumor epithelium segmentation results on the hold-out test set. (left) original image, (middle) expert labelled ground truth, (right) segmentation results. Green pixels show true positives, red false positives and blue false negatives.

5 Discussion

We showed that our algorithm can estimate the M/V-Index comparable to expert level performance. We avoided the need for time-consuming manual labeling of tumor tissue by the innovative use of immunohistochemical stainings as the ground truth. The evaluation of the model on a expert-derived ground truth of the test set serves as a first proof of concept that the M/V-Index can be calculated in an automated, fast and reproducible way. This framework is easily extendable to calculate the M/V-Index on entire WSIs automatically providing even larger time savings for the pathologist and further reducing the potential for inter-observer variability by selecting the region of highest mitotic activity in a computer-aided and more reproducible fashion. In a future

Fig. 4. Results of the manual vs. automatic M/V-Index annotation study with three board-certified pathologist. (left) Epithelium proportion, (right) M/V-Index.

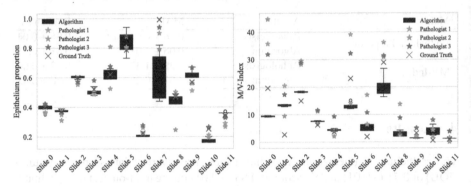

work, this framework can be improved by employing a more precise IHC marker during training, addressing the issue caused by pan-cytokeratin also binding to myoepithelial cells, which is a potential error for the segmentation model.

Acknowledgement. This work was supported by the Bavarian Institute for Digital Transformation (bidt) under the grant "Responsibility Gaps in Human Machine Interaction (ReGInA)"

References

1. Haapasalo H, Pesonen E, Collan Y. Volume corrected mitotic index (M/V-INDEX): the standard of mitotic activity in neoplasms. Pathol Research Practice. 1989;185:551–4.
2. Jannink I, Diest PJV, Baak JP. Comparison of the prognostic value of four methods to assess mitotic activity in 186 invasive breast cancer patients: classical and random mitotic activity assessments with correction for volume percentage of epithelium. Hum Pathol. 1995;26:1086–92.
3. Bulten W, Bandi P, Hoven J, Lotz J, Weiss N, Litjens G et al. Epithelium segmentation using deep learning in H&E-stained prostate specimens with immunohistochemistry as reference standard. Sci Rep. 2019;9.
4. Wilm F, Marzahl C, Breininger K, Aubreville M. Domain adversarial RetinaNet as a reference algorithm for the mitosis domain generalization challenge. Lect Notes Comput Sci. 2022;13166:5–13.
5. Robust quad-tree based registration on whole slide images. Proc MICCAI. 2021;156:181–90.
6. Aubreville M, Stathonikos N, Bertram CA, Klopleisch R, Hoeve N ter, Ciompi F et al. Mitosis domain generalization in histopathology images: the MIDOG challenge. Med Image Anal. 2023;84:102699.

Abstract: Radiomics Processing Toolkit
Role of Feature Computation on Prediction Performance

Jonas R. Bohn[1,2,3,4], Christian M. Heidt[2,5,6], Silvia D. Almeida[1,2,6], Lisa Kausch[1],
Michael Götz[7], Marco Nolden[1,2,5], Petros Christopoulos[2], Stephan Rheinheimer[2,5],
Alan A. Peters[2,5,8], Oyunbileg von Stackelberg[2,5], Hans-Ulrich Kauczor[2,5],
Klaus H. Maier-Hein[1,2,5], Claus P. Heußel[2,5], Tobias Norajitra[1,2]

[1]German Cancer Research Center (DKFZ)
[2]Translational Lung Research Center (TLRC), Member of the German Center for Lung Research
[3]Faculty of Biosciences, Heidelberg University
[4]National Center for Tumor Diseases (NCT), NCT Heidelberg, a partnership between DKFZ and university medical center
[5]University Hospital Heidelberg
[6]Medical Faculty, Heidelberg University
[7]University of Ulm
[8]University Hospital Bern
j.bohn@dkfz-heidelberg.de

Radiomics focuses on extracting and analyzing quantitative features from medical images. Standardizing radiomics is difficult due to variations across studies and centers, making it challenging to identify optimal techniques for any application. Recent works (WORC, Autoradiomics) [1, 2] are introducing radiomics-based frameworks for automated pipeline optimization. Both approaches span the workflow, enabling consistent, and reproducible radiomics analyses. In contrast, finding the ideal solutions for feature extractor and feature selection components, has received less attention. Therefore, we propose the Radiomics Processing Toolkit (RPTK) [3], which adds comprehensive feature extraction and selection components from PyRadiomics and from the Medical Image Radiomics Processor (MIRP) to the radiomics pipeline. We compared RPTK with results from WORC and Autoradiomics and on six different public benchmark data sets. We demonstrate significant improved performance by incorporating the proposed feature processing and selection techniques across all datasets. Additionally, the choice of the feature extractor significantly enhances prediction performance. Our results provide additional guidance in selecting suitable components for optimized radiomics analyses.

References

1. Martijn PAS, Sebastian, Phil T, Milea, Vos M, Guillaume et al. Reproducible radiomics through automated machine learning validated on twelve clinical applications. arXiv preprint server. 2021.
2. Woznicki P, Laqua F, Bley T, Baeßler B. AutoRadiomics: A Framework for Reproducible Radiomics Research. Frontiers in Radiology. 2022;2.
3. Bohn J, Heidt CM, Almeida SD, Kausch L, Götz M, Nolden M et al. RPTK: The Role of Feature Computation on Prediction Performance. Lecture Notes in Computer Sciences. Vol. 14393. MICCAI 2023, Springer Nature, in press 2023.

© Der/die Autor(en), exklusiv lizenziert an
Springer Fachmedien Wiesbaden GmbH, ein Teil von Springer Nature 2024
A. Maier et al. (Hrsg.), *Bildverarbeitung für die Medizin 2024*,
Informatik aktuell, https://doi.org/10.1007/978-3-658-44037-4_38

Towards Unified Multi-modal Dataset Creation for Deep Learning Utilizing Structured Reports

Malte Tölle[1,2,3], Lukas Burger[1,2,3], Halvar Kelm[1,2,3], Sandy Engelhardt[1,2,3]

[1]Department of Internal Medicine III, Heidelberg University Hospital
[2]DZHK (German Centre for Cardiovascular Research), partner site Heidelberg/Mannheim
[3]Informatics for Life Institute, Ruprecht-Karls University Heidelberg
malte.toelle@med.uni-heidelberg.de

Abstract. The unification of electronic health records promises interoperability of medical data. Divergent data storage options, inconsistent naming schemes, varied annotation procedures, and disparities in label quality, among other factors, pose significant challenges to the integration of expansive datasets especially across instiutions. This is particularly evident in the emerging multi-modal learning paradigms where dataset harmonization is of paramount importance. Leveraging the DICOM standard, we designed a data integration and filter tool that streamlines the creation of multi-modal datasets. This ensures that datasets from various locations consistently maintain a uniform structure. We enable the concurrent filtering of DICOM data (i.e. images and waveforms) and corresponding annotations (i.e. segmentations and structured reports) in a graphical user interface. The graphical interface as well as example structured report templates is openly available at https://github.com/Cardio-AI/fl-multi-modal-dataset-creation.

1 Introduction

Deep learning models need vast amounts of training data to obtain the incredible results reported by recent methods. In the realm of medicine, electronic health records (EHR) promise a unified intra- and inter-hospital data representation that improves patient care by providing a timely access to centralized patient's medical records. Such data is comprised of different formats including images, patient history, diagnostic reports, and other clinical domains. In theory, there are many templates that can be followed to ensure interoperability between healthcare providers' data. However, in practice many different data formats and often self defined templates are used that hinder the collection of large scale datasets even in an intra-hospital cohort selection [1]. To complicate above scenario the data of one location is not sufficient for training modern data hungry networks. Training across data from multiple locations is needed, which is impeded by privacy laws. However, to enable a distributed (federated) learning scenario on real world data one must ensure common data formats across all participating locations [2].

Digital imaging and communication in medicine (DICOM) is the internationally accepted standard for communication and storage of medical images and related information across a wide range of medical modalities and disciplines. While originating in the field of imaging it does now also allow for storage and linking of other modalities such as waveforms, text, audio, or speech. Although hospitals around the world have

A. Maier et al. (Hrsg.), *Bildverarbeitung für die Medizin 2024*,
Informatik aktuell, https://doi.org/10.1007/978-3-658-44037-4_39

established an extensive enterprise imaging infrastructure, workflows and software applications based on DICOM often rely on non-standard formats and interfaces for the storage and exchange of data annotations and computational image analysis results [3].

One renowned platform that aims at facilitating the application of algorithms on real world clinical data is Kaapana [4]. In addition to the possibility of deploying algorithms directly in the platform they also provide a graphical filter tool for cohort selection based on the imaging data in the internal picture archiving and communication system (PACS). However, only image related attributes can be filtered and the link to other forms of data (patient letters, diagnoses, geometric relations, etc.) are not included. Multi-modal deep learning schemes have been shown to improve predictive performances across domains [5].

The aim of this work is to provide an application for efficient data integration, matching, and cohort selection for multi-modal deep learning based on real world DICOM data. Data integration refers to the aggregation of diverse data types into a single, coherent framework, while data matching ensures entries can be referenced and linked unambiguously on different levels of the document tree. The contributions of this work are three-fold:

- By leveraging the DICOM standard we integrate data from different sources and modalities into a coherent framework that exceeds the imaging domain by using structured reports (SR).
- We present a method to match and filter the data that is coming from different modalities and linked on different levels in the document tree.
- SRs represent a difficult domain due to their vast amount of templates. We present a method for a unified extraction of the individual important information per template.

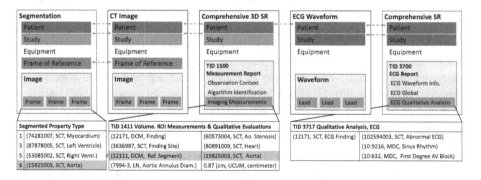

Fig. 1. Data relationships for relevant data to predict pacemaker dependecy after heart valve replacement. Structured Reports can reference e.g. images, waveforms, regions, and segments. Following highdicom we also opt for the general Comprehensive (3D) SR due to its high generalizability [3].

2 Material and methods

To improve understandability we explain our developed tool with a real-world example. Inspired by recent work we envision a scenario where we train a model to predict the risk for an individual patient to receive a pacemaker after undergoing a valve replacement in the heart [6]. First, the individual electrocardiogram (ECG) can provide hints as to whether the patient already has a disturbed stimulus conduction in the heart. Second, imaging modalities such as computed tomography (CT) can provide further information as to whether such an implant might lead to severe consequences for the patient. Important characteristics can be e.g. the geometric relations of the target region in relation to the implant's dimensions as well as the presence and severity of calcification. Last, patient characteristics such as if the patient is a tobacco smoker or a past history of heart diseases or diabetes mellitus can yield further insides (Figure 1).

From the above example three requirements can be derived that a tool for consistent data integration, matching, and cohort selection should fullfil.

- R1 Integration: Consistent representation of data from different formats in an unifying interface.
- R2 Unambiguous Matching: Different data types from the same patient must be matched and queryable together. Concurrently, they must be filterable independent of other types and multiple conditions must be evaluable on the instance level.
- R3 Intuitive Cohort Selection: Graphical visualization and filtering is desirable, while more complicated textual queries should also be possible.

Integrating machine learning models into clinical workflows requires interoperability between existing systems, which can be guaranteed by complying to standards. Although the DICOM standard is mainly used within the imaging departments of hospitals it allows storage of other data types with already defined templates as well.

Structured reports represent a standardized method for the encoding, transmission, and storage of diagnostic reports. In addition to images it also allows the linking of other data types such as e.g. text, audio, time points or other measurements. It allows for a general semantic understanding of data by using universal coded concepts enhancing interoperability [7]. Each SR must have a defined template that consists of a sequence of content items (see Figure 2b). Each content item defines a name-value pair that encodes a domain-specific property or concept. Concept names must follow standard medical ontologies and terminologies such as the Systematized Nomenclature of Medical Clinical Terms (SNOMED CT), which ensures uniqueness and cross domain interpretability [8]. The value can take up to four different types: it can also be a coded concept, it might include a number, comprise one or more sets of points or other graphic data such as surfaces, or can be made up of plain text (Fig. 2a). Other data types such as pixel raster images (secondary capture) are also possible but in here we restrict ourselves initially to the four mentioned data types. However, an extension of our application is straightforward.

Another common data type in radiology are segmentations in which one or multiple structures can be compartmentalized. Each segment can be described by a specific label encoded by a coded concept similar to the name of a content item in SRs that ensures uniqueness. Segments can also be referenced in a SR providing another level of entwinement.

To provide possible integration of our developed filter tool into Kaapana we also opt for Opensearch as the tool of choice for enabling graphical cohort filtering[1]. But our tool can also serve as a stand alone tool which can be linked to any PACS.

A patient can have multiple reports or segmentations, which can contain e.g. different diagnoses or labels for different studies. Filtering these interlinked data types on the same level requires the child element to be aware of its parent due to the possible reference of multiple instances within one object. To ensure a parent document is evaluated at the level of its child, i.e. annotation, we use Opensearch's nested objects. With nested objects we can evaluate whether multiple conditions are true for one instance i.e. our children obtain boundaries. As an example we might want all segmentations that have the left and right ventricle included. Without nested objects we would also receive all instances that have only one of both segmented. To visualize such nested queries one cannot use the default visualizations of Opensearch, one must rather use the declarative language Vega to create custom plots[2].

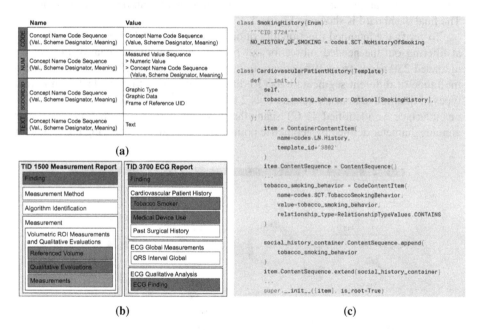

Fig. 2. Schematic overview over structured reports. Each structured report is defined by a template (b). While SRs exhibit highly nested structures, at their core they are comprised of simple data types that are consistent across templates (a). An example of for defining a SR in highdicom is presented in (c).

---

[1]https://opensearch.org/
[2]https://vega.github.io/vega/

3   Results

Our tool allows for the simultaneous filtering of DICOM imaging and waveform modalities and annotations in the form of structured reports and segmentations (R1). The DICOM representation ensures matching on a patient level across time points (R2). In the case of segmentations we visualize all segment descriptions as well as the creator type (R3). Structured report templates exhibit a high degree of sophistication due to their intricately nested structure and the numerous attributes that can be defined [3]. To make the data filterable when uploading the SR's data into Opensearch the user must define, which measurements, geometrical data, qualitative and text attributes shall be queryable by providing the nested path (e.g. for TID 3700 ECG Report: Cardiovascular Patient History - Social History - Tobacco Smoker). As this might be complex at times we believe that it provides the flexibility needed for filtering such a complex data structure as structured reports. The definition of the path to the wanted attributes must be defined once per template, but it can be expanded or contracted at any time (R3). This allows also for the dynamic creation of custom templates if needed, as long as the path to the desired attributes are specified and template is in conformance with the DICOM standard. An example for how to define a custom template can be found in Figure 2c. The final dashboard is shown in Figure 3.

To verify the intended functionality of our tool we uploaded diverse data and aimed at filtering out the needed subset for our pacemaker prediction scenario. In total we uploaded 280 series from 198 patients from three modalities (MRI, CT, ECG), with a multitude of different segmentations (10 different labels). In total we had 12 different types of qualitative items, 4 quantitative, 2 geometric, and 1 free text. With the help of our interface we identified 41 CT scans that have the aorta segmented and the aortic annulus diameter defined by geometric points. By subsequently querying the ECGs for

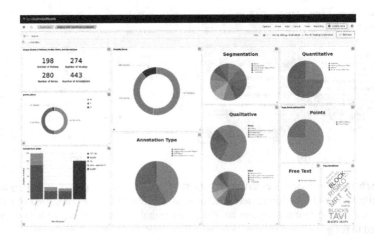

Fig. 3. The created dashboard with the filterable annotation attributes. The type of annotation can be chosen. Segmentations can be queried on individual segment level. Since for qualitative items both name and value are a concept name, we can filter both. For numeric as well as geometric items we filter on the name. When the value is text we incorporate free text search.

which a SR with Cardiac Pacemaker exists, we picked out a further subset of 22 patients. Upon examining pacemaker dependent patients another interesting cohort are patients that have an abnormal ECG but still obtain a valid sinus rhythm. Without nested objects we could not distinguish between the 77 patients that either have a abnormal ECG or a valid sinus rhythm. With nested objects we can filter for the 22 SRs for which both conditions match.

4 Discussion

Annotations in DICOM and especially SRs are a spacious topic; to capture all information that might be potentially recorded they come with high complexity. But utilized appropriately they provide an useful tool for unifying diagnostic reports for physicians, model training, and results leading to interoperability of human and algorithm. Our solution for determining on which attributes to filter the annotations opts for high flexibility as it is applicable to all templates but also the constraint that is must be in conformance with the DICOM standard. We believe our method is a step towards the concurrent filtering and cohort selection of DICOM data and their annotations. SRs still have more inherent complexity than we have covered here. One possible obstacle is that operators do not adhere to the templates. Unwanted items might be uploaded in the process. In addition to obtaining homogenized training data we want to extend the presented concept in future work to also store the model output in a similar consistent manner.

Acknowledgements

This research was supported by grants from the Klaus Tschira Foundation within the Informatics for Life framework, by the DZHK (German Centre for Cardiovascular Research), and by the BMBF (German Ministry of Education and Research).

References

1. Noumeir R. Benefits of the DICOM structured report. J Digit Imaging. 2006;16(4):295–306.
2. Rieke N, Hancox J, Li W, Milletarì F, Roth HR, Albarqouni S et al. The future of digital health with federated learning. NPJ Digit Med. 2020;3(119):2398–6352.
3. Bridge C, Gorman C, Pieper S, Doyle S, Lennerz J, Kalpathy-Cramer J et al. Highdicom: a python library for standardized encoding of image annotations and machine learning model outputs in pathology and radiology. J Digit Imaging. 2022;35(6):1719–37.
4. Scherer J, Nolden M, Kleesiek J, Metzger J, Kades K, Schneider V et al. Joint imaging platform for federated clinical data analytics. JCO Clin Cancer Inform. 2020;4:1027–38.
5. Moor M, Banerjee O, Hossein Abad ZS, Krumholz HM, Leskovec J, Topol EJ et al. Foundation models for generalist medical artificial intelligence. Nature. 2023;616(7956):259–65.
6. Seidler T, Tölle M, André F, Bannas P, Frey N, Friedrich S et al. Federated learning of TAVI outcomes (FLOTO): A collaborative multi-center deep learning initiative. Clin Res Cardiol. 2022.
7. Nobel M, Geel K van, Robben S. Structured reporting in radiology: a systematic review to explore its potential. Eur Radiol. 2022;32:2837–54.
8. Clunie DA. DICOM structured reporting. Bangor: PixelMed, 2000.

Abstract: Comprehensive Multi-domain Dataset for Mitotic Figure Detection

Marc Aubreville[1], Frauke Wilm[2], Nikolas Stathonikos[3], Katharina Breininger[2], Taryn A. Donovan[4], Samir Jabari[2], Robert Klopfleisch[5], Mitko Veta[6], Jonathan Ganz[1], Jonas Ammeling[1], Paul J. van Diest[3], and Christof A. Bertram[7]

[1]Technische Hochschule Ingolstadt, Ingolstadt, Germany
[2]Friedrich-Alexander-Universität Erlangen-Nürnberg, Erlangen, Germany
[3]UMC Utrecht, Utrecht, The Netherlands
[4]Schwarzman Animal Medical Center, New York, USA
[5]Freie Universität Berlin, Berlin, Germany
[6]TU Eindhoven, Eindhoven, The Netherlands
[7]University of Veterinary Medicine, Vienna, Austria
marc.aubreville@thi.de

The density of mitotic figures is a well-established diagnostic marker for tumor malignancy across many tumor types and species. At the same time, the identification of mitotic figures in hematoxylin and eosin-stained tissue slices is known to have a high inter-rater variability, reducing its reproducibility. Hence, mitotic figure identification in tumor tissue is a task worth automating using deep learning models. Additionally, there is high variability in tissue across labs, tumor types, and scanning devices, which leads to a covariant domain shift responsible for reducing the performance of many models. To provide a data foundation for the investigation of robustness and training of robust mitotic figure recognition models alike, we introduced the MIDOG++ dataset [1]. The dataset builds on the training data sets of the MIDOG 2021 and 2022 MICCAI challenges and extends them by two additional tumor types. In total, the dataset features regions of interest with a size of $2mm^2$ from 503 histological specimens across seven different tumor types (breast carcinoma, lung carcinoma, lymphosarcoma, neuroendocrine tumor, cutaneous mast cell tumor, cutaneous melanoma, and (sub)cutaneous soft tissue sarcoma). The annotation database, created from a consensus of three pathologists, aided by a machine learning algorithm to reduce the risk of missing mitotic figures, contains in total 11,937 mitotic figures. In our paper, we have demonstrated that there is a considerable domain gap between individual domains, but also that a combination of multiple domains yields robust mitotic figure detectors across tumor types and scanners.

References

1. Aubreville M, Wilm F, Stathonikos N, Breininger K, Donovan TA, Jabari S et al. Comprehensive multi-domain dataset for mitotic figure detection. Sci Data. 2023;10(1:484).

Assessment of Scanner Domain Shifts in Deep Multiple Instance Learning

Jonathan Ganz[1], Chloé Puget[2], Jonas Ammeling[1], Eda Parlak[3], Matti Kiupel[4],
Christof A. Bertram[3], Katharina Breininger[5], Robert Klopfleisch[2], Marc Aubreville[1]

[1]Technische Hochschule Ingolstadt, Germany
[2]Institute of Veterinary Pathology, Freie Universität Berlin, Germany
[3]Institute of Pathology, University of Veterinary Medicine Vienna, Austria
[4]Department of Pathology and Diagnostic Investigation, Michigan State University
[5]Department of Artificial Intelligence in Biomedical Engineering,
Friedrich-Alexander-Universität Erlangen-Nürnberg, Germany
jonathan.ganz@thi.de

Abstract. Deep multiple instance learning is a popular method for classifying whole slide images, but it remains unclear how robust such models are against scanner-induced domain shifts. In this work, we studied this problem based on the classification of the mutational status of the c-Kit gene from whole slide images of canine mast cell tumors obtained with three different scanners. Furthermore, we investigated the possibility of utilizing image augmentation during feature extraction to overcome domain shifts. Our findings suggest that a notable domain shift exists between models trained on different scanners. Nevertheless, the use of image augmentations during feature extraction failed to address this domain shift and had no positive effect on in-domain performance.

1 Introduction

In recent years, the field of digital pathology has seen vast advances through the application of deep learning algorithms. For some tasks, these algorithms already offer performance comparable to or even exceeding humans [1]. However, the performance of most state-of-the-art methods deteriorates if they are deployed to a data distribution different from the one they were originally trained on. This drop in performance is usually referred to as a domain shift. Domain shifts are caused by covariate shifts between the training and inference data, which can, for example, be caused by a change of the visual representation between both domains. In digital pathology, one reason for visual alterations may be the differences in preparation procedures across different pathology labs [2]. Another source of domain shifts arises from the use of different hardware for digitizing histology slides into whole slide images (WSIs), as scanning the same slide with different scanners produces noticeably different visual representations of the slide [1] (Fig. 1). Consequently, counteracting domain shifts in digital pathology is an active field of research. Another challenge of digital pathology is the sheer size of WSIs, which is regularly in the order of over $100k \times 100k$ pixels. For processing, WSI are divided into patches that are processed individually. To draw conclusions about the entire slide, an aggregation function is needed to combine the information from all the patches. A technique frequently used for this purpose is multiple instance learning (MIL) [3]. In

MIL a WSI is referred to as a bag of instances, and the whole bag is given a label. It is assumed that within a bag, the bag label is present but not all instances are necessarily carrying the bag label. Modern MIL methods employed in the field of WSI classification work in two steps. Firstly, a feature encoder, commonly trained on ImageNet or in a self-supervised fashion on histopathology data, transfers individual slide patches into a latent space representation. Secondly, a MIL model is trained to aggregate these latent features and perform the desired classification task. This approach effectively decreases the computational overhead associated with computing latent space representations of patches [4]. Given the success of MIL in digital pathology, a question that has not been researched extensively is how much such models are affected by scanner-induced domain shifts. This question becomes even more important when considering that online image augmentation cannot be used within the training of the MIL model to increase the robustness of the model due to the use of pre-computed image features. In this work, we investigate the scanner-induced domain shift based on the classification of the mutational status (internal tandem duplication) of the c-Kit exon 11 (c-Kit) gene from slides of canine cutaneous mast cell tumor (CCMCT), one of the most prevalent tumors in dogs. The general feasibility of using deep MIL models to classify such mutations solely based on WSI has already been demonstrated by our group [5]. The presence of a mutation in the c-Kit gene is linked to unregulated cell growth and increased tumor aggressiveness, resulting in a poor prognosis [6]. Furthermore, we investigate whether relatively simple image augmentation techniques applied during feature extraction as described by [7] are suitable to increase the domain robustness of the used models. Our contributions are as follows:

1. We investigate the scanner-induced domain shift on deep multiple instance learning.
2. We show that standard image augmentation applied during feature extraction is insufficient for bridging scanner domain shifts in deep MIL.

2   Methods

In this work, we used the CLAM model introduced by Lu et al. for studying the scanner-induced domain shift. This model has been applied successfully to various problems in digital pathology [4]. Since the model is trained on sets of pre-computed image features,

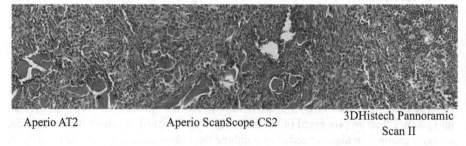

Aperio AT2   Aperio ScanScope CS2   3DHistech Pannoramic
                                                                    Scan II

Fig. 1. Scanning the same slide with different hardware results in considerable visual differences.

the training is performed in two steps. Before the CLAM model is trained, each WSI is split into a set of M patches. Each patch of one WSI is projected into latent space using the feature extractor of a ResNet50 model trained on ImageNet, resulting in $\mathbf{H} \in \mathbb{R}^{M \times C}$ features where $C = 1024$ is the feature dimension of the feature extractor. In the second step, the actual model training is performed on these latent feature vectors. The CLAM model itself consists of a projection layer, an attention module, and a classification layer. The projection layer is a fully connected network with weights $\mathbf{W}_{\mathrm{proj}} \in \mathbb{R}^{512 \times 1024}$ which is used to further compress the patch embeddings. The attention module consists of two linear layers with weights $\mathbf{U} \in \mathbb{R}^{256 \times 512}$ and $\mathbf{Z} \in \mathbb{R}^{1 \times 256}$ with a hyperbolic tangent activation function and a dropout layer in between. For each projected patch feature embedding $\mathbf{h}_m \in \mathbb{R}^{512}$ an attention weight a_m is computed, and the patch embeddings are combined into a slide embedding $\mathbf{b}_{\mathrm{bag}} \in \mathbb{R}^{512}$ by

$$\mathbf{b}_{\mathrm{bag}} = \sum_{m=1}^{M} a_m \mathbf{h}_m$$

The slide embeddings are then forwarded to a classification layer of size $\mathbf{C} \in \mathbb{R}^{K \times 512}$, with K being the number of classes. To encourage the model's learning of class-specific features and constrain the feature space of patch embeddings $\mathbf{h}_m$, a clustering subtask is included in the model. After the first fully connected layer $\mathbf{W}_{\mathrm{proj}}$, a classification layer $\mathbf{W}_{\mathrm{inst},k} \in \mathbb{R}^{2 \times 512}$ is utilized for each class k for clustering the patches into those with strong positive and negative evidence respectively. As no patch-level labels exist, attention scores $\mathbf{h}_m$ are used as pseudo-labels as described in [4]. To enhance variance during training, we applied standard image augmentations during feature extraction as described in [7]. We computed N different versions of each of the M patches, which resulted in $\hat{\mathbf{H}} \in \mathbb{R}^{N \times M \times C}$ features per whole slide image. During training, each time a slide was shown to the model, one of the N patch representations was randomly drawn to construct a feature representation $\tilde{\mathbf{H}} \in \mathbb{R}^{M \times C} \subseteq \hat{\mathbf{H}} \in \mathbb{R}^{N \times M \times C}$ of that slide. To investigate the impact of augmentations on model performance, we utilized two distinct augmentation pipelines with varying degrees of intensity. The light augmentations pipeline includes a color jitter where brightness, saturation, and contrast were randomly changed by a factor λ randomly selected between $1 - \beta \leq \lambda \leq 1 + \beta$ with $\beta = 0.25$. The hue was changed similarly but with $\beta = 0.1$. Color jitter was applied to all patches. Additionally, random blurring and both vertical and horizontal flipping were used with a probability of $p = 0.5$. The heavy augmentations pipeline also uses a color jitter but with $\beta = 0.4$ for all parameters. In addition, vertical and horizontal flipping, random blurring, and additive Gaussian noise are employed with a probability of $p = 0.5$. A 5-fold Monte Carlo cross-validation was performed for each combination of scanner and augmentation pipeline. The same five training, validation, and test splits were utilized for each experiment. 85% of the slides were used for training and validation, and 15% were used for testing.

3 Materials

The study employed three domains comprising identical sections that were each scanned with three different scanners. We used 369 sections of CCMCT collected from the diagnostic archive of the Veterinary Laboratory of the Michigan State University. The first and second domains were scanned at the Institute of Veterinary Pathology of the Free University Berlin using an Aperio ScanScope CS2 and an Aperio AT2, both with a spatial resolution of 0.25 microns per pixel (mpp). The third domain underwent digitization at the University of Veterinary Medicine Vienna with a 3DHistech Pannoramic Scan II slide scanner, which also had a spatial resolution of 0.25 mpp. The mutational status c-Kit gene was determined as part of a prognostic CCMCT panel and was available for all slides. The dataset comprised 173 slides (46.88%) with a negative c-Kit mutation status and 196 slides (53.12%) with a positive c-Kit mutation status.

4   Results

The results of our experiments are presented in Figure 2 (a). Without any augmentations (each first column of Figure 2 (a)), we observed satisfactory in-domain performance for all three scanners, with the models trained on different scanners performing equally well, achieving a mean F1-score of 0.78. In the out-of-domain case, we observed a slight decrease in performance for all combinations of source and target domains. The least decrease occurred in models trained on the AT2 scanner applied to the 3DHistech and those trained on the CS2 scanner applied to the AT2 scanner, with an average

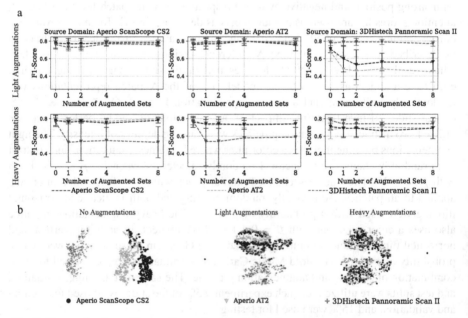

Fig. 2. The results depending on the source domain and the number of augmented sets available during training are shown in (a). A number of zero sets means that no augmentation was used. Each point corresponds to the mean result and standard deviation of a 5-fold Monte Carlo cross-validation. In (b), the UMAP projections of the features of a randomly selected slide to which the different augmentation strategies were applied are shown.

performance drop of 0.01, respectively. The largest drop in performance was observed when models were trained on the 3DHistech scanner. On the slides of the CS2 and AT2 scanners, those models obtained mean ± standard deviation F1-scores of 0.71 ± 0.04 and 0.68 ± 0.11, respectively, resembling a decrease in performance of 0.07 and 0.10. The training with the light augmentation pipeline did not improve the in-domain results when training with the CS2 slide. The out-of-domain performance for the models trained on the AT2 scanned slides improved by 0.03 to an average F1-score of 0.80 ± 0.06 using eight sets. The effect on the slides scanned with the 3DHistech was lower showing an improvement of 0.01 to an F1-score of 0.77 ± 0.03 using four sets. A similar effect was observed for the models that were trained on the slides scanned with the AT2 scanner. For four and eight augmented sets, the mean F1-score increased by 0.02 to 0.80 with a standard deviation of ±0.02 and ±0.04 respectively. The out-of-domain performance on the CS2 and 3DHistech slides increased by 0.04 and 0.03 to an F1-score of 0.80 ± 0.05 and 0.80 ± 0.03, respectively. For the models trained on the slides with the 3DHistech scanner, the results were less favourable. The in-domain performance slightly increased by 0.01, but the out-of-domain performances deteriorated considerably to an average F1-score of 0.56 ± 0.10 for the CS2-scanned slides and to an average F1-score of 0.48 ± 0.09 on the AT2-scanned slides. Similar to the light augmentation pipeline, the more severe augmentations of the heavy augmentation pipeline did not have a beneficial effect on the in-domain performance of the models. For the models trained on the AT2 and 3DHistech slides the in-domain performance even decreased. Furthermore, the stronger augmentation did not lead to better out-of-domain results between the models trained on the CS2 and AT2 slides. The out-of-domain performance of these models on the 3DHistech slides was even lower than with the weaker augmentation. In comparison, the less aggressive light augmentation pipeline delivered better results for the models trained with the CS2 and AT2 scanner data than the more aggressive heavy augmentation pipeline. Compared to the less aggressive augmentation pipeline, the heavy augmentation pipeline led to a less pronounced drop in the results for the models trained with the slides of the 3DHistech scanner. We also observed clear clustering in latent space without augmentation as exemplified by the UMAP plot in Figure 2 (b). The degree of mixing in the latent space is related to the aggressiveness of the augmentation strategy used. The features of the 3DHistech only mix with the features of the other scanners when the most aggressive augmentation is used.

5 Discussion

The results reveal a notable domain shift between models trained on the different domains. This shift appears to be more pronounced between models from different vendors. This is supported by manifold projections as shown in Figure 2 b, which show that the slide digitized with the AT2 and CS2 produced more clustered features compared to the slide digitized with the 3DHistech. Contrary to the results in [7], the in-domain performance did not improve consistently through the use of image augmentations during feature extraction in our experiments. This was regardless of the number of augmented sets per patch that were available during training, and the degree of augmentation that was applied to the patches. A reason for this might be that the ResNet used for feature extraction was trained using augmentations similar to those that we used during feature extraction, which might have made it robust to those permutations. This could explain why the performance has not improved despite the increased number of augmented versions per patch. The variance generated in image space by the augmentation could simply be greater than the variance remaining after the images are projected into the latent space. We did not find that applying augmentations during feature extraction was feasible for bridging the domain gap between models trained on different scanners. Although we observed slight improvements in the out-of-domain performance of AT2 and CS2 scanners, we did not notice such effect for the models trained on 3DHistech slides. This was regardless of the severity of the used augmentation. Additionally, it appears that the ability to generalize between varying scanner domains is not a symmetrical problem. The findings demonstrate that models trained on scanner A can perform well on scanner B, but the reverse is not always the case. This is evident by the out-of-domain results of the models that were trained on the 3DHistech scanner. Additionally, it appears that a proximity of features in latent space alone is not a sufficient criterion for model robustness against domain shift. The results have to be interpreted with care as they only demonstrate the effect of scanner domain shift on one dataset on a selected set of three scanners. Other domain shifts (e.g., staining, laboratory) may behave differently with specific augmentation strategies. Future research can investigate the impact of scanner domain shift on a wider range of classification tasks, incorporating data from additional scanners. Furthermore, this study utilized a basic augmentation approach. A potential next step would be to investigate more advanced augmentation techniques, including stain augmentations or implementing established domain generalization methods such as domain adversarial approaches into the MIL framework.

References

1. Aubreville M, Stathonikos N, Bertram CA, Klopfleisch R, Ter Hoeve N, Ciompi F et al. Mitosis domain generalization in histopathology images: the MIDOG challenge. Med Image Anal. 2023;84:102699.
2. Yagi Y. Color standardization and optimization in whole slide imaging. Diagnostic pathology. Vol. 6. Springer. 2011:1–12.
3. Ilse M, Tomczak J, Welling M. Attention-based deep multiple instance learning. ICML. PMLR. 2018:2127–36.
4. Lu MY, Williamson DF, Chen TY, Chen RJ, Barbieri M, Mahmood F. Data-efficient and weakly supervised computational pathology on whole-slide images. Nat Biomed Eng. 2021;5(6):555–70.
5. Puget C, Ganz J, Ostermaier J, Konrad T, Parlak E, Bertram CA et al. Deep Learning model predicts the c-Kit-11 mutational status of canine cutaneous mast cell tumors by HE stained histological slides. 2024.
6. Webster JD, Yuzbasiyan-Gurkan V, Kaneene JB, Miller R, Resau JH, Kiupel M. The role of c-KIT in tumorigenesis: evaluation in canine cutaneous mast cell tumors. Neoplasia. 2006;8(2):104–11.
7. Zaffar I, Jaume G, Rajpoot N, Mahmood F. Embedding space augmentation for weakly supervised learning in whole-slide images. ISBI. IEEE. 2023:1–4.

Few Shot Learning for the Classification of Confocal Laser Endomicroscopy Images of Head and Neck Tumors

Marc Aubreville[1], Zhaoya Pan[2], Matti Sievert[3], Jonas Ammeling[1], Jonathan Ganz[1], Nicolai Oetter[4], Florian Stelzle[4], Ann-Kathrin Frenken[5], Katharina Breininger[2], Miguel Goncalves[7]

[1]Technische Hochschule Ingolstadt, Ingolstadt, Germany
[2]Friedrich-Alexander-Universität Erlangen-Nürnberg, Erlangen, Germany
[3]Department of Otorhinolaryngology, University Hospital Erlangen, Friedrich-Alexander-Universität Erlangen-Nürnberg, Erlangen, Germany
[4]Department of Oral and Maxillofacial Surgery, University Hospital Erlangen, Friedrich-Alexander-Universität Erlangen-Nürnberg, Erlangen, Germany
[5]RWTH-Aachen University, Aachen, Germany
[7]Department of Otorhinolaryngology, Plastic and Aesthetic Operations, University Hospital Würzburg, Würzburg, Germany
marc.aubreville@thi.de

Abstract. The surgical removal of head and neck tumors requires safe margins, which are usually confirmed intraoperatively by means of frozen sections. This method is, in itself, an oversampling procedure, which has a relatively low sensitivity compared to the definitive tissue analysis on paraffin-embedded sections. Confocal laser endomicroscopy (CLE) is an in-vivo imaging technique that has shown its potential in the live optical biopsy of tissue. An automated analysis of this notoriously difficult to interpret modality would help surgeons. However, the images of CLE show a wide variability of patterns, caused both by individual factors but also, and most strongly, by the anatomical structures of the imaged tissue, making it a challenging pattern recognition task. In this work, we evaluate four popular few shot learning (FSL) methods towards their capability of generalizing to unseen anatomical domains in CLE images. We evaluate this on images of sinunasal tumors (SNT) from five patients and on images of the vocal folds (VF) from 11 patients using a cross-validation scheme. The best respective approach reached a median accuracy of 79.6% on the rather homogeneous VF dataset, but only of 61.6% for the highly diverse SNT dataset. Our results indicate that FSL on CLE images is viable, but strongly affected by the number of patients, as well as the diversity of anatomical patterns.

1 Introduction

Enhanced surgical techniques in the past decade have contributed to increased survival rates for head and neck cancer patients, with precision in tumor excision playing a pivotal role in surgical success [1]. To achieve the fine balance between avoiding too broad excision borders and achieving a complete resection of tumor tissue, frozen sections are taken frequently during surgical removal. The frozen sections provide, however, unsatisfactory levels of sensitivity [2], and extensive sampling carries the additional risk of injuring functionally important anatomical structures, as well as infections and bleeding. Confocal laser endomicroscopy (CLE) has been shown to be a non-invasive, in-vivo, in-situ real time medical imaging modality capable of providing ear-nose-throat (ENT) surgeons with discriminatory features for tumor delineation [3]. CLE enables the depiction of the superficial epithelium, usually to a predetermined depth of 60μm. Since the interpretation of these images can be complex [4], an automatic evaluation of malignancy from CLE images could be a helpful tool for the surgeon both in the intra-operative scenario. The classification of CLE images was shown to be feasible using neural networks [5], the task benefiting from a relatively consistent composition in terms of the malignant entity and the surface epithelium. The classification of CLE images of the sinunasal cavity, however, carries additional challenges. For one, since CLE is not yet an established methodology for the diagnosis of ENT tumors, the number of patients that can be included in pilot studies is limited. This directly leads to a common problem in medical image recognition: Scarcity of training data for machine learning models. This problem is exacerbated by the high diversity of anatomical structures, different pathological entities and concomitant inflammatory and tumoral alterations in the sinunasal cavity, which leads to a high data diversity in CLE images. Problems like these, with high data variability and a low number of cases can be solved using few shot learning (FSL) methods, as recent success in the field of CLE demonstrates [6]. FSL is a metric learning paradigm that seeks to find a latent space representation for measuring the similarity or dissimilarity of samples, enabling highly generalizable separation of classes. In this work, we show the principal viability of FSL methods on CLE data of head and neck tumors. We assess this on multiple anatomical locations, including tumors of the oral cavity and the vocal folds, as well as sinunasal tumors. It is the first attempt at FSL from CLE images in the head and neck region.

2   Materials

We used three datasets, each from a different domain of CLE images. Ground truth was established by the gold standard of histopathology. All datasets share that they

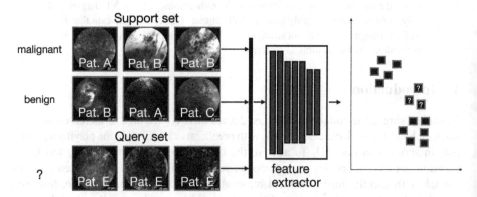

Fig. 1. We consider CLE malignancy classification a few shot learning task with episodic training. Patients are selected to belong to the support set or the hold out (query) set.

patient and anatomical location and a less pronounced clustering with histology (Fig. 2), highlighting the high data diversity of the task.

3 Methods

We compare multiple state-of-the-art FSL methods that are commonly used in similar scenarios. Training was always performed in 5-fold cross-validation schemes. All methods utilize a deep convolutional network as feature extractor and we used Adam as optimizer with a learning rate of 10^{-4}.

3.1 Preprocessing

CLE has a circular field of view, representing the physical cross-section of the fiber. Reflections and other effects occur at the peripheral region of this field of view and additionally, there is a strong gradient introduced by the field of view, which does not help model convergence. Therefore, we restricted the model's input to the inner rectangle of the circle. Additionally, we used standard augmentation (arbitrary rotation, flipping, blurring, sharpness adjustments) and resizing to 224×224 and normalization as training image transforms.

3.2 Few shot learning methods

FSL methods are commonly trained and evaluated using episodic training. Therein, a mini-batch that is fed to the model consists of a fixed number of support images with corresponding labels and query images that represent new samples to classify for the model and assess the potential to generalize based on these few samples from the query set. We used a five-shot setup, i.e. using five samples per class per mini-batch in the support set, and ten-fold evaluation, i.e. using ten samples per class (if available) for the query set. We used 500 episodes for training and 500 episodes for the evaluation of each method. Commonly, images used in FSL are assumed to be independent. However, since a high correlation of frames within patients must be expected, the split between images was carried out on the patient level, i.e. the patient of the test set was not part of the support set. Each of the selected FSL methods relies on having a feature extractor that was trained on a related task. For this, we used a ResNet18 feature extractor, pre-trained on ImageNet, which we trained on the OC dataset on the same FSL task, and used the VF and SNT dataset as hold out sets of a different domain. Hypothesizing stronger generalization if the feature extractor was trained on a more diverse dataset, we also trained the feature extractor on the combined OC/VF dataset and evaluated it on the SNT dataset. In addition to the full dataset evaluation, we also provide a dataset ablation using a random subset of five patients from the VF dataset to be able to compare the properties of both datasets using similar patient counts. We evaluated the use of four different approaches for FSL: prototypical networks [7], the SimpleShot method [8], relation networks [9], and matching networks [10]. Prototypical networks [7] determine a single representative (*prototype*) feature vector for each class in the support set and optimize the feature extractor to minimize intra-class L2 distance and maximize inter-class L2 distance. During inference, the L2 distance of the samples of the query set are determined and the class with smallest distance is chosen. The SimpleShot method is motivated by the nearest neighbor approach and very similar, but employs a cosine distance in latent space instead of an L2 distance [8]. Relation networks learn the latent space discrimination function by using a network that combines the current feature vector with the class prototypes to provide a relation score [9]. Matching networks go one step further by attempting to learn a mapping from the extracted features (of a possibly imperfectly matching feature extractor) to a new representation where the problems are better separable given the support set [10].

4 Results

As shown in Fig. 3, all FSL methods show similar performance on the task. We reached a median accuracy of 77.0%, 79.6%, 78.4%, and 78.5% for prototypical networks, SimpleShot, relation networks, and matching networks on the VF dataset, respectively. When evaluated on the 5-patient subset dataset ablation, we find a median accuracy of 72.5%, 76.1%, 70.2%, and 84.8%, respectively. Overall, while all methods perform well on the full VF dataset, we find a considerable increase in result variability if the number of patients is reduced. Furthermore, the application in the SNT domain yields reduced performance across all methods (median accuracy of 59.1%, 46.4%, 50.0% and 42.3%, respectively, when trained on OC dataset), with all of them benefiting from the

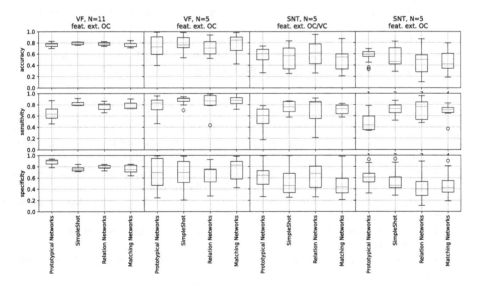

Fig. 3. Results of all methods on the four conditions: The full vocal folds (VF) dataset with 11 patients, an ablated random 5 patient subset thereof, and the sinunasal tumor (SNT) dataset. Training of the feature extractor was carried out on the oral cavity (OC) dataset, or, in one case on the joint OC+VF dataset.

extended OC/VF dataset used for training the feature extractor (60.4%, 56.9%, 61.6%, and 54.4%,respectively).

5 Discussion

Our work confirms the findings of Zhou et al. [6] that FSL is, in principle, a highly capable method for the CLE imaging modality. Furthermore, we successfully demonstrated that FSL methods possess the inherent capability to achieve robust generalization across diverse anatomical domains. The results also indicate, however, that even though FSL methods are specifically targeted at samples with sparse data coverage, they would in fact benefit strongly from larger data sets. We conclude that the considerable performance drop between the evaluation on the SNT dataset and the VF dataset is likely caused by a much higher data diversity, stemming from the increased anatomical diversity found within the sinonasal cavity, as also underlined by the visual clustering of patients in Fig. 2. Results from human raters in our group revealed an accuracy, sensitivity and specificity of 86.9%, 90,6%, and 84.6%, respectively, by human experts on a similar data set. This suggests a notable potential for further improvement with larger datasets.

References

1. Sharma RK et al. Conditional and overall disease-specific survival in patients with paranasal Sinus and nasal cavity cancer: improved outcomes in the endoscopic era. J Rhinol Allergy. 2022;36(1):57–64.
2. Layfield EM et al. Frozen section evaluation of margin status in primary squamous cell carcinomas of the head and neck: a correlation study of frozen section and final diagnoses. Head Neck Pathol. 2018;12(2):175–80.
3. Sievert M et al. Konfokale Laser-Endomikroskopie des Kopf-Hals-Plattenepithelkarzinoms: eine systematische Übersicht. Laryngo Rhino Otologie. 2021;100(11):875–81.
4. Liu J et al. Learning curve and interobserver agreement of confocal laser endomicroscopy for detecting precancerous or early-stage esophageal squamous cancer. PloS One. 2014;9(6):e99089.
5. Aubreville M et al. Transferability of deep learning algorithms for malignancy detection in confocal laser endomicroscopy images from different anatomical locations of the upper gastrointestinal tract. BIOSTEC. Springer. 2019:67–85.
6. Zhou J, Dong X, Liu Q. Boosting few-shot confocal endomicroscopy image recognition with feature-level MixSiam. Biomed Opt Express. 2023;14(3):1054–70.
7. Snell J, Swersky K, Zemel R. Prototypical networks for few-shot learning. Adv Neural Inf Process Syst. 2017;30.
8. Wang Y et al. Simpleshot: revisiting nearest-neighbor classification for few-shot learning. arXiv preprint arXiv:1911.04623. 2019.
9. Sung F et al. Learning to compare: relation network for few-shot learning. CVPR. 2018:1199–208.
10. Vinyals O, Blundell C, Lillicrap T, Wierstra D et al. Matching networks for one shot learning. Adv Neural Inf Process Syst. 2016;29.

Computational Ontology and Visualization Framework for the Visual Comparison of Brain Atrophy Profiles

Devesh Singh, Martin Dyrba

Deutsches Zentrum für Neurodegnerative Erkrankungen (DZNE), Rostock, Germany
martin.dyrba@dzne.de

Abstract. Alzheimer's disease (AD) accounts for more than two-thirds of all dementia cases. Existing MRI volumetry tools summarize pathology found within brain MRI scans. However, they often lack methods for aggregating information at different brain abstraction levels, and lack an intuitive visualizations. We propose a computational pipeline for quantifying hierarchical volumetric deviations and generating interactive summary visualizations. We collected N=3115 MRI scans from five different data cohorts. We used the FastSurferCNN tool to obtain brain region segmentations and estimate their raw volumes. First, we created a semantic model, encoding hierarchical anatomical relationships in the web ontology language (OWL) model and a computational framework for aggregating volumetric deviations. Second, we developed a visualization framework, providing interactive visual 'sunburst' summary plots. The summary plots can highlight mean-group or single-subject atrophy profiles, enhancing visual comparison of atrophy profiles with different AD phases. Our pipeline could assist clinicians in discovering brain pathologies or subgroups in an interpretable and reliable manner.

1 Introduction

The most common cause of dementia is Alzheimer's disease (AD), which accounts for more than two-thirds of all dementia cases. The progression of AD leads to regional volumetric changes in the brain, specifically there is gray matter volume reduction (atrophy) in the medial temporal lobe. The volumetric loss and cortical thinning are structural pathologies visible in T1-weighted MRI scans, which can be observed already in the early stages of AD.

Within the informatics domain, there have been studies representing the brain at the level of anatomical regions of interest (ROIs), and establishing relationships among these ROIs in a formal model, which is termed as 'ontology'. However, some of the ontologies derived by text mining from scientific documents lack an explicit mapping between the ROIs [1]. There are other ontological studies which explicitly represent relationships amongst ROIs, created under the Foundational Model of Anatomy (FMA) framework [2]. The FMA framework captures the spatial and taxonomical relationships amongst anatomical entities. However, the FMA lacks computational aspects which could allow to aggregate pathological information at different levels of abstraction.

There are several applications for MRI volumetry, which aim to assist clinicians in the evaluation of brain MRI scans [3]. These tools typically report percentile scores in a tabular manner or as radar plots. However, these tools only report few selected ROIs, defined a priori by the manufacturer targeted towards a specific disease. Notably, these

© Der/die Autor(en), exklusiv lizenziert an
Springer Fachmedien Wiesbaden GmbH, ein Teil von Springer Nature 2024
A. Maier et al. (Hrsg.), *Bildverarbeitung für die Medizin 2024*,
Informatik aktuell, https://doi.org/10.1007/978-3-658-44037-4_43

tools lack a generalizable framework for reporting and aggregating disease pathology information at different levels of brain abstractions. Hence, these tools lack intuitive and generalizable methods of visualizing these hierarchical findings.

The goal of our study was to create a comprehensible disease exploration pipeline. Extending the current tools, we propose a novel interpretation pipeline by combining computational ontological methods for aggregating pathological information, and visual summary reports to enhance disease comprehensibility across the whole brain at once. Our study also aimed to utilize resulting summary reports for highlighting both group characteristics of disease stages as well as single-subject atrophy profiles.

2   Materials and methods

In our study, T1-weighted volumetric MRI scans were obtained from five study sources: The Alzheimer's Disease Neuroimaging Initiative (ADNI), study phases ADNI2 and ADNI3; the Australian Imaging, Biomarker & Lifestyle Flagship Study of Ageing (AIBL); the DZNE Longitudinal Study on Cognitive Impairment and Dementia (DEL-CODE); and the European DTI Study on Dementia (EDSD). The data from all cohorts was pooled. Wherever scans from multiple time points were available, we considered only the first MRI scan. Our study included N=3115 MRI scans in total, with 1434 healthy control (HC) participants, 1132 people with mild cognitive impairment (MCI), and 549 patients with dementia due to Alzheimer's disease (AD).

We applied the convolutional neural network based, FastSurferCNN [4] brain segmentation pipeline as a preprocessing step: The MRI scans in native space were segmented into anatomical ROIs (Fig. 1a), and for each the volume measurements were estimated. FastSurferCNN follows the Desikan–Killiany–Tourville (DKT) atlas containing 100 different anatomical ROIs.

2.1   Semantic modeling

We built the computational ontology framework in Python using the *owlready2* package. In alignment with the FMA framework, we developed an OWL ontology capturing membership relationships among ROIs using the Protégé modeling software [5]. In our computational anatomy framework, the 100 anatomical ROIs, i.e. the output of the segmentation pipeline, are first initialized as base-level ROIs (here also termed as 'child-ROI') and then aggregated recursively (here termed as 'parent-ROI') with increasing abstraction level. In the ontology (Fig. 1b), child-ROIs are first aggregated within the respective lobe, then within the hemisphere, then within the forebrain or hindbrain concepts, and lastly representing the whole brain as root node.

Subsequently, for each subject, we quantify the volume deviation from the healthy control participants for each ROI. We utilized the w-score measure for this purpose [6], calculated by: $w = (Observed\ Vol - Expected\ Vol)\ /\ std\ dev(Control's\ residuals)$.

To get the expected volume of the ROIs, we trained linear regression (LR) models including covariates like age, sex, brain size (total intracranial volume) and MRI field strength. The LR models were trained in a computationally and memory efficient manner, where the parent-ROI's LR coefficients were derived by adding the constituent child-ROI's LR coefficients. The computational framework was implemented in Python using the *scikit-learn* package for training the LR models and the *owlready2* package's SPARQL engine to process the ontology queries.

2.2 Summary plots

We propose so-called 'sunburst charts' for summarizing volumetric deviation scores. The sunburst summary charts were realized with Plotly, a data visualization platform for Python. Here, the hierarchical anatomical membership concepts were visualized as concentric rings, with each ring representing a level of abstraction. Using a custom color scale, the gradual increment in color intensity marks the incremental pathological volumetric findings. The lower levels of deviations were represented by shades of yellow. The higher levels of volumetric deviations, marking a pathological finding with considerable deviations from normal levels, were represented either in green hues, marking enlargement or were represented either in red hues, marking atrophy. To allow quick and easy visual comparison, it was required that the summary charts were kept constant across multiple samples and group mean profiles. Thus, we chose to represent all ROIs in the outermost ring in a constant size, irrespective of their anatomical volume.

The implementation of our pipeline is available via GitHub[1].

3 Results

3.1 Semantic modeling

For encoding the a priori neuroanatomical structure, we developed an OWL ontology as illustrated in Figure 1. To encode parent-child relations amongst ROIs, we modeled child-ROIs as subclasses of parent-ROIs. From the FastSurferCNN segmentation tool, we got 100 ROIs which represent the child-ROI classes in the ontology. We defined 24 new parent classes, which represent the aggregated ROIs at higher abstraction levels. We directly store model parameters of the trained or inferred linear regression (LR) model coefficients in the ontology as data annotations of the associated ROI classes. The w-scores of each subject and every ROI level are also stored in the ontology, with LR coefficients being stored in the classes and w-scores being stored in the instances.

3.2 Summary plots

The sunburst summary plots enable the representation of pathology across all brain regions and aggregation levels at once. In the group mean summary plots illustrated in Figure 2, we see a sequential decrease of the w-scores of the temporal lobe in concordance with the severity of atrophy levels generally marked with AD progression, i.e. slight atrophy of medial temporal lobe in mild cognitive impairment and strong atrophy in dementia due to AD.

In Figure 3, we show a subject-level summary plot for ADNI3 participant ID 6650 - a 76-year-old male suffering from mild dementia due to AD, with 16 years of education and a mini-mental state examination (MMSE) score of 23. The atrophy patterns are primarily localized in the bilateral temporal lobes, highlighted in dark orange and red.

---

[1]https://github.com/martindyrba/CompOntoVisFramework

4 Discussion

We proposed a pipeline for quantifying and reporting brain atrophy findings from MRI scans. Both components of our pipeline, i.e. the computational ontology and visualization framework, were developed in a modular fashion and can easily be modified according to the use-case's needs. Within the semantic model, the ontology can be adapted to other segmentation tools and brain atlases. The hierarchy and levels of the ROI aggregation can also be adapted by updating the ontology OWL file. Similarly, it is possible to alter the visualizations of the summary plot tools.

To our knowledge, all the existing open-source neuroanatomical ontologies either lack a precise definition of parent-child ROI relationship when derived using text-mining methods, or lack a computational component for aggregating the volumetric pathology. The existing MRI volumetry reporting tools lack intuitive and generalizable methods for visualizing these hierarchical findings. The novelty of the proposed disease exploration pipeline lies in incorporating a computationally efficient mechanism for the quantification of volumetric deviations by explicitly encoding parent-child relations between the brain regions, and intuitive visualization of the same. We propose a computational

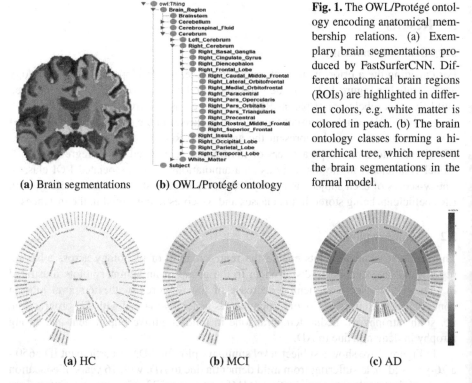

Fig. 1. The OWL/Protégé ontology encoding anatomical membership relations. (a) Exemplary brain segmentations produced by FastSurferCNN. Different anatomical brain regions (ROIs) are highlighted in different colors, e.g. white matter is colored in peach. (b) The brain ontology classes forming a hierarchical tree, which represent the brain segmentations in the formal model.

(a) Brain segmentations   (b) OWL/Protégé ontology

(a) HC   (b) MCI   (c) AD

Fig. 2. Summary plots, illustrating average w-scores across all the ROIs, highlighting group differences between AD stages: (a) HC - Healthy Controls, (b) MCI - Mild Cognitive Impairment, (c) AD - Dementia due to Alzheimer's disease. Refer to Figure 3 for larger text elements.

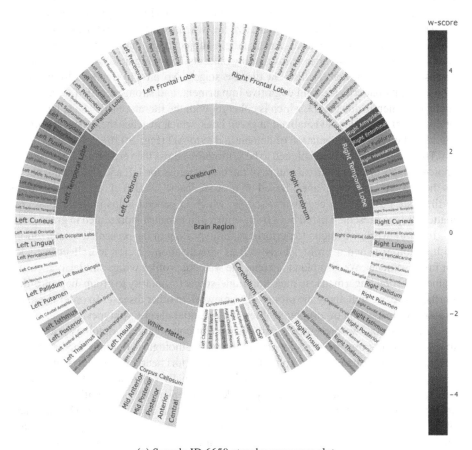

(a) Sample ID 6650 atrophy summary plot.

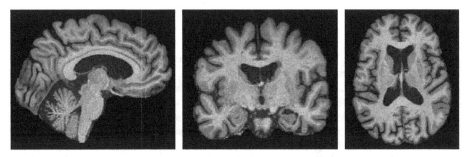

(b) Sample ID 6650 T1-weighted MRI scan.

Fig. 3. (a) Single-subject sunburst chart and (b) the corresponding MRI scan for the ADNI3 participant ID 6650 with mild dementia due to Alzheimer's disease. Refer to the GitHub repository for an interactive online version: https://github.com/martindyrba/CompOntoVisFramework.

framework for calculating deviations from normal volumetric levels with w-scores for each ROI. The computations were realized as efficient as possible by inferring the parent-ROI's regression model coefficients from the child-ROI's regression models.

The sunburst plots efficiently summarize the w-scores across the whole brain regions at once, both for group means as well as single-subject data, enabling fast visual exploration and inspection of large neuroimaging datasets. From Figure 2, we see the gradual disease progression across different disease stages: No atrophy for healthy controls, slight atrophy patterns for mild cognitive impairment, and stronger medial temporal atrophy in dementia due to AD, which is coherent with the literature [6]. The enlargement of the lateral ventricles is visualized in green hues, which matches the expected patterns found in the typical presentation of dementia due to AD (Fig. 2c) [6].

The summary plots were aligned to be symmetric across the vertical axis. This design choice reflects the symmetrical nature of the brain, across the left and right hemispheres on the coronal and axial planes. Based on user feedback, we also chose different colors to illustrate positive and negative w-scores, which in general helps in separating gray matter atrophy presented in red hues from ventricular expansion presented in green hues.

In future work, we intend to perform usability testing of the presented visualizations with radiologists and neurologists as well as visualization experts, to collect feedback for improvements. We also plan to extend the w-score profiles with a similarity measure framework, creating a metric to measure single-subject similarity to group mean profiles. Furthermore, we will apply the proposed framework to other diseases in order to enable explorative inspection of atrophy profiles and potential disease subtypes.

In conclusion, we presented a two-component computational ontology framework to systematically quantify and report volumetric pathological findings for brain MRI scans. Our semantic ontology explicitly encodes a priori neuroanatomical relationships amongst brain regions and implements computationally efficient calculation of volumetric deviation. Our summary plots provide a convenient way to intuitively visualize volumetric deviations at different hierarchical abstraction levels at once. The summary plots can be applied to visualize either single-subject or aggregated group-average characteristics. Overall, our pipeline enables an automated and efficient approach for reporting pathological brain atrophy findings.

References

1. Doms A, Jakonienė V, Lambrix P, et al. Ontologies and text mining as a basis for a semantic web for the life sciences. Reason Web. 2006:164–83.
2. Rosse C, Mejino JL. A reference ontology for biomedical informatics: the foundational model of anatomy. J Biomed Inform. 2003;36(6):478–500.
3. Pemberton HG, Zaki LA, Goodkin O, et al. Technical and clinical validation of commercial automated volumetric MRI tools for dementia diagnosis: a systematic review. Neuroradiol. 2021;63(11):1773–89.
4. Henschel L, Conjeti S, Estrada S, et al. Fastsurfer: a fast and accurate deep learning based neuroimaging pipeline. Neuroimage. 2020;219:117012.
5. Musen MA. The protégé project: a look back and a look forward. AI Matters. 2015;1(4):4–12.
6. Jack CR, Petersen RC, Xu YC, et al. Medial temporal atrophy on MRI in normal aging and very mild Alzheimer's disease. Neurol. 1997;49(3):786–94.

Abstract: Denoising of Home OCT Images using Noise-to-noise Trained on Artificial Eye Data

Marc Rowedder[1], Timo Kepp[2], Tobias Neumann[3], Helge Sudkamp[3], Gereon Hüttmann[4], Heinz Handels[1,2]

[1]Institute of Medical Informatics, University of Lübeck, Lübeck, Germany
[2]German Research Center for Artificial Intelligence, Lübeck, Germany
[3]Visotec GmbH, Lübeck, Germany
[4]Institute of Biomedical Optics, University of Lübeck, Lübeck, Germany
marc.rowedder@uni-luebeck.de

Optical coherence tomography (OCT) established as an essential part of the diagnosis, monitoring and treatment programs of patients suffering from wet age-related macular degeneration (AMD). To further improve disease progression monitoring and just-in-time therapy, home OCTs such as the innovative self-examination low-cost full-field OCT (SELFF-OCT) are developed, enabling self-examination by patients due to its technical simplicity and cost efficiency, but coming at the cost of reduced image quality indicated by a low signal-to-noise ratio (SNR). Although deep learning denoising methods based on convolutional neural networks (CNN) or generative adversarial networks (GAN) achieve state-of-the-art denoising performance in improving the SNR for better image interpretability, they usually require noise-free images for training, which are not available for OCT imaging or can only be approximated by repeated scanning followed by complex and error-prone registration and multi-frame averaging processes. To circumvent this drawback, we propose a denoising approach in this work based on utilizing paired SELFF-OCT images acquired from the retina of an artificial eye to train a Noise2Noise (N2N) network by repeatedly mapping one noisy image to another noisy realization of the same image. Training of the network is performed with a small amount of data comprising only two OCT volumes. The performance of the proposed approach is evaluated by denoising unseen SELFF-OCT images from the retina of the artificial eye as well as real human eyes, utilizing standard image quality assessment (IQA) metrics like peak signal-to-noise ratio (PSNR) and structure similarity index measure (SSIM) as well as non-reference quality metrics. The qualitative and quantitative results of the evaluation verify the effectiveness of the proposed N2N approach by an improved SNR, while important structural information in the scans is preserved. Furthermore, the results reveal a superior denoising performance of the proposed approach compared to the application of conventional OCT denoising methods like block-matching and 3D filtering (BM3D) and probability-based non-local means (PNLM) [1].

References

1. Rowedder M, Kepp T, Neumann T, Sudkamp H, Hüttmann G, Handels H. Denoising of home OCT images using Noise2Noise trained on artificial eye data. Proc SPIE. 2024. Accepted.

© Der/die Autor(en), exklusiv lizenziert an
Springer Fachmedien Wiesbaden GmbH, ein Teil von Springer Nature 2024
A. Maier et al. (Hrsg.), *Bildverarbeitung für die Medizin 2024*,
Informatik aktuell, https://doi.org/10.1007/978-3-658-44037-4_44

Abstract: Metal-conscious Embedding for CBCT Projection Inpainting

Fuxin Fan[1], Yangkong Wang[1], Ludwig Ritschl[2], Ramyar Biniazan[2], Marcel Beister[2], Björn Kreher[2], Yixing Huang[3], Steffen Kappler[2], Andreas Maier[1]

[1]Fakultät für Pattern Recognition, FAU Erlangen-Nürnberg
[2]Siemens Healthcare GmbH, Forchheim
[3]Department of Radiation Oncology, Universitätsklinikum Erlangen, FAU Erlangen-Nürnberg
fuxin.fan@fau.de

The existence of metallic implants in projection images for cone-beam computed tomography (CBCT) introduces undesired artifacts which degrade the quality of reconstructed images. In order to reduce metal artifacts, projection inpainting is an essential step in many metal artifact reduction algorithms. In this work, a hybrid network combining the shift window (Swin) vision transformer (ViT) and a convolutional neural network is proposed as a baseline network for the inpainting task. To incorporate metal information for the Swin ViT-based encoder, metal-conscious self-embedding and neighborhood-embedding methods are investigated [1]. Both methods have improved the performance of the baseline network. Furthermore, by choosing appropriate window size, the model with neighborhood-embedding could achieve the lowest mean absolute error of 0.079 in metal regions and the highest peak signal-to-noise ratio of 42.346 in CBCT projections. At the end, the efficiency of metal-conscious embedding on both simulated and real cadaver CBCT data has been demonstrated, where the inpainting capability of the baseline network has been enhanced.

References

1. Fan F, Wang Y, Ritschl L, Biniazan R, Beister M, Kreher B et al. Metal-conscious embedding for CBCT projection inpainting. IEEE ISBI. 2023:1–5.

Abstract: Self-supervised Pre-training for Dealing with Small Datasets in Deep Learning for Medical Imaging
Evaluation of Contrastive and Masked Autoencoder Methods

Daniel Wolf[1,2], Tristan Payer[1], Catharina S. Lisson[2], Christoph G. Lisson[2], Meinrad Beer[2], Michael Götz[2,3], Timo Ropinski[1,3]

[1]Visual Computing Research Group, Institute of Media Informatics, Ulm University, Germany
[2]Experimental Radiology Research Group, Department for Diagnostic and Interventional Radiology, Ulm University Medical Center, Germany
[3]These two authors contributed equally to this work
daniel.wolf@uni-ulm.de

Deep learning in medical imaging has the potential to minimize the risk of diagnostic errors, reduce radiologist workload, and accelerate diagnosis. Training such deep learning models requires large and accurate datasets, with annotations for all training samples. However, in the medical imaging domain, annotated datasets for specific tasks are often small due to the high complexity of annotations, limited access, or the rarity of diseases. To address this challenge, deep learning models can be pre-trained on large image datasets without annotations using methods from the field of self-supervised learning. After pre-training, small annotated datasets are sufficient to fine-tune the models for a specific task. The most popular self-supervised pre-training approaches in medical imaging are based on contrastive learning. However, recent studies in natural image processing indicate a strong potential for masked autoencoder approaches. Our work [1] compares state-of-the-art contrastive learning methods with the recently introduced masked autoencoder approach "SparK" for convolutional neural networks (CNNs) on medical images. Therefore, we pre-train on a large unannotated CT image dataset and fine-tune on several CT classification tasks. Due to the challenge of obtaining sufficient annotated training data in medical imaging, it is of particular interest to evaluate how the self-supervised pre-training methods perform when fine-tuning on small datasets. By experimenting with gradually reducing the training dataset size for fine-tuning, we find that the reduction has different effects depending on the type of pre-training chosen. The SparK pre-training method is more robust to the training dataset size than the contrastive methods. Based on our results, we propose the SparK pre-training for medical imaging tasks with only small annotated datasets.

References

1. Wolf D, Payer T, Lisson CS, Lisson CG, Beer M, Götz M et al. Self-supervised pre-training with contrastive and masked autoencoder methods for dealing with small datasets in deep learning for medical imaging. Nat Sci Rep. 2023;13(1):20260.

Abstract: Enhanced Diagnostic Fidelity in Pathology Whole Slide Image Compression via Deep Learning

Maximilian Fischer[1,2,3], Peter Neher[1,2,11], Peter Schüffler[6,7], Shuhan Xiao[1,4], Silvia Dias Almeida[1,3], Constantin Ulrich[1,2,12], Alexander Muckenhuber[6], Rickmer Braren[8], Michael Götz[1,5], Jens Kleesiek[9,10], Marco Nolden[1,11], Klaus Maier-Hein[1,3,4,11,12]

[1]German Cancer Research Center (DKFZ) Heidelberg, Division of Medical Image Computing
[2]German Cancer Consortium (DKTK)
[3]Medical Faculty, Heidelberg University
[4]Faculty of Mathematics and Computer Science, Heidelberg University
[5]Clinic of Diagnostics and Interventional Radiology, Section Experimental Radiology, Ulm University Medical Centre
[6]TUM School of Medicine and Health, Institute of Pathology, Technical University of Munich
[7]TUM School of Computation, Information and Technology, Technical University of Munich
[8]Department of Diagnostic and Interventional Radiology, Faculty of Medicine, Technical University of Munich
[9]Institute for AI in Medicine (IKIM), University Medicine Essen
[10]German Cancer Consortium (DKTK), partner site Essen
[11]Pattern Analysis and Learning Group, Department of Radiation Oncology, Heidelberg University Hospital
[12]National Center for Tumor Diseases (NCT)
maximilian.fischer@dkfz-heidelberg.de

Accurate diagnosis of disease often depends on the exhaustive examination of whole slide images (WSI) at microscopic resolution. Efficient handling of these data-intensive images requires lossy compression techniques. This paper investigates the limitations of the widely-used JPEG algorithm, the current clinical standard, and reveals severe image artifacts impacting diagnostic fidelity. To overcome these challenges, we introduce a novel deep-learning (DL)-based compression method tailored for pathology images. By enforcing feature similarity of deep features between the original and compressed images, our approach achieves superior Peak Signal-to-Noise Ratio (PSNR), Multi-Scale Structural Similarity Index (MS-SSIM), and Learned Perceptual Image Patch Similarity (LPIPS) scores compared to JPEG-XL, Webp, and other DL compression methods. Our method increases the PSNR value from 39 (JPEG80) to 41, indicating improved image fidelity and diagnostic accuracy. This work was published on the International Workshop on Machine Learning in Medical Imaging [1].

References

1. Fischer M, Neher P, Schüffler P, Xiao S, Ulrich C, Muckenhuber A et al. Enhanced diagnostic fidelity in pathology whole slide image compression via deep learning. Mach Learn Med Imaging. 2023.

Abstract: Self-supervised CT Dual Domain Denoising using Low-parameter Models

Fabian Wagner[1], Mareike Thies[1], Laura Pfaff[1], Oliver Aust[2], Sabrina Pechmann[3], Daniela Weidner[2], Noah Maul[1], Maximilian Rohleder[1], Mingxuan Gu[1], Jonas Utz[4], Felix Denzinger[1], Andreas Maier[1]

[1]Pattern Recognition Lab, FAU Erlangen-Nürnberg, Germany
[2]Department of Rheumatology and Immunology, FAU Erlangen-Nürnberg, Germany
[3]Fraunhofer Institute for Ceramic Technologies and Systems IKTS, Germany
[4]Department AIBE, FAU Erlangen-Nürnberg, Germany
fabian.wagner@fau.de

Computed tomography (CT) is routinely used for three-dimensional non-invasive imaging. Numerous data-driven image denoising algorithms were proposed to restore image quality in low-dose acquisitions. However, considerably less research investigates methods already intervening in the raw detector data due to limited access to suitable projection data or correct reconstruction algorithms. In this work, we present an end-to-end trainable CT reconstruction pipeline that contains denoising operators in both the projection and the image domain and that are optimized simultaneously without requiring ground-truth high-dose CT data [1]. In addition to experiments with shallow convolutional neural networks, we use trainable bilateral filter layers as known denoising operators [2]. These custom filter layers only require gradient-based optimization of four parameters, each with well-defined effect on the filtering operation. Our experiments reveal that including an additional projection denoising operator in the CT reconstruction pipeline improved the overall denoising performance by 82.4–94.1 %/12.5–41.7 % (PSNR/SSIM) on abdomen CT and 1.5–2.9 %/0.4–0.5 % (PSNR/SSIM) on X-ray Microscopy data relative to the low-dose baseline. We have publicly released our helical CT reconstruction framework, Helix2Fan [3], which includes a raw projection rebinning step to render helical projection data suitable for differentiable fan-beam reconstruction operators and end-to-end learning. Additionally, the trainable bilateral filter layers employed in this study have been contributed to the medical open network for artificial intelligence (MONAI).

References

1. Wagner F, Thies M, Pfaff L, Aust O, Pechmann S, Weidner D et al. On the benefit of dual-domain denoising in a self-supervised low-dose CT setting. Proc IEEE. 2023.
2. Wagner F, Thies M, Gu M, Huang Y, Pechmann S, Patwari M et al. Ultralow-parameter denoising: trainable bilateral filter layers in computed tomography. Med Phys. 2022;49(8).
3. Wagner F, Thies M, Gu M, Huang Y, Pechmann S, Patwari M et al. Helix2Fan: helical to fan-beam CT geometry rebinning and differentiable reconstruction of DICOM-CT-PD projections. https://github.com/faebstn96/helix2fan. 2023.

© Der/die Autor(en), exklusiv lizenziert an
Springer Fachmedien Wiesbaden GmbH, ein Teil von Springer Nature 2024
A. Maier et al. (Hrsg.), *Bildverarbeitung für die Medizin 2024*,
Informatik aktuell, https://doi.org/10.1007/978-3-658-44037-4_48

Comparative Analysis of Radiomic Features and Gene Expression Profiles in Histopathology Data using Graph Neural Networks

Luis C. Rivera Monroy[1,2], Leonhard Rist[1], Martin Eberhardt[2], Christian Ostalecki[2], Andreas Bauer[2], Julio Vera[2], Katharina Breininger[3], Andreas Maier[1]

[1]Pattern Recognition Lab, Friedrich-Alexander-Universität Erlangen-Nürnberg, Erlangen, Germany
[2]Department of Dermatology, Universitätsklinikum Erlangen, Erlangen, Germany
[3]Department Artificial Intelligence in Biomedical Engineering, FAU Erlangen-Nürnberg, Erlangen, Germany
luis.rivera@fau.de

Abstract. This study leverages graph neural networks to integrate MELC data with Radiomic-extracted features for melanoma classification, focusing on cell-wise analysis. It assesses the effectiveness of gene expression profiles and Radiomic features, revealing that Radiomic features, particularly when combined with UMAP for dimensionality reduction, significantly enhance classification performance. Notably, using Radiomics contributes to increased diagnostic accuracy and computational efficiency, as it allows for the extraction of critical data from fewer stains, thereby reducing operational costs. This methodology marks an advancement in computational dermatology for melanoma cell classification, setting the stage for future research and potential developments.

1 Introduction

In post-genomic research, a primary objective is elucidating the relationship between molecular networks and their corresponding cells or tissues. These networks, crucial for specific cellular functions, depend on proteins being precisely positioned, temporally synchronized, and in the correct concentration for effective interactions [1].

Understanding and constructing protein networks by measuring and describing local interactions is vital for deeper understanding of diseases. A significant advancement in this field has been the development of imaging technologies, such as fluoroscopy, which marked a breakthrough by enabling the affinity analysis of multiple proteins. However, the capacity of these technologies to represent the complexity of cellular networks is limited [2]. Addressing this, methods like multi-epitope-ligand cartography (MELC) have enhanced the depth of tissue characterization through iterative staining, enabling more comprehensive analysis [3, 4].

MELC represents an improvement over traditional imaging techniques by providing detailed tissue characterization at a cellular level. When combined with machine learning, MELC enables detailed cell-wise classification based on gene expression profiles, offering invaluable insights for medical research, including treatment effects and prognosis evolution [5, 6].

© Der/die Autor(en), exklusiv lizenziert an
Springer Fachmedien Wiesbaden GmbH, ein Teil von Springer Nature 2024
A. Maier et al. (Hrsg.), *Bildverarbeitung für die Medizin 2024*,
Informatik aktuell, https://doi.org/10.1007/978-3-658-44037-4_49

Recent advancements in oncology have leveraged Radiomics combined with machine learning for precision diagnostics. Studies by Liang et al., Pattarone et al., Gomez et al., and Mercaldo et al. highlight the significant role of Radiomics in cancer research, providing new diagnostic and predictive tools through machine-learning classifiers [7–10].

In melanoma, the most lethal skin cancer, prognosis traditionally depends on expert analysis of clinical history and histopathology images [11]. Albrecht et al. emphasize the importance of feature standardization in mathematical models for melanoma assessment, considering the subtype diversity and the need for detailed lesion characterization [12]. Graph-based methods are emerging, combining biological parameters with various domain features for a more generalized approach.

This study investigates semi-supervised cell classification in MELC pathology samples by focusing on two types of features: gene expression profiles derived from the multiplex digital image and Radiomics. These features are utilized in both traditional machine learning models and a graph neural network to evaluate their comparative performance. Following the methodology outlined by our previous work [5], this research also incorporates dimensionality reduction techniques to assess their impact on classification accuracy, mainly when applied in conjunction with Graph Neural Networks.

2 Materials and methods

2.1 Dataset

This investigation evaluated the proposed methodology using a dataset designed for cell-wise classification, comprising tissue samples from suspected melanoma cases. The dataset, included specimens from 27 cases, 20 of which were confirmed melanoma instances, with the remainder being healthy tissue samples [5]. Each specimen was processed following the MELC protocol, which involved incubation with affinity reagents, application of fluoroscope-coupled antibodies, capturing images through immunofluorescence microscopy, and gently bleaching the staining agents, allowing for the application of up to 100 different staining agents. In this study, the samples were exposed to 80-85 antigens, and their fluorescent responses were digitized.

The resulting images were digitally captured for analysis, each with a high resolution of 0.45 $\mu m/pixel$ and dimensions of 2018×2018 pixels. In cases where tumors were identified, expert segmentation was performed by a medical professional, thus maintaining consistency with the approach established in our previous work and facilitating a direct comparison and follow-up of the findings.

2.2 Graph structure

In our 2023 study, we demonstrated the effective use of graph-based models to encapsulate complex cellular data, specifically in melanoma [5]. This research utilized Cellpose [13] for cell segmentation, employing the MELC technique to analyze cellular structures. Two distinct graph representations were explored: the first, grounded in feature similarity and spatial proximity, adheres to the methodology established by Wolf et al.

[14]; the second utilizes cell spatial coordinates, aligning with the approach of Palla et al. [15], and adopts a neighborhood size as defined in our previous publication [5].

In these models, individual cells are conceptualized as nodes within a graph, with a typical sample containing approximately 2,080 cells. The relationships between these cells, or edges, are delineated based on the aforementioned criteria of similarity or proximity. For training, the graph is structured to comprise 40,500 nodes and 202,500 edges, providing a comprehensive framework for analyzing cellular interactions in melanoma.

2.3   Dimensionality reduction

Integrating Radiomic features into neighborhood graph-based approaches significantly enhances cell classification in histopathological analysis. These features include first-order intensity statistics, shape-based descriptors, and complex texture features. Notably, texture features from the gray level co-occurrence matrix (GLCM) and the gray level run length matrix (GLRLM) provide a detailed characterization of cellular attributes [16]. GLCM analyzes the spatial relationship of pixel intensities, while GLRLM focuses on the length of consecutive pixels having the same intensity in an image. When applied as node attributes in graphs, these features impart a nuanced understanding of each cell, addressing challenges like initialization sensitivity and suboptimal local minima in graph optimization [17].

Furthermore, advanced dimensionality reduction techniques such as uniform manifold approximation and projection (UMAP) and t-distributed stochastic neighbor edging (tSNE) enhance this process. These techniques effectively compress high-dimensional data, facilitating the creation of detailed yet computationally efficient neighborhood graphs [18, 19]. This combination of image analysis and graph-based modeling improves cell classification accuracy and provides deeper insights into biological structures in histopathological images [20]. The resulting graph models, enriched with Radiomic data, become potent tools for identifying patterns in cell populations, enhancing diagnostic precision and research in histopathology [18, 19].

2.4   Graph random neural network

In the domain of semi-supervised learning for graph-structured data, the graph random neural networks (GRAND) architecture, as introduced by Feng et al. (2020), has demonstrated notable efficacy, particularly in weakly supervised tasks, robust performance, and efficient training [21]. This architecture addresses critical limitations inherent in traditional graph neural networks (GNNs), such as over-smoothing, non-robustness, and inadequate generalization in scenarios with sparse labeled nodes. GRAND distinguishes itself by strategically decoupling feature propagation from transformation, a design choice that mitigates complexity and over-smoothing issues prevalent in conventional GNNs. Central to its success in graph-structured data analysis, GRAND's methodology integrates a random propagation strategy using DropNode to create perturbed feature matrices, enhancing robustness and employing consistency regularization to maintain uniform classification confidence across nodes and their neighborhoods.

2.5 Experimental design

In this study, we adhered to the methodology for performance evaluation as outlined by our previous work, employing a data split of 70% for training, 10% for validation, and 20% for testing [5]. This distribution was designed to ensure a balanced representation of healthy and melanoma tissues across each dataset segment. The optimization of hyperparameters was methodically conducted on the training set, utilizing a Bayesian search strategy.

We employed XGBoost and Random Forest for baseline comparisons, widely recognized as standard machine-learning algorithms for handling tabular data. The graph neural network (GNN) training followed the original authors' implementation guidelines and a similar approach to hyperparameter optimization [21]. Our analysis aims to compare the efficacy of two distinct types of features: gene expression profiles derived from multi-array imaging and Radiomic-generated features, which encompass first-order intensity statistics, shape-based descriptors, and complex texture features. This comparative study is designed to elucidate these feature sets' relative strengths and applications in the context of our machine learning models. An overview of the proposed pipeline can be seen in Figure 1.

3 Results

As outlined in Figure 2, a discernible trend indicates enhanced performance in node classification for melanoma cells when utilizing Radiomic features combined with UMAP for training. This observation is drawn from a comparative evaluation of two feature types in the GNN framework and their interactions with various dimensionality reduction techniques.

4 Discussion

The analysis of our results, as detailed in Figure 2, demonstrates that graph representations incorporating cell spatial locations outperform those based on gene expression

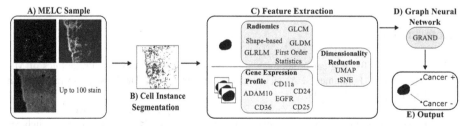

Fig. 1. Computational Pipeline for MELC Data-Based Cell Classification. A) Input: Multiple MELC sample images. B) Semi-supervised cell instance segmentation. C) Feature Extraction: Radiomic features and Gene expression profiling. D) Features encoded in a GRAND. E) Output: Classification of cells as cancer positive or negative.

Fig. 2. Comparative Analysis of Gene Expression Profiles and Radiomic Features in Training Graph Convolutional Neural Networks. This table summarizes the results of training graph convolutional neural networks using two distinct data sources: gene expression profiles derived from images and features extracted via Radiomics.

	Method	Feature Type	Dimensionality Reduction	Accuracy	F1-Score	AUROC
Tabular	XGBoost	Gene Expression	-	0.71	0.75	0.78
		Radiomics	-	0.74	0.77	0.79
	Random Forest	Gene Expression	-	0.74	0.70	0.66
		Radiomics	-	0.74	0.72	0.68
Graph Neural Network	Feature Neighborhood	Gene Expression	-	0.65	0.75	0.73
			UMAP	0.83	0.82	0.89
			tSNE	0.60	0.77	0.71
		Radiomics	-	0.70	0.76	0.75
			UMAP	0.84	0.84	**0.91**
			tSNE	0.63	0.79	0.73
	Spatial Neighborhood	Gene Expression	-	0.79	0.69	0.70
			UMAP	0.87	0.90	0.88
			tSNE	0.78	0.70	0.71
		Radiomics	-	0.82	0.71	0.73
			UMAP	**0.89**	**0.92**	0.90
			tSNE	0.77	0.68	0.68

profiles alone. This finding supports the importance of spatial context in cell classification. We observed that methods using tabular profiles and feature graphs show similar performance, attributed to their comparable information encoding strategies.

In dimensionality reduction, UMAP emerges as the superior technique, aligning with previous findings on its ability to capture spatial patterns and cellular neighborhoods effectively [5]. Conversely, tSNE focuses on maintaining feature correlations, offering value but less impacting classification performance.

A pivotal discovery in our study is the consistent effectiveness of Radiomic features over direct gene expression profiles from digital pathological samples. This trend is consistent across various methods and types of dimensionality reduction, and Radiomic features achieve enhanced results when combined with these techniques. Addressing limitations in staining agent selection, Radiomic-extracted features emerge as a viable solution, extracting relevant biological features for melanoma cell classification. This research marks an advancement in computational dermatology, suggesting new avenues for more precise and efficient melanoma cell classification techniques.

References

1. Schubert W. Topological proteomics, toponomics, MELK-technology. Proteomics of Microorganisms: Fundamental Aspects and Application. Berlin, Heidelberg: Springer Berlin Heidelberg, 2003:189–209.
2. Gao L, Lin F, Han D, Jiang J, Yang C, Zhuang Z et al. Quantitative fluorescence resonance energy transfer analysis on the direct interaction of activation-2b with histone H3/Switch-3B protein in arabidopsis mesophyll protoplasts. J Fluoresc. 2021:981–8.
3. Ruetze M, Gallinat S, Wenck H, Deppert W, Knott A. In situ localization of epidermal stem cells using a novel multi epitope ligand cartography approach. Integr Biol. 2010;2(5-6):241–9.

4. Bonnekoh B, Böckelmann R, Pommer A, Malykh Y, Philipsen L, Gollnick H. The CD11a binding site of Efalizumab in psoriatic skin tissue as analyzed by multi-epitope ligand cartography robot technology: introduction of a novel biological drug-binding biochip assay. Skin Pharmacol Physiol. 2006;20(2):96–111.
5. Rivera Monroy LC, Rist L, Eberhardt M, Ostalecki C, Baur A, Vera J et al. Employing graph representations for cell-level characterization of melanoma MELC samples. 2023 IEEE 20th International Symposium on Biomedical Imaging (ISBI). 2023:1–5.
6. Lazic D, Kromp F, Kirr M, Mivalt F, Rifatbegovic F, Halbritter F et al. Single-cell landscape of bone marrow metastases in human neuroblastoma unraveled by deep multiplex imaging. bioRxiv. 2020:2020–9.
7. Liang W, Wang B, Tao J, Peng M, Tu X, Qiu X et al. A machine learning–based multidimensional model integrating clinical, radiomics, and cell-free DNA methylation biomarkers for the classification of pulmonary nodules. J Clin Oncol. 2023;41(16_suppl):3070–0.
8. Pattarone G, Acion L, Simian M, Mertelsmann R, Follo M, Iarussi E. Learning deep features for dead and living breast cancer cell classification without staining. Sci Rep. 2021;11(1):10304.
9. Gómez OV, Herraiz JL, Udías JM, Haug A, Papp L, Cioni D et al. Analysis of cross-combinations of feature selection and machine-learning classification methods based on [18F] F-FDG PET/CT radiomic features for metabolic response prediction of metastatic breast cancer lesions. Cancers (Basel). 2022;14(12):2922.
10. Mercaldo F, Brunese MC, Merolla F, Rocca A, Zappia M, Santone A. Prostate gleason score detection by calibrated machine learning classification through radiomic features. Appl Sci. 2022;12(23):11900.
11. Chopra A, Sharma R, Rao UN. Pathology of melanoma. Surg Clin. 2020;100(1):43–59.
12. Albrecht M, Lucarelli P, Kulms D, Sauter T. Computational models of melanoma. Theor Biol Med Model. 2020;17(1):1–16.
13. Pachitariu M, Stringer C. Cellpose 2.0: how to train your own model. Nat Methods. 2022;19(12):1634–41.
14. Wolf FA, Angerer P, Theis FJ. SCANPY: large-scale single-cell gene expression data analysis. Genome Biol. 2018;19:1–5.
15. Palla G, Spitzer H, Klein M, Fischer D, Schaar AC, Kuemmerle LB et al. Squidpy: a scalable framework for spatial omics analysis. Nat Methods. 2022;19(2):171–8.
16. Griethuysen JJ van, Fedorov A, Parmar C, Hosny A, Aucoin N, Narayan V et al. Computational radiomics system to decode the radiographic phenotype. Cancer Res. 2017;77(21):e104–e107.
17. Ardizzoni S, Saccani I, Consolini L, Locatelli M. Local optimization of MAPF solutions on directed graphs. 2023.
18. Wang HY, Zhao Jp, Zheng CH. SUSCC: secondary construction of feature space based on UMAP for rapid and accurate clustering large-scale single cell RNA-seq data. Interdisip Sci. 2021;13:83–90.
19. Do VH, Canzar S. A generalization of t-SNE and UMAP to single-cell multimodal omics. Genome Biol. 2021;22(1):1–9.
20. Pati P, Jaume G, Fernandes LA, Foncubierta-Rodríguez A, Feroce F, Anniciello AM et al. Hact-net: A hierarchical cell-to-tissue graph neural network for histopathological image classification. Uncertainty for Safe Utilization of Machine Learning in Medical Imaging, and Graphs in Biomedical Image Analysis. Springer. 2020:208–19.
21. Feng W, Zhang J, Dong Y, Han Y, Luan H, Xu Q et al. Graph random neural networks for semi-supervised learning on graphs. Adv Neural Inf Process Syst. 2020;33:22092–103.

Magnetisation Reconstruction for Quantum Metrology

Kartikay Tehlan[1,2], Michele Bissolo[3], Riccardo Silvioli[3], Johannes Oberreuter[1,4],
Andreas Stier[3], Nassir Navab[1], Thomas Wendler[1,2]

[1]Chair for Computer Aided Medical Procedures and Augmented Reality, TUM School of
Computation, Information and Technology, Technical University of Munich, Garching, Germany
[2]Clinical Computational Medical Imaging Research, Department of Interventional and
Diagnostic Radiology and Neuroradiology, University Hospital Augsburg, Augsburg, Germany
[3]Walter Schottky Institute and TUM School of Natural Sciences, Technical University of
Munich, Garching, Germany
[4]Machine Learning Reply GmbH
k.tehlan@tum.de

Abstract. Widefield nitrogen-vacancy (NV) magnetometry presents a promising
method for the detection of cancer biomarkers, offering a new frontier in medical
diagnostics. The challenge lies in the inverse problem of accurately reconstructing
magnetisation sources from magnetic field measurements, a task complicated by
the noise sensitivity of the data, and the ill-posed nature of the inverse problem. To
address this, we employed a physics informed neural network (PINN) on 2D magnetic materials, combining the strengths of convolutional neural networks (CNN)
with underlying physical laws of magnetism. The physics informed loss during
the training of the neural network constrains the parameter space to physically
plausible reconstructions. The physics-constraining results in improved accuracy
and noise robustness. This paves the way for understanding the requirements for
the development of such models for quantum sensing in biomedicine.

1 Introduction

Recent advancements in biomedical sensing, particularly through the use of nitrogen-
vacancy (NV) center-based sensors in diamonds, have significantly expanded the diagnostic capabilities for various health conditions. These sensors stand out for their
exceptional sensitivity and precision, especially in detecting deep brain magnetic signals, such as the detection of paramagnetic molecules in the midbrain, which is crucial
for understanding and diagnosing neurological conditions like Parkinson's disease. NV
centers offer a non-invasive and precise alternative for probing intricate biological systems at the microscopic scale [1, 2]. For instance, magnetic fields generated by neuronal
activity or microscopic magnetic particles within cells can be detected and imaged using
widefield NV magnetometry [3]. This capability could revolutionize our approach to
understanding neural dynamics or tracking intracellular processes.

However, translating the raw magnetic field data obtained from NV centers into
clear, interpretable biomedical information poses a significant challenge. This process
inherently involves an ill-posed inverse problem, where the objective is to reconstruct
the source of magnetic fields (e.g., neural activity or intracellular dynamics) from the
sensor readings. For this we use a physics informed neural network (PINN) [4], and

scrutinise the physics informed network's efficacy through a range of metrics, including mean squared error and standard deviation, alongside robustness to noise.

We employed two-dimensional (2D) materials, specifically chromium sulphur bromide (CrSBr) [5], as a proxy for biological tissues in our experiments. The choice of 2D materials over actual biological tissues was driven by several pragmatic factors. Firstly, 2D materials like CrSBr exhibit well-characterized magnetic properties such as its Curie temperature, magnetisation domains and layer dependence with applications in development of storage devices and quantum sensors. Secondly, the use of 2D materials circumvents the challenges associated with sourcing and handling biological tissues. Synthetic datasets are used for validating our methodology in a controlled and reproducible manner. Ground truth magnetisation from the simulated CrSBr samples are used to generate magnetic field values at the position of the NV centers using analytical equations, exploiting the similarity of CrSBr samples to cuboidal geometries [6]. The generated magnetic field and position mask of the 2D samples are used as the input to the neural network, and the output magnetisation is compared with the ground truth.

1.1 Related work

Applications of NV centers in understanding biological processes are rapidly expanding, including NMR and thermometry, cellular pH measurement, and nanorheometry [7–9]. In the realm of imaging biomagnetism, NV centers have significant diagnostic applications for brain injuries and disorders like dementia and epilepsy [10], and are appealing due to development of wearable MEG devices that do not require shielding, and are suitable for children [1]. Another application lies in the imaging of cells labelled with magnetic particles. The high sensitivity and spatial resolution of widefield NV magnetometers make them well-suited for detecting magnetic fields in a variety of biological samples, including those relevant for cancer biomarker identification [11].

But once these biomagnetic signals are acquired, their analyses require reconstruction of the magnetic moments and surface currents that generated the magnetic fields. Analytical (Fourier transform), numerical (gradient descent, Gauss-Newton method), and finite element methods (FEM) (micromagnetics libraries such as Ubermag [12]) techniques used to address the inverse problem of magnetisation reconstruction are usually sensitive to noise, require complex priori information or solve iteratively and are very slow to converge [13–15].

Deep learning methods are effective tools for ill-posed inverse problems in 2D/3D image data analyses[16]. We can also incorporate the known physics (in this case, the laws of magnetism) into the training process, which makes the learning physics-guided, significantly improving the solution's accuracy, interpretability and generalizability. Physics informed neural networks map the physical laws to the neural network through an additional term in the loss function, which signifies the differential equation's residual when computed on the neural network's output. However, PINNs might require significant knowledge to implement effectively [4, 17].

The use of PINNs has been explored in fluid dynamics and geophysics, however, their application in the domain of magnetism, particularly for the inverse problem of magnetisation reconstruction, remains largely unexplored. Only very recently have similar approaches involving PINNs have been implemented [18], however, this untrained approach does not follow the training-validating-inference routine of deep learning, and is therefore not suitable for conventional predictions.

2 Materials and methods

2.1 Dataset

To overcome the constraints of limited physical samples of CrSBr, we generated synthetic data for the neural network, ensuring a training dataset with known magnetisation ground truths. The simulated CrSBr samples are placed 100nm away from the NV Centers, and the magnetic field strength is generated in the three Cartesian axes from the provided ground truth magnetisation of the sample. The dataset consisted of 2000 samples of CrSBr, which was split 80-10-10 in training, validation and testing datasets.

The magnetisation magnitude ($1e5$ A/m), orientation ($0 - 2\pi$ rad), and number of antiferromagnetic layers ($1 - 3$) are normalised to $[0, 1]$ range. The resolution of the dataset is chosen as 500×500 pixels, since the resolution scales linearly with the time taken to calculate the magnetic field with Ubermag.

Pre-processing also involves adding noise to the input data for robustness. Poisson noise to model the photo-luminescence noise and additive gaussian noise to model the other sources of noise are used. Poisson noise was added to the magnetic field H using the numpy library, $H_{Noisy} = H + n_p(H)$. The gaussian noise was added to the input signal through a normal distribution with the desired variance ϵ^2, $H_{Noisy} = H + \mathcal{N}(0, \epsilon^2)$.

The boundary conditions, namely the continuous normal component of the magnetic field at the boundary in the absence of surface currents, and zero magnetisation outside the magnetic sample, are satisfied through the magnetic field generation algorithm, and loss function respectively.

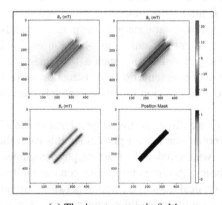

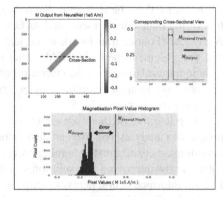

(a) The input magnetic field   (b) The output reconstructed magnetisation

Fig. 1. Example 4 channel input (Magnetic field vector and position mask), and output (3 channels of reconstructed M - magnitude, orientation, and number of layers). For the output, a cross-sectional view is shown (top right) as well as a distribution of pixel values showing the reconstructed values against the ground truth, and the resulting error. The x-axis and y-axis in the input/output images are pixel positions.

2.2 Method

Due to the advantages of the U-Net [19] style of CNNs, an encoder-decoder style of architecture was chosen [12]. Encodings were done by MaxPooling, and decoding through ConvTranspose. Skip connections for interpolation, and residual connections for modelling differential equations were added. Activation ELU with exponentially decaying learning rate ($\alpha = 0.99$, initial $lr = 1e$-3) was selected. The network was trained in approx 300 epochs with early stopping. Batch normalisation fixed the comparatively larger errors in reconstruction on the shorter edges of the rectangular samples. The physics informed loss was calculated for pseudorandom $n/4$ batches every 10th epoch - since this is a CPU intensive process. The batch size was also limited to 4 due to the CPU memory requirements.

2.3 Loss function

Even in presence of external magnetic fields, we are interested in the field generated by the given magnetisation. The relations between magnetisation M and magnetic field strength H are governed by Maxwell's and Landau-Lifshitz-Gilbert differential equations. The neural network predicted magnetisation (M_{NN}) can be used to calculate the magnetic field (H_{Calc}) through micromagnetic libraries such as Ubermag. The physics-informed loss function ($\mathcal{L}_{Phy}$) can be defined to capture the discrepancy between the magnetic field computed directly from the network's output (H_{Calc}), and the magnetic field obtained from the experimental/simulated data (H_{IN})

$$\mathcal{L}_{MSE} = \frac{1}{n}(M_{NN} - M_{GT})^2 , \mathcal{L}_1 = |M_{NN} - M_{GT}| , \mathcal{L}_{Phy} = \frac{1}{n}(H_{Calc} - H_{IN})^2$$

These losses were weighted to have similar error values for each loss.

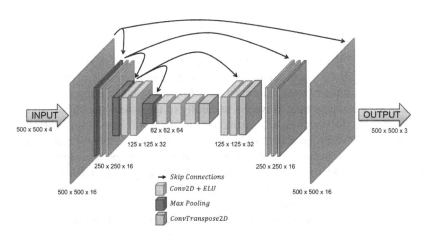

Fig. 2. The architecture of the neural network showing the skip connections.

Tab. 1. Comparison of reconstruction accuracy at Threshold MSE 10% for networks trained with and without physics informed loss (*Phy*) with addition of Gaussian noise with different variances.

Noise Level SD	Reconstruction w/ Phy	Accuracy w/o Phy
No added noise	0.6103	0.3247
0.5 (0.33% of Signal)	0.6097	0.2369
10 (6.66% of Signal)	0.5587	0.1596
20 (13.33% of Signal)	0.5583	0.1018

2.4 Evaluation

Mean square error (MSE) and its standard deviation (SD) over all the pixels in the reconstructed magnetisation across the samples in the dataset are used to evaluate the reconstruction and its dispersion quantitatively. Additionally, an accuracy metric with a threshold MSE is defined as the proportion of pixels in the image with reconstruction MSE less than the threshold value which is application specific. Here we have chosen a small arbitrary threshold of 10% to observe the effects of the physics informed loss.

3 Results

The MSE and SD for networks trained with and without physics informed loss on the test data were 0.0046(0.0067) and 0.0076(0.0098) respectively. The accuracy for these networks at threshold MSE of 10% were 0.6103 and 0.3247 respectively.

The physics informed model reached a higher accuracy of pixels with MSE less than 10% compared to the non physics informed model. The former is also robust to added Gaussian noise with a standard deviation 20.

4 Discussion

In this paper we have demonstrated an approach to integrate physics principles with the advantages of CNNs to address the ill-posed inverse problem of magnetisation reconstruction from measured magnetic fields. Approaches such as incorporating known operators [20] can help to improve the reliability of the underlying physics outside the PINNs' training distributions, and expand beyond magnetic fields from CrSBr samples.

While the PINNs robustness to added noise shows its potential for real-world quantum metrology applications, it still needs evaluation with larger and more diverse synthetic datasets. Validating the effectiveness of physics informed models with data from real magnetic samples, to comprehensively capture the magnetic phenomenon, along with real noise, measurement effects due to point spread functions, and heterogeneity of the datasets, would be highly beneficial in assessing the capabilities of these models, particularly accuracy and reliability, making them suitable for applications in the biomedical field.

References

1. Aslam N, Zhou H, Urbach EK, Turner MJ, Walsworth RL, Lukin MD et al. Quantum sensors for biomedical applications. Nature Reviews Physics. 2023;5(3):157–69.
2. Sulzer D, Cassidy C, Horga G, Kang UJ, Fahn S, Casella L et al. Neuromelanin detection by magnetic resonance imaging (MRI) and its promise as a biomarker for Parkinson's disease. NPJ Parkinsons Dis. 2018;4(1):11.
3. Hong S, Grinolds MS, Pham LM, Le Sage D, Luan L, Walsworth RL et al. Nanoscale magnetometry with NV centers in diamond. MRS Bulletin. 2013;38(2):155–61.
4. Raissi M, Perdikaris P, Karniadakis GE. Physics informed deep learning (part i): data-driven solutions of nonlinear partial differential equations. arXiv preprint arXiv:1711.10561. 2017.
5. Doherty MW, Manson NB, Delaney P, Jelezko F, Wrachtrup J, Hollenberg LC. The nitrogen-vacancy colour centre in diamond. Phys Rep. 2013;528(1). The nitrogen-vacancy colour centre in diamond:1–45.
6. Engel-Herbert R, Hesjedal T. Calculation of the magnetic stray field of a uniaxial magnetic domain. J Appl Phys. 2005;97(7).
7. Kuwahata A, Kitaizumi T, Saichi K, Sato T, Igarashi R, Ohshima T et al. Magnetometer with nitrogen-vacancy center in a bulk diamond for detecting magnetic nanoparticles in biomedical applications. Sci Rep. 2020;10(1):2483.
8. Wu Y, Weil T. Recent developments of nanodiamond quantum sensors for biological applications. Adv Sci. 2022;9(19):2200059.
9. Belser S, Hart J, Gu Q, Shanahan L, Knowles HS. Opportunities for diamond quantum metrology in biological systems. Appl Phys Lett. 2023;123(2).
10. Poghosyan V, Rampp S, Wang ZI. Magnetoencephalography (MEG) in epilepsy and neurosurgery. Front Hum Neurosci. 2022;16:873153.
11. Glenn DR, Lee K, Park H, Weissleder R, Yacoby A, Lukin MD et al. Single-cell magnetic imaging using a quantum diamond microscope. Nat Methods. 2015;12(8):736–8.
12. Beg M, Lang M, Fangohr H. Ubermag: towards more effective micromagnetic workflows. IEEE Trans Magn. 2022;58(2):1–5.
13. Meltzer AY, Levin E, Zeldov E. Direct reconstruction of two-dimensional currents in thin films from magnetic-field measurements. Phys Rev Appl. 2017;8:064030.
14. Broadway D, Lillie S, Scholten S, Rohner D, Dontschuk N, Maletinsky P et al. Improved current density and magnetization reconstruction through vector magnetic field measurements. Phys Rev Appl. 2020;14:024076.
15. Feldmann DM. Resolution of two-dimensional currents in superconductors from a two-dimensional magnetic field measurement by the method of regularization. Phys Rev B. 2004;69:144515.
16. Goodfellow I, Bengio Y, Courville A. Deep learning. MIT Press, 2016.
17. Karniadakis GE, Kevrekidis IG, Lu L, Perdikaris P, Wang S, Yang L. Physics-informed machine learning. Nat Rev Phys. 2021;3(6):422–40.
18. Dubois A, Broadway D, Stark A, Tschudin M, Healey A, Huber S et al. Untrained physically informed neural network for image reconstruction of magnetic field sources. Phys Rev Appl. 2022;18:064076.
19. Ronneberger O, Fischer P, Brox T. U-net: convolutional networks for biomedical image segmentation. Medical Image Computing and Computer-Assisted Intervention–MICCAI 2015: 18th International Conference, Munich, Germany, October 5-9, 2015, Proceedings, Part III 18. Springer. 2015:234–41.
20. Maier AK, Syben C, Stimpel B, Würfl T, Hoffmann M, Schebesch F et al. Learning with known operators reduces maximum error bounds. Nat Mach Intell. 2019;1(8):373–80.

Improving Segmentation Models for AR-guided Liver Surgery using Synthetic Images

Michael Schwimmbeck, Serouj Khajarian, Stefanie Remmele

Research Group Medical Technologies, University of Applied Sciences Landshut, Germany
s-mschw8@haw-landshut.de

Abstract. AR-guided open liver surgery is a field of intense research. However, due to the lack of RGB-D videos of the surgery scene, there are not any solutions for automatic real-time tracking and registration of the virtual models to the patient's anatomy, yet. We provide the first proof of concept for generating synthetic liver surgery images using surgery phantoms with a 3D print of a real liver. Thus, the RGB-D camera of an AR device captures realistic depth patterns. The RGB images of the phantom are enriched by realistic liver textures using image synthesis methods. We use these data to augment training data for RGB-D segmentation. Furthermore, we compare three common image synthesis methods that are based on generative adversarial networks (GANs) in demo setting for this purpose. We evaluate our synthetic data by measuring the performance of an RGB-D segmentation model for porcine liver images. Results show that we can outperform models trained only on real data by 3 % to 4 % when using a GauGAN approach. Furthermore, we observe biases due to overuse of synthetic data for augmentation factors higher than 50 %. Results propose a novel phantom-based concept for data synthesis in AR-guided surgery and serve as guidance for future technical improvements.

1 Introduction

Liver resections are particularly challenging when tumors or metastases are located close to hilar structures or major vessels. Due to the complex anatomy of the liver, it is difficult to correctly localize tumors during open surgery. However, vessel injury as well as an operative trauma should be avoided as far as possible. Furthermore, accurate tumor localization maximizes healthy liver residual volume [1].

To address these issues, computer-assisted surgical navigation systems are a subject of increasing research interest. In particular, the use of augmented reality (AR) has been suggested as a promising approach in open surgery to cope with the above-mentioned challenges. AR offers the possibility to project a model of anatomical structures and their interior structures onto the surgical area during interventions in-situ. Consequently, the map for the intervention and any additional guidance is displayed directly on the target organ [2]. The surgeon thus does not need to look back and forth between different views to mentally fuse the pre-operative CT-scan with the live-view of the intervention. Different types of hardware have been considered for this purpose e.g., smartphones, tablets or head-mounted displays (HMDs) like the Microsoft HoloLens or the Magic Leap [3]. Consequently, the accuracy of an intervention is determined by the hardware but also by the registration and tracking algorithms in use.

© Der/die Autor(en), exklusiv lizenziert an
Springer Fachmedien Wiesbaden GmbH, ein Teil von Springer Nature 2024
A. Maier et al. (Hrsg.), *Bildverarbeitung für die Medizin 2024*,
Informatik aktuell, https://doi.org/10.1007/978-3-658-44037-4_51

Ma et al. [3] compare numerous state-of-the-art registration and tracking techniques in the field of surgery of which a fair amount is marker-based. Deep Learning based tracking offers a markerless approach, but requires a high amount of data with accurate semantic segmentation masks for model training. In laparoscopic liver interventions, video capturing is an intrinsic part of the intervention and a few open datasets, like videos of the Cholec80 dataset [4], are available to the community, supporting rapid technical improvements in this field of research. Due to the limited number of patients included in these studies, data shortage is still an issue, motivating the use of generative adversarial networks (GANs) for the synthesis of additional images and thus the enhancement of the training data [5].

The automatic registration of virtual models to the real anatomy in AR apps requires depth information of the scene in addition to the RGB images. Tracking of organs in RGB-D streams, in return, needs training of models with RGB-D data of open surgeries. However, open surgeries are typically not recorded by video devices and certainly not by depth cameras and thus open data are just not available. Therefore, up to date, automatic liver tracking and registration methods for AR-guided liver surgery do not exist at all. The lack of data is an even more challenging topic than in minimal invasive laparoscopic procedures.

Recently, Pfeiffer et al. [5] have suggested to even further increase laparoscopic data by anatomic models from CT segmentations and rendering software to generate artificial laparoscopic videos. These are textured with image-to-image translation, again using the above-mentioned open data for synthesis. In theory, the depth stream could be synthesized from these data as well. However, depth information are highly error-prone. Artifacts i.e., signal loss and smoothing, appear at the transition of objects. The modeling of open surgery scenes and the sensor noise would need a relevant amount of real data as well, so that this approach is not applicable here.

2 Materials and methods

The main idea of this work is to solve these issues with a novel phantom-based synthesis approach. We increase the amount of training data for the RGB-D model by recording images of liver surgery phantoms that contain a 3D print of a real liver. Using the final AR device for recording thus delivers realistic depth streams of the surgery scene. We also use image-to-image translation in order to enrich the images with realistic liver textures. The plain and unique color of the print filament further facilitates labeling and image translation. For this, we further compare three different GAN-based approaches (CycleGAN [6], an MUNIT extension by Pfeiffer et al. [5] (referred to as MUNIT+ in the following), GauGAN [7]) in a demo setting for the translation of phantom images into realistically-looking liver images. The methods are compared investigating the performance of a liver segmentation model trained on these data. The concept of data generation for model training is depicted in Fig. 1.

2.1 Data recording, synthesis, depth stream mapping

Unpaired image-to-image translation converts a source image domain into a target image domain [6]. Therefore, we built two phantoms - one for each domain. The phantom simulating the source domain consists of a realistically-looking replication of a simple clinical setup for open liver surgery. It contains real surgery cloths, colorized bandages, 3D-printed abdominal spreaders and a 3D-printed liver phantom that has anatomic reference to a human liver based on the 3D-IRCAD data [8]. As we need semantic segmentation labels for each training image, the liver phantom was designed in unique red colorization to make labeling effort as low as possible. In the target domain phantom, a porcine liver that has a similar texture compared to human livers replaces the 3D-printed liver phantom. Sample images showing both phantoms are presented in column 1 and 5 in Figure 2.

All data were captured with Microsoft HoloLens 2 by using Photo/Video RGB camera stream and depth stream. For both synthesis and segmentation training, we recorded 250 frames for each phantom that were extended to 1,000 samples each using classical data augmentation methods (e.g., rotation and brightness variation).

We trained all three synthesis models for 100 epochs with a batch size of 1. For MUNIT+, we changed the weight of the MS-SSIM loss within the loss function to 10 (A -> B) and 6 (B -> A) in order to improve structural preservation during image translation. We trained CycleGAN and GauGAN with their original settings. CycleGAN and MUNIT+ are trained for direct image-to-image translation based on the above mentioned 1000 images from the source and target domain, each. GauGAN synthesis generates a liver segment from a binary labelmap. It is trained on 100 porcine liver images and additional liver labelmaps. This time, the porcine liver was placed on a homogeneous background to facilitate manual labeling. The final image is generated by replacing the phantom segment in the input image by the synthetic GauGAN output.

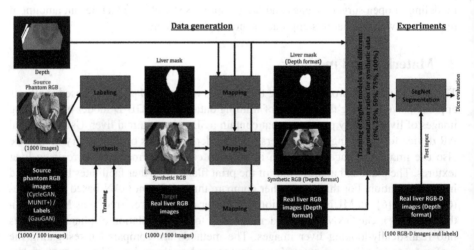

Fig. 1. HoloLens-recorded RGB images and depth stream frames are used to increase the amount of training data for an RGB-D segmentation model with realistically-looking liver surgery images. The use of a uni-color 3D print of a real liver results in realistic depth streams and facilitates the generation of labels. After image synthesis with different GAN-based models, the generated images are transformed to the format of the depth stream and are used to train an RGB-D SegNet segmentation model with different augmentation ratios.

2.2   Segmentation experiments

The above-mentioned work of Pfeiffer et al. [5] evaluates the benefit of the synthetic data by measuring the improvement of the segmentation performance (dice scores) for tracking in laparoscopy. We follow this approach and design a series of experiments to show the influence of the synthetic RGB-D training data relative to real RGB-D training data on the performance of a segmentation network. Therefore, we use 1,000 images each generated by one of the three synthesis methods.

After texture synthesis, the synthetic liver images are projected to the HoloLens RGB-D stream format using conversion functions provided by the HoloLens 2 sensor streaming application (HL2SS) [9]. Together with the corresponding depth frame and label they serve as training data for segmentation. Another 1000 real porcine liver RGB-D frames are recorded and labeled manually for segmentation quality comparison.

A SegNet architecture [10] with a binary Cross-Entropy loss function was employed for segmentation. We trained the model for 100 epochs in all cases with a batch size of 25 and split data in 80/20 percentage training/validation split manner. For further analysis, the model is trained using only real data to establish a reference. The experiments include augmenting the real dataset with the synthetic images with different ratios (25 % - 50 % - 75 % - 100 %). To test the trained models, we acquire an additional real dataset containing 100 images of a target domain phantom using a different porcine liver. The dataset includes images showing the liver from different perspectives, thus simulating a real application of the models. The semantic segmentation masks predicted for the test images were then compared to ground-truth segmentation masks. We calculate the achieved gain in terms of an averaged dice score for each model on the test dataset and compare the results to the reference model.

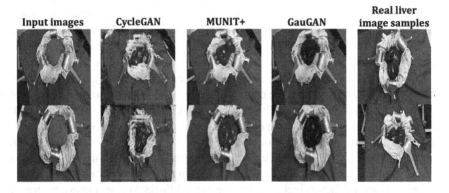

Fig. 2. Column 1 shows image translation input images and column 2-4 the translation output of CycleGAN, MUNIT+ and GauGAN. For comparison, column 5 pictures some sample images of another real porcine liver.

Tab. 1. Comparison of averaged dice scores for all trained models. In addition, experiment 1 serves as reference due to being trained only on real data.

ID	Ratio: Real data	Ratio: Synthetic data	CycleGAN	MUNIT+	GauGAN
1	100 %	0 %	0.85 ± 0.04	0.85 ± 0.04	0.85 ± 0.04
2	0 %	100 %	0.51 ± 0.23	0.70 ± 0.15	0.75 ± 0.12
3	100 %	25 %	0.71 ± 0.07	0.78 ± 0.10	0.88 ± 0.05
4	100 %	50 %	0.57 ± 0.09	0.85 ± 0.06	0.89 ± 0.04
5	100 %	75 %	0.65 ± 0.14	0.69 ± 0.09	0.77 ± 0.08
6	100 %	100 %	0.78 ± 0.11	0.76 ± 0.11	0.77 ± 0.10

3 Results

We present the averaged dice scores for all experiments in Table 1. In contrast to the other two methods, GauGAN synthesis increases segmentation performance by 3 % to 4 % for 25 % and 50 % augmentation factors, respectively. Higher augmentation ratios decrease segmentation performance in our experiments. Synthetic data generated using CycleGAN and MUNIT+ cannot outperform reference scores.

Exemplary image translations using CycleGAN, MUNIT+ and GauGAN are depicted in Figure 2. The synthetic images differ in colorization. Furthermore, several structural artifacts occur in CycleGAN translations while colorization artifacts affect MUNIT+ translations. GauGAN translations demonstrate a high label fidelity.

4 Discussion

The results demonstrate that we are able to improve semantic liver segmentation by 3 % to 4 % with the synthetic images of GauGAN and provide a new concept for mitigating data shortage in AR-guided liver surgery. Other approaches, like [5] using laparoscopy images, achieve performance improvements up to 14 % when augmenting with synthetic data. However, for this preliminary proof of concept we use 10 times less synthetic data.

GauGAN has a very accurate label fidelity, since only the already labeled liver structure was synthesized instead of the complete image. This is due to the basic functionality of GauGAN that is trained on labelmaps. However, this comes with a higher preparation effort for labeling compared to the other two approaches. CycleGAN synthesis imitates the (target) porcine liver outlines and thus distorts the structure of the liver. Images generated using the MUNIT+ model preserve the original phantom structures (input image) better compared to the images generated using the CycleGAN model. This can be attributed to several factors including the use of the MS-SSIM loss supporting structural preservation in the MUNIT+ model [5]. We suspect occurring structural distortions to mitigate scores.

Regarding colorization, livers synthesized by GauGAN appear to be darker than real livers. This is due to GauGAN training data being acquired in a setting where the liver is situated outside the phantom. This makes livers easier to label but goes along with different recording settings. MUNIT+ synthesizes a main liver color being closer to reference but meets colorization artifacts at edges of structures. While the colorization appears more realistic, CycleGAN output images contain noise artifacts that appear due to inappropriate data regarding the amount and diversity for this approach.

It is important to note that the main focus of this work was to prove the benefit of the concept of phantom-based RGB-D synthesis rather than an end-to-end optimization of the entire workchain. The demo setting using porcine livers and a limited number of samples allowed for a preliminary decision on appropriate synthesis models for further development with reasonable effort for training data generation and labeling. In Artificial Intelligence (AI)-supported and AR-guided liver surgeries, the amount of real images will always be limited in comparison to synthetic data. Furthermore, considering evaluation, biases due to overuse of synthetic data in augmentation need to be avoided, especially in applications with high data shortage, as in our case.

Future work will determine how to adapt the synthesized images to real surgery scenes. This involves examining the necessary amount of real data and methods of augmentation as well as the number of training epochs to further reduce translation artifacts at image synthesis. Specifically, reducing artifacts generated by MUNIT+ could further increase the segmentation performance. Additionally, few-shot GANs might contribute to our problem as they work primarily on foreign domain data and use only a very limited number of images from the target domain for synthesis [11].

References

1. Orcutt ST, Anaya DA. Liver resection and surgical strategies for management of primary liver cancer. Cancer Control. 2018;25(1):1073274817744621.
2. Kumar RP, Pelanis E, Bugge R, Brun H, Palomar R, Aghayan DL et al. Use of mixed reality for surgery planning: assessment and development workflow. J Biomed Inform. 2020;112:100077.
3. Ma L, Huang T, Wang J, Liao H. Visualization, registration and tracking techniques for augmented reality guided surgery: a review. Phys Med Biol. 2022.
4. Twinanda AP, Shehata S, Mutter D, Marescaux J, De Mathelin M, Padoy N. Endonet: a deep architecture for recognition tasks on laparoscopic videos. IEEE Trans Med Imaging. 2016;36(1):86–97.
5. Pfeiffer M, Funke I, Robu MR, Bodenstedt S, Strenger L, Engelhardt S et al. Generating large labeled data sets for laparoscopic image processing tasks using unpaired image-to-image translation. Med Image Comput Comput Assist Interv. Springer. 2019:119–27.
6. Zhu JY, Park T, Isola P, Efros AA. Unpaired image-to-image translation using cycle-consistent adversarial networks. Proc IEEE Int Conf Comput Vis. 2017:2223–32.
7. Park T, Liu MY, Wang TC, Zhu JY. Semantic image synthesis with spatially-adaptive normalization. Proc IEEE Comput Soc Conf Comput Vis Pattern Recognit. 2019:2337–46.
8. Soler L, Hostettler A, Agnus V, Charnoz A, Fasquel J, Moreau J et al. 3D image reconstruction for comparison of algorithm database: a patient specific anatomical and medical image database. IRCAD, Strasbourg, France, Tech. Rep. 2010;1(1).
9. Dibene JC, Dunn E. HoloLens 2 sensor streaming. arXiv preprint arXiv: 2211.02648. 2022.
10. Badrinarayanan V, Kendall A, Cipolla R. Segnet: a deep convolutional encoder-decoder architecture for image segmentation. IEEE Trans Pattern Anal Mach Intell. 2017;39(12):2481–95.
11. Liu MY, Huang X, Mallya A, Karras T, Aila T, Lehtinen J et al. Few-shot unsupervised image-to-image translation. Proc IEEE Int Conf Comput Vis. 2019:10551–60.

Application of Active Learning-based on Uncertainty Quantification to Breast Segmentation in MRI

Kai Geißler[1], Markus Wenzel[1,2], Susanne Diekmann[1], Heinrich von Busch[3], Robert Grimm[3], Hans Meine[1]

[1]Fraunhofer Institute for Digital Medicine MEVIS, Bremen, Germany
[2]Constructor University Bremen, Bremen, Germany
[3]Siemens Healthineers AG, Erlangen, Germany
kai.geissler@mevis.fraunhofer.de

Abstract. In medical image segmentation with deep learning, large amounts of annotated data are needed to train precise models. Such annotations are time-consuming and costly to create, since medical experts need to ensure their quality. Active learning techniques may reduce the expert effort. In this work, we compare different sample selection strategies for training a model for breast segmentation in MR images using 3D U-Nets: We evaluate two uncertainty-based approaches that compute the voxel-wise entropy or epistemic uncertainty based on a Bayesian neural network approximated via Monte Carlo dropout and compare them against a random selection as baseline. We find that both uncertainty-based approaches improve over the baseline in the earlier iterations, but lead to a similar performance in the long run. In early iterations they are 2-4 active learning iterations ahead of the "random selection" strategy, which corresponds to one or several days of saved annotation time. We also assess how well the different uncertainty measures correlate with the segmentation quality and find that epistemic uncertainty is a better surrogate measure than the commonly used plain entropy.

1 Introduction

Active learning (AL) is a machine learning paradigm that aims to improve the perfor-mance and reduce the annotation effort for machine learning algorithms by selectively querying the most informative samples for annotation. One potential application of AL is in the field of medical imaging, where manual annotations of large datasets are costly and time-consuming to create because medical experts are required to properly capture anatomical structures. For instance, segmenting the breast region in magnetic resonance imaging (MRI) is one such challenging task due to the variability in breast appearance and ambiguous anatomy in some regions. Breast masks can be leveraged to provide re-gions of interest for tumor segmentation [1] or to compute the amount of fibroglandular tissue as well as background parenchymal enhancement in the breast [2].

Some approaches for sample selection in AL are based on the uncertainty estimated for each sample [3, 4] while others try to find samples which are representative for the dataset. There are also approaches which combine both ideas.

Different ways have been proposed to estimate the uncertainty of deep neural net-works, like using the raw model outputs, model ensembles [5], test time augmentation

© Der/die Autor(en), exklusiv lizenziert an
Springer Fachmedien Wiesbaden GmbH, ein Teil von Springer Nature 2024
A. Maier et al. (Hrsg.), *Bildverarbeitung für die Medizin 2024*,
Informatik aktuell, https://doi.org/10.1007/978-3-658-44037-4_52

[6] or Monte Carlo dropout [7]. Monte Carlo dropout sampling can be seen as an approximation of Bayesian neural networks (BNN), computing a posterior distribution over the model outputs. During training, the model is trained using dropout layers without any further modifications. During inference, different dropout masks are used to sample the models' posterior distribution.

Based on these samples there are different ways to compute the voxel-wise uncertainty of the image, such as entropy, variance or variation ratio over the samples [3]. For segmentation tasks there are also structure level measures like the volume variation coefficient and the mean pairwise Dice score between the predictions [8].

[9] introduced an uncertainty decomposition into aleatoric and epistemic uncertainty. Aleatoric uncertainty captures uncertainty inherent to the data, like measurement or labeling errors, and can only be reduced by higher quality data, while epistemic uncertainty captures the uncertainty in the model parameters which can be reduced by more data. The latter is the quantity of interest for AL, where the goal is to reduce the uncertainty of the model as quickly as possible and with as little data as possible, to obtain a well performing model.

Our goal with this study is to validate the applicability of Monte Carlo dropout for AL to the imaging domain of breast MRI and to test if we can improve over measuring uncertainty with the commonly used entropy by using its decomposition into aleatoric and epistemic uncertainty.

2 Materials and methods

2.1 Data

The data used is a fully anonymized, proprietary collection of pre-contrast axial 3D T1-weighted breast MR images, retrospectively collected from four different institutions. Six different acquisition protocols including fat-suppressed (FS) as well as non fat-suppressed imaging are used in total, covering five scanner models at 1.5 T and 3 T from Siemens Healthcare and GE. Voxel sizes range from 0.43-1.02 mm in-plane and from 1.2-2.5 mm in slice direction. In total, 185 image volumes with corresponding breast masks are used with approximately 30 images per protocol type. Breast masks were created by a radiologist, a radiological technologist and a scientific assistant after an introduction by the radiologist. We randomly select 40% of cases for testing and use the remaining data for training and validation as described in the following section.

2.2 Active learning experiment setup

The model architecture is based on the 3D U-Net. It uses 5 levels and has one dropout layer before two convolutional layers at each level in the up- and downpath except for the highest level. A dropout rate of 0.2 is used for all dropout layers. In preliminary experiments, we found our results to be insensitive to moderate changes in these settings. The models use padded convolutions, 6 base filters and instance normalization.

We use the sum of categorical cross entropy and Dice loss as loss function and use an Adam optimizer. We apply a cosine annealing learning rate scheduler starting with a learning rate of 10^{-3}, train for 20000 steps and use a batch size of 2. For data augmentation, the batch generators library is used.

As usual in organ segmentation targeting large structures, we downsample the images and use a resolution of $240 \times 240 \times 112$ voxels. Image values are normalized by linearly mapping their 2% and 98% percentiles to 0 and 1, respectively.

For the AL experiment, five cases are selected from the training data pool in each iteration. Four of these are added to the training data and one is added to the validation data, because one also wants to increase the validation data as the number of annotated cases increases. The different model families start off with the same five cases and the same trained model in the first iteration to eliminate random differences caused by different starting conditions. For the uncertainty-based models the cases are selected to be the five cases with the highest respective uncertainty score in this model iteration. For the BNN approximation, we draw 20 dropout samples per inference. Due to long training times (about a day per model), we carry out each AL experiment only once.

When sampling a set of predictions, there are several ways to combine these into voxel-wise uncertainties, such as entropy, variation ratio, variance over the samples and margin between the highest and second highest class probability, as well as the decomposition into aleatoric and epistemic uncertainty. In addition one can choose different ways to aggregate the voxel-wise uncertainties into one for the image volume, e.g. averaging all the uncertainties in the volume or averaging them only within a mask of the foreground object, like it is done in [4].

3 Results

3.1 Selecting an uncertainty measure for active learning

Since AL experiments are costly to run for segmentation tasks, we need to select a subset of the uncertainty measures and aggregations methods beforehand to reduce the number of possible combinations to evaluate. To do so, we train one 3D U-Net on all available data in the training pool, compute Dice scores on the testing set and assess the relation between the Dice scores and uncertainty measures visually and quantitatively.

As a concise summary of this analysis, we present Spearman's rank correlation coefficient in Table 1. In the unmasked case, we do not find any strong correlation. Averaging only within a dilated segmentation mask, we find good correlation for the epistemic uncertainty, variation ratio, variance and the margin.

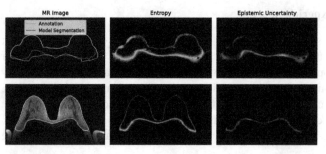

Fig. 1. Two example images with corresponding uncertainty maps. Most uncertainty can be observed at the segmentation contour, especially at the border between breast and pectoralis muscle as well as the axilla region.

Tab. 1. Spearman's correlation coefficient between Dice score and uncertainty measure for models trained on full training data pool. Uncertainty measures are either averaged over the full image or restricted to the dilated segmentation mask. Cases with a strong correlation (magnitude ≥ 0.6) are marked in bold.

Masked	Entropy	Epistemic	Aleatoric	Margin	Variation Ratio	Variance
No	0.30	-0.17	0.36	0.29	0.04	-0.20
Yes	-0.52	**-0.66**	-0.34	**-0.61**	**-0.74**	**-0.68**

Hence, we use the masked uncertainty measures for the following AL experiment, because they show stronger correlations. From these, we select entropy because it is commonly used in related work, and epistemic uncertainty because of its strong theoretical justification. Example results for these measures are presented in Figure 1.

3.2 Active learning experiment

We assess segmentation quality over the course of our AL iterations using the Dice score and average symmetric surface distance. Their results are presented graphically in Figure 2. We will focus on the Dice score in the following since the average surface distance showed a development analogous to the Dice score. From iteration 1 on, the epistemic uncertainty approach yields better results than the random one, and from iteration 2 also the entropy based approach yields better results than the random selection. Both uncertainty based approaches show very similar performance over the whole experiment. In iteration 7, the performance of the random sampling approach reaches the performance of the uncertainty based approaches. To rate which improvements are significant, we perform a quantile regression on the 5th percentile of the Dice scores for each AL iteration. We find that the entropy (epistemic uncertainty) based approach has significant improvements ($p<0.001$) in iteration 2, 3 and 6 (2, 3, 5 and 6 resp.) over the random baseline.

The uncertainty based approaches are 2-4 iterations ahead of the baseline in terms of model performance in early iterations. This translates to 10-20 volumes less to be annotated compared to random acquisition. Depending on the efficiency of the annotation process, this can save one or more days of annotation time. The final performance is very similar across the different strategies.

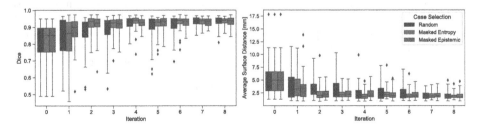

Fig. 2. Dice score and average surface distance evaluated on test data for different AL strategies.

These observations confirm prior findings [4] that random selection of cases is already a strong baseline, but uncertainty-based selection allows to improve over it, especially with respect to outliers (poorly performing cases).

3.3 Correlation of uncertainty and segmentation quality over time

If we use an uncertainty measure to select data in AL settings, it is important that this measure is a good predictor for the respective improvement in segmentation quality when using it to select the next training cases. Based on the assumption that the improvement is largest when adding cases that currently have the lowest Dice score, we compute the Spearman's rank correlation coefficient between the current Dice scores and the uncertainty measures. This is done for all acquisition strategies and for each iteration. Again, we compute the correlations for the average entropy and epistemic uncertainty within a dilated breast mask.

The correlations are presented in Figure 3. What may appear surprising at first, is that the observed correlation between the Dice score and the uncertainty measures decreases in later AL iterations. However, the segmentation quality increases with each iteration, so that the distribution of Dice scores gets closer to the optimum and much narrower (Fig. 2). Since both Dice scores and uncertainty measures are subject to measurement errors, at least part of which do not scale with the absolute values, this reduces the signal-to-noise ratio. Therefore, in later iterations, small variations in the Dice coefficients easily change the rank order and severely affect Spearman's correlation coefficient.

If we compare the correlations of entropy and epistemic uncertainty with the Dice scores we observe that the correlations decrease faster for the entropy. This means the epistemic uncertainty continues to be better at ranking the cases by their segmentation quality.

From these observations we conclude that epistemic uncertainty indeed better captures model uncertainty than the more commonly used entropy, even though this improvement did not translate to earlier performance improvements in our specific AL setting. Additionally, qualitative inspection of the model uncertainty (Fig.1) indicates that epistemic uncertainty better captures regions in which segmentation errors happen.

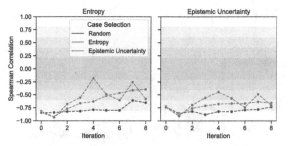

Fig. 3. Correlation of Dice score and different uncertainty measures over AL iterations. Shaded areas mark different levels of correlation of Spearman's rank correlation coefficient, brighter areas revealing stronger correlation.

4 Discussion

We evaluated two uncertainty-based AL strategies, both of which showed an improvement over the random case selection baseline using a 3D U-net model to segment the breast in MRI volumes. Specifically, in early iterations the uncertainty based strategies are 2-4 iterations ahead of the baseline in terms of model performance, which corresponds to 10-20 cases less to be annotated. In the long run, the uncertainty based approaches reach the same performance as the baseline.

We could not observe significant differences in model performance between strategies based on entropy and epistemic uncertainty, yet the correlation between estimated uncertainties and Dice scores was stronger for the epistemic uncertainty. This indicates that the epistemic uncertainty is better suited than the more commonly used entropy to find cases on which the model does not perform well yet to guide AL procedures.

Acknowledgement. We thank our clinical partners Dieter Szolar (Diagnostikum Graz, Austria), Sabine Ohlmeyer (Universitätsklinikum Erlangen, Germany), Edyta Szurowska (Medical University of Gdansk, Poland) and Uwe Fischer (Diagnostic Breast Center Göttingen, Germany) for providing the data for this study. We also thank Sophia Winkler and Christiane Engel for their efforts with creating annotations and Felix Thielke for his support on several parts of the implementation.

References

1. Zhang J, Saha A, Zhu Z, Mazurowski MA. Hierarchical convolutional neural networks for segmentation of breast tumors in MRI with application to radiogenomics. Proc IEEE. 2018;38(2):435–47.
2. Nam Y, Park GE, Kang J, Kim SH. Fully automatic assessment of background parenchymal enhancement on breast MRI using machine-learning models. J Magn Reson Imaging. 2021;53(3):818–26.
3. Gal Y, Islam R, Ghahramani Z. Deep bayesian active learning with image data. Proc ICML. 2017:1183–92.
4. Chlebus G, Schenk A, Hahn HK, Van Ginneken B, Meine H. Robust segmentation models using an uncertainty slice sampling-based annotation workflow. Proc IEEE. 2022;10:4728–38.
5. Lakshminarayanan B, Pritzel A, Blundell C. Simple and scalable predictive uncertainty estimation using deep ensembles. Adv Neural Inf Process Syst. 2017;30.
6. Wang G, Li W, Aertsen M, Deprest J, Ourselin S, Vercauteren T. Aleatoric uncertainty estimation with test-time augmentation for medical image segmentation with convolutional neural networks. Neurocomputing. 2019;338:34–45.
7. Gal Y, Ghahramani Z. Dropout as a bayesian approximation: representing model uncertainty in deep learning. Proc IEEE. 2016:1050–9.
8. Roy AG, Conjeti S, Navab N, Wachinger C. Inherent brain segmentation quality control from fully convnet monte carlo sampling. Proc IEEE. 2018:664–72.
9. Kendall A, Gal Y. What uncertainties do we need in bayesian deep learning for computer vision? Adv Neural Inf Process Syst. 2017;30.

Guidance to Noise Simulation in X-ray Imaging

Dominik Eckert[1], Magdalena Herbst[1], Julia Wicklein[1], Christopher Syben[1],
Ludwig Ritschl[1], Steffen Kappler[1], Sebastian Stober[2]

[1] Siemens Healthcare GmbH, Forchheim, Germany
[2] Otto von Guericke University, Magdeburg, Germany
dominik.eckert@siemens-healthineers.com

Abstract. In medical imaging, noise is an inherent occurring signal corruption, especially for the X-ray imaging where dose exposure to the patient should be minimal. Besides potential image degeneration, which may hinder accurate diagnoses, the noise can have negative impact on signal processing and evaluation algorithms, especially in deep learning (DL) methods. Furthermore, for the training of DL based noise reduction or to bolster DL methods against degeneration due to unseen types of noise or noise levels, it is inevitable to have a thorough and correct noise simulation available. This paper introduces a comprehensive noise simulation method that integrates the strengths of existing techniques into a more complete solution. Simultaneously, our approach aims to minimize the reliance on device-specific measurements and data, by proposing an automatic detector gain estimation.

1 Introduction

X-ray imaging comes with the specialty of ionizing radiation and therefore a balance between applied dose (should be minimal) and meaningful imaging need to be found. Therefore, a thorough understanding of the effects that lead to noise is necessary. The noise primarily originates from three sources: scintillator material interactions, detector electronic noise and photon randomness. The scintillator is responsible for converting the X-ray photons into visible light. This light spreads within the scintillator layers and therefore alters the nose characteristic in the images [1, 2]. In the detector, the light is converted into electric signals, which are affected by electronic noise, typically manifesting as Gaussian noise. However, on static recordings electronic noise is insignificant and is often neglected in most simulations [3]. The most important effect comes from the randomness of the arriving photons, which is challenging for the noise simulation as the noise itself depends on the actual signal and the other noise effects. Furthermore, the measured signal intensities are linearly related to the number of photons and not the actual photon count. As most noise simulations depend on the precise number of photons, there exist a necessity to estimate or measure this linear dependency.

In the field of X-ray imaging, numerous noise simulation methods have been proposed [4–6]. We will compare the state-of-the-art studies based on their methodology, the process of detector gain determination, the requirement for additional measurements (particularly the recording of flatfield images), the incorporation of existing noise, and the simulation of scintillator blurring. We provide a summary in Table 1. Baath et al. [5] developed a method that assumes knowledge of the noise power spectrum (NPS) of

Tab. 1. Comparative Analysis of Different Methods for Noise Simulation in X-ray Imaging. *Methodology:* The approach upon which the simulation is based. *Gain:* Specifies whether the Detector Gain is simulated. *Flatfield:* Indicates whether a Flatfield measurement is required. *Existing-Noise:* States whether existing noise is considered in the simulation. *Scintillator:* Denotes whether scintillator blurring is considered in the simulation.

Reference	Methodology	Gain	Flatfield	Existing-Noise	Scintillator
Bath et al. [5]	NPS	not needed	yes	implicit	implicit
Cesarelli et al. [9]	Poisson	-	no	-	no
Borges et al. [6]	Anscombe	measured	yes	measured	no
Hariharan et al. [8]	Anscombe	manually	no	manually	calibrated
Proposed Method	Poisson	automatically	no	analytical	empirically

two flatfield images at two dose levels. The known NPS is used to generate a noise image which, when added to the original image, simulates the noise characteristics at the lower dose level. Borges et al. [6] introduced a novel approach by adding the noise in the Anscombe domain [7]. This method involves acquiring two flatfield images at different radiation doses and modeling the noise based on the local variance of these images. Hariharan et al. [8] exploit the generalized Anscombe transformation to also account for electornic noise. They manually measure the existing noise on flat patches of the image, which is used for the simulation to calculate the existing variance, and add the missing noise in Anscombe domain to the image. Furthermore, the account for scintillator blurring, by convolving with a gaussian kernel, and determine it's sigma with measurements on the NPS. Cesarelli et al. [9] propose a different approach that directly simulates Poisson noise. They estimate an increase in Poisson noise by adding Gaussian noise with mean zero and variance dependent on the expected pixel intensity. Our proposed method also directly simulates Poisson noise but differs from Cesarelli et al.'s approach by exploiting the SNR to analytically considering the existing noise, and doing an automatic detector gain measurement to avoid having to carry out additional measurements.

2 Noise simulation

Since the noise is directly related to the X-ray dose, i.e., a reduction in the dose leads to a reduction in the average intensity and at the same time to an increase in the noise, the relationship between the two effects must be handled correctly in the simulation. Dose reduction simulations on acquired X-ray images can be done by reducing the mean and enhancing the noise. However, for correct simulations, the average intensity and the existing noise level must be determined via the detector gain. In addition, the effect of scintillator blurring on the noise characteristic must be taken into account. The three consecutive steps for a noise simulation on acquired images are depicted in Figure 1.

2.1 Poisson distribution

Before we delve into the simulation, it's crucial to understand the properties of the Poisson distribution [10]. These properties are not only necessary for estimating the detector gain but also for simulating additional noise. The Poisson distribution describes the probability that z photons arrive at one detector pixel depending on the mean arrival rate λ of one pixel

$$P(z|\lambda) = \frac{\lambda^z e^{-\lambda}}{z!} \quad \text{with} \quad \sigma^2 = \mu = \lambda \tag{1}$$

Hence, the randomness is pixel dependent. Furthermore, we can utilize two specific properties of the Poisson distribution for the simulation First, for the mean value μ and the variance σ^2 of the distribution,applies, and second it can be approximated by a normal distribution, whose mean and variance equals λ [11]

$$P(z|\lambda) \approx N_0(\mu_0 = \lambda, \sigma_0^2 = \lambda) \tag{2}$$

2.2 Detector gain estimation

In X-ray imaging, pixel intensities i are altered by photon conversion to visible light, but remain proportional to the photon count via $z = k \cdot i$. The detector gain k allows conversion back to average photon counts. Using equation 1, which states $\sigma = \mu$, k can be determined. For the transformed image $k \cdot i$, we have $k^2 \sigma_i = k\mu_i$. Solving for k yields

$$k = \frac{\sigma_i^2}{\mu_i} \tag{3}$$

We propose two methods for estimating the parameters σ_i^2 and μ_i: To estimate the parameters σ_i^2 and μ_i we propose an algorithmic estimation: The image has to be divided into patches and those with minimal entropy (indicating an absence of anatomy) must be selected. On these patches, the variance and mean can be measured, and with that k can be calculated. The final estimation of k is then the mean of these values. Alternatively, areas with an absence of anatomy can be also selected by hand, if no automatic procedure is needed.

In our simulation, we applied the algorithmic estimation using patches of size 15×15 and calculated k for the 10 patches with the lowest entropy.

2.3 Reducing the number of arriving photons or enhancing the noise

Dose reduction, such as noise simulation, can be conceptualized as scaling the mean photon arrival rate λ by a factor α^2. Scaling λ with α^2 also results in the scaling of the signal-to-noise ratio (SNR) by α, since the SNR is defined as $\text{SNR} = \frac{\mu}{\sigma} = \frac{\lambda}{\sqrt{\lambda}} = \sqrt{\lambda}$

$$\text{SNR}_\alpha = \alpha \frac{\mu_0}{\sigma_0} = \alpha \sqrt{\lambda} \tag{4}$$

| Detector Gain | > | Noise Enhancement | > | Scintillator Blurring |

Fig. 1. The three steps of dose reduction / noise simulation.

By utilizing Equation 2, pixel-specific Gaussian noise $N_p(0, \sigma_x^2)$ can be introduced to modify the SNR to SNR_α. However, the appropriate amount of σ_x^2 must be determined by setting

$$\frac{\mu_0}{\sqrt{\sigma_0^2 + \sigma_x^2}} \overset{!}{=} \sqrt{\alpha}\frac{\mu_0}{\sigma_0} \tag{5}$$

Rearranging the formula results in $\sigma_x^2 = (\frac{1}{\alpha} - 1)\sigma_0^2$, or equivalently, $(\frac{1}{\alpha} - 1)\lambda$. Therefore, the pixel-specific Gaussian noise to be added is solely dependent on the mean photon arrival rate. We estimate λ for each pixel by applying a median filter to the photon-count image.

In addition to adjusting the noise characteristics, the number of photons must also be modified. To achieve the downscaled number of photons, equation 1 must be satisfied. Consequently, the image must be scaled, and a new scaling factor k can be derived as follows:

$$k = \frac{\sigma_x^2 + \sigma_0^2}{\mu_0} = \frac{\lambda(\frac{1}{\alpha} - 1) + \lambda}{\lambda} = \frac{1}{\alpha} \tag{6}$$

2.4 Scintillator blurring

In X-ray systems, scintillators convert incoming X-ray radiation into visible light. However, light scattering within the scintillator can cause light to hit neighboring pixels, introducing a correlation of information between them. Hence, the Poisson noise characteristics is altered [1, 2, 12]. To account for this spreading effect, the simulated Poisson noise needs to be convolved with a Gaussian kernel defined by σ_s [12]. In our algorithm, we empirically chose σ_s to be 0.6 pixel, a value that depends on the scintillator material and thickness. Given that the pixel size of our detector is 0.296 mm, σ_s can be also be expressed in mm as 0.177 mm.

3 Results

To evaluate our proposed method, we captured chest X-Ray images of the same phantom from 8 different positions. Each position was imaged twice, first with a lower dose (80.9 kV and 2.0 mAs) and then with a higher dose (80.9 kV and 8.0 mAs). The low dose image served as the ground truth, while the high dose image was used for dose reduction simulation.

We compared our method, which accounts for existing noise, with a simpler approach that adds Poisson noise without this consideration. We measure the differences between ground truth standard deviation and the the simulated noise standard deviation, $\sigma(\text{sim.}) - \sigma(\text{gt})$. The measured results are presented in Table 2 and one image is depicted in Figure 2. This comparison was conducted to assess the impact of considering existing noise in the image on the simulation accuracy, which is the calculation of Section 2.3.

We examined the necessity of simulating scintillator blurring. Without blurring, noise tends to cover all frequencies equally, resulting in a more white noise. The scintillator, acting as a low-pass filter, dampens higher frequencies. This experiment was

Tab. 2. The difference between the ground truth low dose standard deviation and the simulated image standard deviation is presented.

Image	1	2	3	4	5	6	7	8	mean
Proposed Sim.	1.58	0.44	0.79	-0.52	1.44	0.49	-2.12	-2.21	-0.013 ± 1.38
Simple Sim.	-2.75	-5.15	-5.60	-3.65	-0.99	-2.08	-7.60	-5.19	-4.13 ± 2.02

conducted to understand the effect of scintillator blurring on the noise spectrum. The resulting NPSs are shown in Figure 3 and the resulting images are depicted in Figure 2.

4 Discussion and conclusion

In this study, we introduced an automated noise simulation pipeline capable of estimating the detector gain, accounting for existing noise in the ground truth, and considering scintillator blurring. Our findings underscore the importance of considering pre-existing noise in images, as demonstrated by the first experiment. The second experiment further highlighted the significance of simulating scintillator blurring, which brings the NPS closer to that of the ground truth by acting as a low-pass filter that dampens high frequencies.

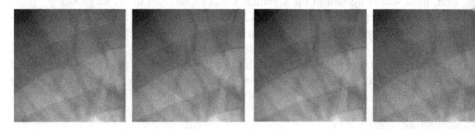

Fig. 2. From left to right: low dose ground truth image; image with our noise Simulation; simple noise simulation; image without scintillator blurring.

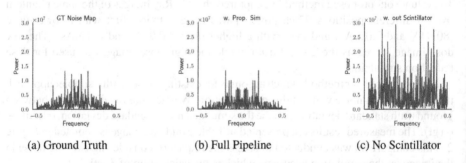

(a) Ground Truth   (b) Full Pipeline   (c) No Scintillator

Fig. 3. Noise Power Spectrum of: (a) the ground truth noise map, (b) the noise map simulated with the full pipeline, and (c) the noise map simulated with the pipeline, but without scintillator blurring.

Despite these experiments, our method calls for more detailed investigations, particularly concerning detector gain estimation. In our study, we tried to be as device independent as possible. Hence, we determined the detector blurring σ_s empirically. Uncertainties in parameters such as σ_s or the detector gain can be integrated into the training of neural networks, which might lead to more generalized models. If a more device specific method is necessary, we would advise to apply Hariharan et. al [8] or Baath et. al [5].

Disclaimer. The concepts and information presented in this paper are based on research and are not commercially available.

References

1. Luckner C, Herbst M, Weber T, Beister M, Ritschl L, Kappler S et al. High-speed slot-scanning radiography using small-angle tomosynthesis: investigation of spatial resolution. Med Phys. 2019;46(12):5454–66.
2. Li G, Luo S, Yan Y, Gu N. A method of extending the depth of focus of the high-resolution X-ray imaging system employing optical lens and scintillator: a phantom study. Biomed Eng Online. 2015;14(1):1–14.
3. Bushberg JT, Boone JM. The Essential Physics of Medical Imaging. Lippincott Williams & Wilkins, 2011.
4. Eckert D, Wicklein J, Herbst M, Dwars S, Ritschl L, Kappler S et al. Deep learning based tomosynthesis denoising: a bias investigation across different breast types. J Med Imaging. 2023;10(6):64003–3.
5. Båth M, Håkansson M, Tingberg A, Månsson LG. Method of simulating dose reduction for digital radiographic systems. Radiat Prot Dosimetry. 2005;114(1-3):253–9.
6. Borges LR, Oliveira HCd, Nunes PF, Bakic PR, Maidment AD, Vieira MA. Method for simulating dose reduction in digital mammography using the anscombe transformation. Med Phys. 2016;43(6Part1):2704–14.
7. Makitalo M, Foi A. Optimal inversion of the Anscombe transformation in low-count Poisson image denoising. IEEE Trans Image Process. 2010;20(1):99–109.
8. Hariharan SG. Novel Analytical and Learning-based Image Processing Techniques for Dose Reduction in Interventional X-ray Imaging. PhD thesis. Technische Universität München, 2023.
9. Cesarelli M, Bifulco P, Cerciello T, Romano M, Paura L. X-ray fluoroscopy noise modeling for filter design. Int J Comput Assist Radiol Surg. 2013;8:269–78.
10. Poisson SD. Recherches sur la probabilité des jugements en matière criminelle et en matière civile precédées des règles générales du calcul des probabilités par sd poisson. Bachelier, 1837.
11. Hubbard W. The approximation of a poisson distribution by a gaussian distribution. Proc IEEE. 1970;58(9):1374–5.
12. Oppelt A. Imaging Systems for Medical Diagnostics: Fundamentals, Technical Solutions and Applications for Systems Applying Ionizing Radiation, Nuclear Magnetic Resonance and Ultrasound. John Wiley & Sons, 2006.

Automated Lesion Detection in Endoscopic Imagery for Small Animal Models

Thomas Eixelberger[1,4], Qi Fang[2], Bisan A. Zohud[2], Ralf Hackner[1,4], Rene Jackstadt[3], Michael Stürzl[2], Elisabeth Naschberger[2], Thomas Wittenberg[1,4]

[1]Chair for Visual Computing, Friedrich-Alexander-Universität Erlangen-Nürnberg
[2]Division of Molecular and Experimental Surgery, Universitätsklinikum Erlangen
[3]German Cancer Research Center (DKFZ), Heidelberg
[4]Fraunhofer Institute for Integarted Circuits IIS, Erlangen
thomas.eixelberger@fau.de

Abstract. Murine animal models are routinely used in research of gastrointestinal diseases, for example to analyze colorectal cancer or chronic inflammatory bowel diseases. By using suitable (miniaturized) endoscopy systems, it is possible to examine the large intestine of mice with respect to inflammatory, vascular or neoplastic changes without the need to sacrifice the animals. This enables the acquisition of high-resolution colonoscopy image sequences that can be used for the visual examination of tumors, the assessment of inflammation or the vasculature. Since the human resources for analyzing a multitude of videos, are limited, an automated evaluation of such image data is desirable. Video recordings ($n = 49$) of mice with and without colorectal cancer (CRC) were employed for this purpose and scored by clinical experts. The videos contained mice with tumors in 33 cases and 16 are pathologically normal. For the automatic detection of neoplastic changes (e.g. polyps), a deep neural network based on the YOLOv7-tiny architecture was applied. This network was previously trained on >36,000 human colon images with neoplasias visible in all frames. On test data with human images, the precision of the network is Prec = 0.92, and Rec = 0.90. The network was applied to the mouse data without any changes. To avoid false-positive detections a color-based method was added to differentiate between stool residues and polyps. With the framework for the detection of neoplastic changes and classification of stool residues, we achieve results of Prec = 0.90, Rec = 0.98, F1 score = 0.94. Without the detection of stool residues, the values were dropping to Prec = 0.65 and Rec = 0.98, as 19 occurrences of stool are incorrectly classified as tumors. Our network trained on human data for neoplasia detection is able to accurately detect tumors in the murine colon. An additional module for the separation of stool residues is essential to avoid integration of wrongly positive cases.

1 Introduction

Murine animal models of gastro-intestinal diseases have been introduced and established as key tools to investigate the mucosal immune system, cancer development as well as colitis in the gut [1–3]. Furthermore, such models are also used for the evaluation of novel medication. Overall, such murine animal models have fundamentally contributed to obtain knowledge of the pathogenesis of various diseases in the past, but also have

© Der/die Autor(en), exklusiv lizenziert an
Springer Fachmedien Wiesbaden GmbH, ein Teil von Springer Nature 2024
A. Maier et al. (Hrsg.), *Bildverarbeitung für die Medizin 2024*,
Informatik aktuell, https://doi.org/10.1007/978-3-658-44037-4_54

been used as model systems of mucosal immune responses by investigating the interplay of different immune cells. Nevertheless, in order to analyze tumor development, Inflammatory bowel disease (IBD) or physiological changes of the colon tissue the animals have to be sacrificed at the endpoint. Hence, colonoscopy of mice has been established as a new non-destructive protocol for medical and immunological research to examine the colon for inflammatory, vascular or neoplastic changes [4, 5].

For this purpose, mice with colonic tumors or IBD are anesthetized and examined with a rigid endoscope, introduced via the anus, while the colon is insufflated with air. Subsequently, high resolution (HD) colonoscopy image sequences can be acquired which are used for visual inspection to score tumors or the grade of IBD.

As the resources required to conduct such animal experiments, including the reading time to evaluate the thus acquired colonoscopic videos are limited, an automated assessment of such large scale image data is needed. As recently, new methods using deep learning approaches have been introduced to support endoscopists in routine colonoscopic screening and to increase the adenoma detection rate (ADR), it is of interest, if and how such deep learning approaches for polyp detection [6–8] are applicable and useful for the assessment of similar image data obtained from small animals.

2 Materials and methods

2.1 Preparation protocol

Both female and male mice were used. All mice were housed in specific pathogen–free conditions and were routinely screened for pathogens according to Federation of European Laboratory Animal Science Associations (FELASA) guidelines. The experiments were approved by the government of central Franconia according to the current guidelines for animal experiments. All mice had ad libitum access to a standard diet and water. Mice were orthotopically injected in the colon wall with syngenic CRC tumor cells (VAKPT organoids) using a high-resolution mini-endoscopy instrument (Karl-Storz) under anesthesia with isoflurane. Afterwards, the mice were monitored weekly until the endpoint (week 6) using mini-endoscopy and videos were captured during this follow up. Figure 1 depicts the recording setup used for the mice colonoscopy.

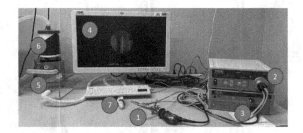

Fig. 1. Experimental setup of the colonoscopy mini-endoscope. (1) camera head with rigid endoscope, (2) light source, (3) endoscopy system with USB storage, (4) monitor, (5) Plexiglas chamber to narcotise the mice with Isoflurane gas, (6) absorption filter for the gas and (7) Falcon tube.

2.2   Data

We received n_{seq} = 49 colonoscopic videos of mice, prepared by and captured with the protocol and device as described above. Within this data collection n_{tumor} = 33 videos contained at least one tumor, while n_{normal} = 16 were pathologically normal.

In total, the collected videos have a length of t_{total} = 51:11 minutes. The average length is t_μ = 1:03 minutes, with a standard deviation t_σ = 57 seconds. The median length is t_{median} = 42 seconds, with a minimum video duration of t_{min} = 11 seconds and a maximum of t_{max} = 4:48 minutes. All videos have a framerate of 30 frames per second and a resolution of 1920 × 1080 pixels. Example frames of the received videos can be found in Figure 2.

2.3   Detection algorithm

For the automatic detection of tumorous regions in the colonoscopy videos we used a pre-trained YOLOv7-tiny architecture and two additional image processing steps.

2.3.1   YOLOv7-tiny architecture. The 'You Only Look Once' (YOLO) architecture is an one-stage detector network for real-time object detection. It combines both localization and classification of objects depicted in the images in one single neural network. Wang et al. [9] have presented a new YOLO version in 2022. The tiny version of the YOLOv7 architecture is optimized to run on edge devices. The model size has been reduced from 36.9 million to 6.2 million parameters. Additionally, the tiny version uses leaky rectified linear units (ReLUs) as activation functions in contrast to the regular version, which uses sigmoid linear units (SiLU). Wang et al. [9] have shown that the tiny version is nearly 180% faster than the normal version, but has only a 13% decrease in the average precision (AP). The YOLOv7-tiny architecture was trained with 36,596 human coloscopic images from the public dataset LDPolyp [10] and a private dataset [11]. The learning-rate was 0.01 and the stochastic gradient descent (SGD) optimizer was used.

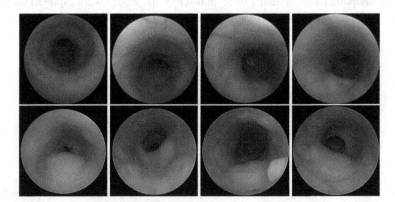

Fig. 2. Top row: examples of colonoscopic frames from inflamed mice without tumors; bottom row: examples with tumors by cell injected organoids.

The Precision after 200 epochs on different public datasets (Kvasir, CVC-ClinicDB, ETIS-Larib, and PICCOLO) with an intersection over union of 30% is 0.92, the Recall 0.90, and the F1-score = 0.91.

2.3.2 Pre- and post-processing. Some of the videos include parts with fecal debris ('stool') which are often rated as tumors within the neural network. To prevent these false positive detections, we calculate the median pixel value of the hue channel inside the detected bounding box. If the median hue value is in the range between 50 and 70 (being related to 'yellow'), the bounding box is rated as 'stool' and not as 'polyp'.

Almost all investigated videos include parts where the endoscope is located outside of the mouse body. Nevertheless, the used neural network is not able to identify these parts as outside and yields to false results in these sections. To identify valid section inside the colon the color of the frames are used. Specifically, only video parts with a continues impression of 'red' are labeled as inside the mouse colon. Hence, only the inside parts are analysed by the neural network. During the continuous analysis of a colonoscopy video the neural network sometimes makes false detections in single frames or cannot detect anything in single frames. In order to minimize these faults, we used the SORT algorithm, suggested by Bewley et al. [12]. Thus, the detection of a polyp is valid, when it is detected over at least 5 consecutive frames, while possible missing detections are interpolated using the Kalman filter of the SORT algorithm, respectively.

2.4 Evaluation parameters

For the evaluation we used the neural network in a Nvidia TensorRT environment and achieved a mean processing time of 30 ms per frame using an Intel i7, 16 GB RAM and a Nvidia 1050Ti. The video frames were cropped and down-scaled to a size of 640 × 640 pixels. We used a confidence value of $c = 0.2$ and an non-maximum suppression of 0.05. The SORT algorithm used an minimum overlap between successive bounding boxes of 50% and a minimum of 5 successive bounding boxes must succeed this value to be rated as positive.

3 Results

In Table 1 the results of the neural network (YOLOv7-tiny) with and without the stool detector are listed. TP stands for 'true positive', FP as false positive, and FN for 'false negative'. A detection is labelled as TP when the automatic approach detects a tumor in the sequence, which has been confirmed by the expert, as FP when the algorithm did not find a tumor, but which was indicated by the expert, and as FP when the algorithm finds a tumor, which has not been labelled by the expert. Furthermore, values for Precision, Recall, and the F1-Score are calculated using Precision $= TP/(TP+FP)$, Recall $= TP/(TP+FN)$, and $F1 = (2 \cdot \text{Precision} \cdot \text{Recall})/(\text{Precision} + \text{Recall})$.

Figure 3 shows four examples of correctly (TP) detected tumors by the YOLOv7-tiny network (top row) and four examples (bottom row) of incorrect detections (FP) and one missing detection of tumor. Using the image-processing steps described above, the FP detections of 'stool' are corrected afterwards.

Tab. 1. Results of the neural network with and without the stool detector.

Method	TP	FP	FN	Precision	Recall	$F1$-Score
YOLOv7-tiny	41	22	1	0.651	0.976	0.781
YOLOv7-tiny with stool detection	57	6	1	0.905	0.983	0.942

4 Discussion

An automatic lesion detection for mice colon was investigated by employing a pretrained YOLOv7-tiny based neural network. According to Table 1 the network (originally developed for the detection of humane polyps) is capable to find polyps also in mice colon but too often classifies fecal debris as tumor. With the addition of an image-processing based 'stool' detector, the Precision rises significant and delivers satisfying results. The automatic detection fails in three cases when colon folds have the same shape as polyps (Fig. 3 bottom row last image) and in three cases the color of the fecal debris is not in the range of the 'stool' detector. Another elementary part is the SORT tracking algorithm which robustly eliminates single false detections.

Further work will evaluate the proposed detection approach on a wider range of colonoscopic video sequences of murine animal models with other endoscopic cameras as well as a variation of depicted lesions.

Acknowledgement. This work has partially been supported by the German Research Society (DFG) under the Grant TRR/SFB 305, sub projects B08 (to EN) & Z1 (to TW).

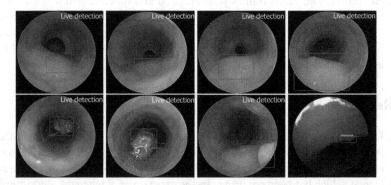

Fig. 3. Top row: correctly detected tumors; Bottom row: falsely detected tumors. The first two images show fecal debris, the third detected stool instead of the injected tumor in the center of the image, and the last shows normal colon mucosa.

References

1. Chen C, Neumann J, Kühn F, Lee SM, Drefs M, Andrassy J et al. Establishment of an endoscopy-guided minimally invasive orthotopic mouse model of colorectal cancer. Cancers (Basel). 2020;12(10):3007.
2. Rosenberg DW, Giardina C, Tanaka T. Mouse models for the study of colon carcinogenesis. Carcinogenesis. 2009;30(2):183–96.
3. Taketo MM, Edelmann W. Mouse models of colon cancer. Gastroent. 2009;136(3):780–98.
4. Becker C, Fantini MC, Neurath MF. High resolution colonoscopy in live mice. Nat Protoc. 2006;1(6):2900–4.
5. Becker C, Fantini MC, Wirtz S, Nikolaev A, Kiesslich R, Lehr HA et al. In vivo imaging of colitis and colon cancer development in mice using high resolution chromoendoscopy. Gut. 2005;54(7):950–4.
6. Wittenberg T, Raithel M. Artificial intelligence-based polyp detection in colonoscopy: where have we been, where do we stand, and where are we headed? Visc Med. 2020;36(6):428–38.
7. Krenzer A, Banck M, Makowski K, Hekalo A, Fitting D, Troya J et al. A real-time polyp-detection system with clinical application in colonoscopy using deep convolutional neural networks. J Imaging. 2023;9(2).
8. Ghose P, Ghose A, Sadhukhan D, Pal S, Mitra M. Improved polyp detection from colonoscopy images using finetuned YOLO-v5. Multimed Tools Appl. 2023.
9. Wang CY, Bochkovskiy A, Liao HYM. YOLOv7: trainable bag-of-freebies sets new state-of-the-art for real-time object detectors. 2022.
10. Ma Y, Chen X, Cheng K, Li Y, Sun B. LDPolypVideo benchmark: a large-scale colonoscopy video dataset of diverse polyps. Proc MICCAI. 2021:387–96.
11. Eixelberger T, Wolkenstein G, Hackner R, Bruns V, Mühldorfer S, Geissler U et al. YOLO networks for polyp detection: a human-in-the-loop training approach. Curr Dir Biomed Eng. 2022;8(2):277–80.
12. Bewley A, Ge Z, Ott L, Ramos F, Upcroft B. Simple online and realtime tracking. Processing IEEE. 2016:3464–8.

Ultrasound to CT Image-to-image Translation for Personalized Thyroid Screening

Carl A. Noack[1], Francesca De Benetti[1], Kartikay Tehlan[1,2], Nassir Navab[1], Thomas Wendler[1,2,3]

[1]Chair for Computer Aided Medical Procedures and Augmented Reality, Technische Universität München, Garching, Germany
[2]Clinical Computational Medical Imaging Research, Department of Interventional and Diagnostic Radiology and Neuroradiology, University Hospital Augsburg, Augsburg, Germany
[3]Institute of Digital Health, University Hospital Augsburg, Neusaess, Germany
francesca.de-benetti@tum.de

Abstract. The use of 2D scintigraphy in the screening for thyroid pathologies is widespread, however its diagnostic value is limited because the activity of multiple thyroid lesions cannot be effectively resolved. Combining the scintigraphy with a CT would allow to simulate 3D SPECT and thereby increase the diagnostic value of the screening. However, during screening programs ultrasound is preferred to CT, because of its widespread availability and harmlessness. Therefore, tools to translate the thyroid ultrasound to CT are needed. In this perspective, we propose to translate ultrasound images of the thyroid into synthetic CT images using a GAN-based architecture. Our proposed approach results in a higher anatomical consistency between the input US and the output synthetic CT compared to the baseline. The synthetic CTs exhibit a realistic HU distribution compared to real CTs and maintain realistic appearance as indicated by the Fréchet Inception Distance.

1 Introduction

In 2021, more than 63.000 people were diagnosed with thyroid pathologies in Germany [1]. The screening for thyroid pathologies is conventionally done with ultrasound imaging (US), followed by technetium-99m (^{99m}Tc) pertechnetate scintigraphy in cases of suspicious lesions and low levels of serum thyroid-stimulating hormone [2]. Despite being an established imaging modality, the diagnostic value of scintigraphy is limited because it only provides a 2D projection of the region of interest (ROI). This is particularly a problem in patients with multiple thyroid lesions because the activity of each lesion cannot be effectively resolved. The use of single proton emission tomography (SPECT) would solve this problem, but its use in screening is limited due to the low image quality and the radiation burden [3].

Using tools such as GATE [4], 3D SPECT can be simulated using a CT volume and the radioactivity distribution in the ROI. Projecting the SPECT onto a plane and comparing it to the real 2D scintigraphy would ensure that the simulated SPECT represents the real uptake in the patient. In the simulation, the CT describes the anatomy of the ROI as well as the density and chemical composition of the tissue, which is effectively encoded in the hounsfield units (HU). However, during screening, CT is not used because it is costly and involves ionizing radiation. For this reason, it would be desirable to convert the thyroid US acquired during screening to a CT-like volume, which will be used as input of the SPECT simulation. Given that the imaging principles of both US and CT rely on tissue densities (in the form of acoustic impedance and speed of sound in the case of the US), we can assume that the translation from one to the other is possible [5]. To the best of our knowledge, this is the first paper proposing:

- an unpaired I2IT approach from real US to synthetic CT (sCT)
- a generator loss formulation for generative adversarial networks (GAN) to enforce structural anatomical consistency and realistic HU values in the generated images

1.1 Related work

The conversion of images between different "styles" is conventionally known as image-to-image translation (I2IT). Recently, GAN-based architectures have been widely used for I2IT due to their ability to learn from unpaired data. In medical imaging, GANs have been used for cross-modality I2IT (such as from MRI to CT) and denoising [6].

Only limited research tackles the problem of converting US into another modality. Vedula el al. trained a supervised CNN architecture to translate 2D US to sCT images [5]. To obtain US-CT image pairs needed for supervised training, they simulated US from the CT images. This is a big limitation as they did not consider real US.

An unsupervised I2IT approach from US to MR of the fetal brain was proposed by Jiao et al. [7], who used a network based on CycleGAN to ensure the structural similarity of the generated synthetic MR images. Yet, MR is not quantitative in nature and has more common information with US than CT, so their approach would not be as suitable.

2 Materials and methods

2.1 Dataset and preprocessing

Due to the lack of publicly available paired US/CT data, we used unpaired data.

We obtained 16 3D US volumes of both lobes of the thyroid from the SegThy dataset [8], which includes also the segmentations for the thyroid, the jugular veins and the carotid arteries. An expert annotator labeled the trachea, the background (i.e., where there is no information), and the remaining tissue. Finally, the US volumes were normalized to the [0, 1] range. The US labels were used to generate label-based sCT ($_{LB}$sCT) by assigning a HU value (mean) to all pixels of a label. The label-specific HU value has been computed from the original CT (Tab. 1). We chose not to simulate US from CT for paired data as our target application is transforming real US.

Despite the large number of CT datasets available online, to our knowledge, none of them includes healthy CT volumes of the head-and-neck region. Therefore, we acquired CT data from 52 patients treated at Klinikum Rechts der Isar (Munich, Germany) between September 2019 and January 2023 (ethic approval 244/19S), which showed no abnormalities in the thyroid region. In each CT scan, we cropped a ROI around the thyroid using anatomical landmarks (C4 and T1 vertebrae and the trachea) as guidance.

Tab. 1. Label-wise HU given by mean μ and standard deviation σ calculated from a random subset of 12 real CT volumes.

ROI	HU ($\mu \pm \sigma$)
Thyroid	168.5 ± 50
Blood (jugular vein, carotid artery)	196 ± 58
Soft tissue	-24.5 ± 82

Finally, the CT volumes were clipped to a range of [-1000, 1000] HU and normalized to the [-1, 1] range.

An expert annotator labeled thyroid, trachea, carotid arteries, and jugular veins in 4 CT volumes (for a total of 295 slices), which will be used during the evaluation.

Due to the limited amount of data, we used a 2D (slice by slice) approach. Therefore, we extracted 2D axial slices from our volumes and obtained a total of 4256 US slices and 1301 CT slices. The slices were resampled to be of size 256 × 256.

Although GANs are very good at modifying the style of an image, they are prone to hallucinations and geometric distortions in the synthetic image [9]. In order to limit the hallucinations in the region without US information and let the network focus on the ROI, we masked the real CT images during training using the "background" label of the US image (Fig. 1).

2.2 Method

The generator, following the implementation by Kong et al. [10], consists of an encoder with three 2D convolutional blocks, then nine ResNet blocks, and finally a decoder with two 2D up-convolutional blocks. Instance normalization and ReLU were used. A 2D padding layer, followed by a convolutional layer and a hyperbolic tangent (to ensure outputs $\in [-1, 1]$), were placed after the decoder to produce the sCT image.

The discriminator is based on PatchGAN [11], which assesses individual patches instead of the full image. This enforces sharper outputs, accurate modelling of high-frequencies details and reduced artifacts [12]. The network consists of one 2D convolutional layer followed by a LeakyReLU, three 2D blocks including padding, downsampling, convolution, batch normalization, and LeakyReLU, and, finally, a 2D convolu-

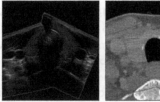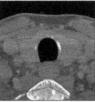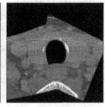

Fig. 1. Input US (left), original CT (center), masked CT (right), with outline of the background label based on the US.

tional layer that returns the prediction of size 30 × 30, where an entry of 1 is associated with a patch predicted to be real and 0 otherwise.

2.3 Loss function

As adversarial loss, which is the fundamental loss in a GAN, we use the formulation from Least Squares GAN [13]. In our case, the adversarial loss for the generator $\mathcal{L}_{adv}$ is then defined as

$$\mathcal{L}_{adv} = MSE(\mathcal{D}(\hat{b}), \mathbf{1}^{30 \times 30})$$

where $\mathcal{D}(\hat{b})$ is the discriminator's prediction on the synthetic image $\hat{b}$ that is output by the generator and $\mathbf{1}^{30 \times 30}$ is the target (ones, i.e., prediction indicates image to be real, as the generator's loss should be low when it is able to fool the discriminator).

To ensure structural consistency and realistic HU, we evaluated the use of an additional generator loss term, which we call "label-based CT loss" and define as

$$\mathcal{L}_{CT} = MSE(sCT, _{LB} CT)$$

The total generator loss is then: $\mathcal{L}_G = \mathcal{L}_{adv} + \lambda \mathcal{L}_{CT}$, where $\lambda = 20$ at epoch 0 increases by 1 in each epoch until $\lambda = 40$. By incrementing λ, we counteract the growing dominance of $\mathcal{L}_{adv}$ over $\mathcal{L}_{CT}$ during training.

The PatchGAN discriminator loss $\mathcal{L}_{\mathcal{D}}$ is defined as

$$\mathcal{L}_{\mathcal{D}} = MSE(\mathcal{D}(b), \mathbf{1}^{30 \times 30}) + MSE(\mathcal{D}(\hat{b}), \mathbf{0}^{30 \times 30})$$

where $\mathcal{D}(b)$ is the discriminator's prediction on the real image b and $\mathbf{1}^{30 \times 30}$ is its corresponding target (low discriminator loss for correctly indicating real/synthetic).

2.4 Evaluation

We evaluated our models on one complete US volume (157 slices), which was excluded from the training data.

The *structural consistency* between the anatomical structures in the original US image and the sCT image is crucial. To measure this, we trained a segmentation model (with the same architecture as the generator, but with 4 ResNet blocks) on real CT and $_{LB}$sCT images. At test phase, we used this model to segment the trachea, the jugular veins, the carotid arteries, the background, and the remaining tissue in the sCT. We then measured the Dice score (DSC ↑) between the resulting segmentation and the segmentation of the original US. Since sCTs with good structural consistency result in segmentations close to the US segmentation, we use DSC as metric of structural consistency.

We used the fréchet inception distance (FID ↓) to evaluate the *realism* of our model [14], i.e. its performance in generating realistic CT images. FID captures the similarity between two datasets (synthetic and real) by measuring the Fréchet distance between distributions of extracted, vision-relevant features from both datasets and has been found to be consistent with human judgment [15]. Another crucial aspect is the correct prediction of the HU in the sCT, because they represent the density and the chemical composition of the tissues. To evaluate this, we compared the normalized, averaged histograms of the real CT images and the sCT ones in terms of correlation C (↑) [16].

3   Results

The baseline method (with $\mathcal{L}_G = \mathcal{L}_{\text{adv}}$) achieves DSC = 0.72±0.023 and FID = 1.49 whereas the proposed method (with $\mathcal{L}_G = \mathcal{L}_{\text{adv}} + \mathcal{L}_{CT}$) results in DSC = 0.77±0.025 and FID = 0.43. Visual inspection of the sCT generated by the proposed method confirms that sCT look realistic and the anatomy is preserved (Fig. 2). In terms of artifacts, the baseline model hallucinates and generates bright bone-like structures around the trachea. This is not visible in the proposed model. Moreover, in most slices, the two models generate a black region above the trachea, in correspondence with the misalignment of the two sides of the 3D US. Regarding the realism of the predicted HU, the proposed method resulted in a correlation of $C = 0.85$, which is considered satisfactory.

4   Discussion

To the best of our knowledge, we presented the first I2IT approach to translate US slices into synthetic CT (sCT) slices. It is based on a GAN architecture and employs an auxiliary label-based sCT ($_{LB}$sCT) to ensure the structural similarity between the input US and the predicted sCT, and enforces realistic HU. Due to the limited data, our proposed approach is 2D. However, it can be easily applied to 3D data.

The translation from US to CT involves (1) learning to translate the contrast in the US images (due to reflection of the US waves) to the contrast in the CT (due to attenuation), and (2) dealing with information missing in US (due to total reflection or

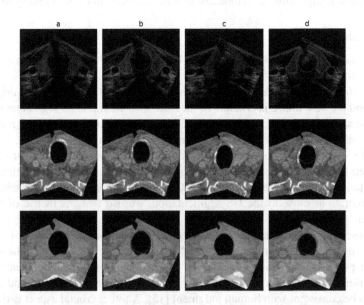

Fig. 2. (a) and (c): examples of US (top), sCT (baseline) and sCT (proposed method). (b) and (d): (a) and (c), respectively, with the contours of thyroid, jugular veins, and carotid arteries.

depth attenuation). To address this, (1) we introduced the label-based sCT and (2) masked the regions where US lacks information. These approaches suit our target application but may be insufficient for others.

Overall, our method demonstrates greater anatomical accuracy than the conventional I2I GANs. Additionally, it ensures realism, as evidenced by the FID. We believe that, as result, this method can play a crucial role in the target application of estimating 3D SPECT images from 2D scintigraphy and 3D US for personalized thyroid diagnostics.

References

1. Schilddrüsenerkrankungen in deutschen Krankenhäusern | Statista — de.statista.com.
2. Russ G, Bonnema SJ, Erdogan MF, Durante C, Ngu R, Leenhardt L. European Thyroid Association guidelines for ultrasound malignancy risk stratification of thyroid nodules in adults: the EU-TIRADS. Eur Thyroid J. 2017.
3. Ahmed N, Niyaz K, Borakati A, Marafi F, Birk R, Usmani S. Hybrid SPECT/CT imaging in the management of differentiated thyroid carcinoma. Asian Pac J Cancer Prev. 2018.
4. Jan S, Santin G, Strul D, Staelens S, Assié K, Autret D et al. GATE: a simulation toolkit for PET and SPECT. Phys Med Biol. 2004.
5. Vedula S, Senouf O, Bronstein AM, Michailovich OV, Zibulevsky M. Towards CT-quality ultrasound imaging using deep learning. arXiv preprint arXiv:1710.06304. 2017.
6. Chen J, Chen S, Wee L, Dekker A, Bermejo I. Deep learning based unpaired image-to-image translation applications for medical physics: a systematic review. Phys Med Biol. 2023.
7. Jiao J, Namburete AI, Papageorghiou AT, Noble JA. Self-supervised ultrasound to MRI fetal brain image synthesis. IEEE Trans Med Imaging. 2020.
8. Krönke M, Eilers C, Dimova D, Köhler M, Buschner G, Schweiger L et al. Tracked 3D ultrasound and deep neural network-based thyroid segmentation reduce interobserver variability in thyroid volumetry. Plos One. 2022.
9. Cohen JP, Luck M, Honari S. Distribution matching losses can hallucinate features in medical image translation. Proc MICCAI. Springer. 2018.
10. Kong L, Lian C, Huang D, Hu Y, Zhou Q et al. Breaking the dilemma of medical image-to-image translation. Adv Neural Inf Process Syst. 2021.
11. Zheng C, Cham TJ, Cai J. The spatially-correlative loss for various image translation tasks. Proc IEEE/CVF CVPR. 2021.
12. Isola P, Zhu JY, Zhou T, Efros AA. Image-to-image translation with conditional adversarial networks. Proc IEEE CVPR. 2017.
13. Mao X, Li Q, Xie H, Lau RY, Wang Z, Paul Smolley S. Least squares generative adversarial networks. Proc IEEE ICCV. 2017.
14. Hoyez H, Schockaert C, Rambach J, Mirbach B, Stricker D. Unsupervised image-to-image translation: a review. Sensors. 2022.
15. Heusel M, Ramsauer H, Unterthiner T, Nessler B, Hochreiter S. GANs trained by a two time-scale update rule converge to a local nash equilibrium. Adv Neur Inf Proc Syst. 2017.
16. Bityukov S, Maksimushkina A, Smirnova V. Comparison of histograms in physical research. Nucl Energy Technol. 2016.

Abstract: Multistage Registration of CT and Biopsy CT Images of Lung Tumors

Anika Strittmatter[1,2], Alexander Hertel[3], Steffen Diehl[3], Matthias F. Froelich[3], Stefan O. Schoenberg[3], Sonja Loges[4], Tobias Boch[4], Daniel Nowak[5], Alexander Streuer[5], Lothar R. Schad[1,2], Frank G. Zöllner[1,2]

[1]Computer Assisted Clinical Medicine, Medical Faculty Mannheim, Heidelberg University
[2]Mannheim Institute for Intelligent Systems in Medicine, Medical Faculty Mannheim, Heidelberg University
[3]Department of Radiology and Nuclear Medicine, Mannheim University Medical Centre, Medical Faculty Mannheim, Heidelberg University
[4]Department of Personalised Oncology, Mannheim University Medical Centre, Medical Faculty Mannheim, Heidelberg University
[5]Department of Hematology and Oncology, Mannheim University Medical Centre, Medical Faculty Mannheim, Heidelberg University
anika.strittmatter@medma.uni-heidelberg.de

The research project "Radiomics enhanced CT-guided targeted biopsy in lung cancer" utilises pre-calculated intratumoural heterogeneity areas to perform CT-guided biopsies of lung tumors. This involves the fusion of CT images acquired during preliminary examinations and their radiomics maps with biopsy CT images to detect potential intratumoral heterogeneity areas, requiring registration of the corresponding images. So, we developed a multistage registration approach with rigid preregistration. The dataset comprises 13 thorax CT volumes recorded during preliminary examinations (called CT images) and 13 narrow CT volumes (6 slices) acquired during biopsies (called biopsy CT images) of 13 patients with lung tumors. In some cases, due to the intervention, patients were lying on their side during the biopsy, whereas they were lying on their back during the preliminary examination. Rigid preregistration was initially performed to correct large rotations and translations. The rotation was determined using bounding boxes and ITK-Snap was used to estimate corresponding slices in the images. The preregistered CT images were then registered to the biopsy CT images using a SimpleElastix multistage algorithm, including rigid, affine, and deformable transformations. The transformations from the rigid preregistration and SimpleElastix were then applied to the radiomics maps. The results demonstrate that the multistage registration resulted in high structural similarity and overlap of lung tumors in the CT and biopsy CT images, enabling "virtual biopsies" and extraction of quantitative radiomics features of the exact puncture site [1].

References

1. Strittmatter A, Hertel A, Diehl S, Froelich MF, Schoenberg SO, Loges S et al. A multistage registration of CT and biopsy CT images of lung tumors. Proc 6th Conf on Image-Guided Interventions. 2023:17–8.

Abstract: Spatiotemporal Illumination Model for 3D Image Fusion in Optical Coherence Tomography

Stefan B. Ploner[1,2], Jungeun Won[2], Julia Schottenhamml[1], Jessica Girgis[3], Kenneth Lam[3], Nadia Waheed[3], James G. Fujimoto[2], Andreas Maier[1]

[1]Pattern Recognition Lab, Friedrich-Alexander-Universität Erlangen-Nürnberg, Germany
[2]Research Laboratory of Electronics, Massachusetts Institute of Technology, USA
[3]Department of Ophthalmology, New England Eye Center, USA
stefan.ploner@fau.de

Optical coherence tomography (OCT) is a non-invasive, micrometer-scale imaging modality that has become a clinical standard in ophthalmology. By raster-scanning the retina, sequential cross-sectional image slices are acquired to generate volumetric data. In-vivo imaging suffers from discontinuities between slices that show up as motion and illumination artifacts. We present a new illumination model that exploits continuity in orthogonally raster-scanned volume data [1]. Our novel spatiotemporal parametrization adheres to illumination continuity both temporally, along the imaged slices, as well as spatially, in the transverse directions. Yet, our formulation does not make inter-slice assumptions, which could have discontinuities. This is the first optimization of a 3D inverse model in an image reconstruction context in OCT. Evaluation in 68 volumes from eyes with pathology showed reduction of illumination artifacts in 88% of the data, and only 6% showed moderate residual illumination artifacts. The method enables the use of forward-warped motion corrected data [2], which is more accurate, and enables supersampling and advanced 3D image reconstruction in OCT [3, 4].

References

1. Ploner S, Won J, Schottenhamml J, Girgis J, Lam K, Waheed N et al. A spatiotemporal illumination model for 3d image fusion in optical coherence tomography. 2023 IEEE 20th International Symposium on Biomedical Imaging (ISBI). 2023:1–5.
2. Ploner S, Chen S, Won J, Husvogt L, Breininger K, Schottenhamml J et al. A spatiotemporal model for precise and efficient fully-automatic 3D motion correction in OCT. Medical Image Computing and Computer Assisted Intervention: MICCAI 2022. Ed. by Wang L, Dou Q, Fletcher PT, Speidel S, Li S. Cham: Springer Nature Switzerland, 2022:517–27.
3. Won J, Yaghy A, Ploner S, Takahashi H, Reimann M, Girgis JM et al. Motion correction and volume merging of ultrahigh resolution OCT enable 3D visualization and longitudinal tracking of hyperreflective foci. ARVO Imaging in the Eye Conference 2023, Invest. Ophthal. & Vis. Sci. Vol. 64. (9). 2023:PP0018–PP0018.
4. Ploner S, Won J, Yaghy A, Lam K, Girgies J, Schottenhamml J et al. Advanced volume rebuilding overcomes quilting, stretching, and banding image artifacts in orthogonally-scanned OCT. ARVO Annual Meeting 2023, Invest. Ophthal. & Vis. Sci. Vol. 64. (9). 2023:2371–1.

© Der/die Autor(en), exklusiv lizenziert an
Springer Fachmedien Wiesbaden GmbH, ein Teil von Springer Nature 2024
A. Maier et al. (Hrsg.), *Bildverarbeitung für die Medizin 2024*,
Informatik aktuell, https://doi.org/10.1007/978-3-658-44037-4_57

Abstract: Gradient-based Geometry Learning for Fan-beam CT Reconstruction

Mareike Thies[1], Fabian Wagner[1], Noah Maul[1,2], Lukas Folle[1], Manuela Meier[1,2], Maximilian Rohleder[1,2], Linda-Sophie Schneider[1], Laura Pfaff[1,2], Mingxuan Gu[1], Jonas Utz[3], Felix Denzinger[1,2], Michael Manhart[2], Andreas Maier[1]

[1]Pattern Recognition Lab, FAU Erlangen-Nürnberg
[2]Siemens Healthcare GmbH, Erlangen
[3]Department AIBE, FAU Erlangen-Nürnberg
mareike.thies@fau.de

Incorporating computed tomography (CT) reconstruction operators into differentiable pipelines has proven beneficial in many applications. Such approaches usually focus on the projection data and keep the acquisition geometry fixed. However, precise knowledge of the acquisition geometry is essential for high quality reconstruction results. Here, the differentiable formulation of fan-beam CT reconstruction is extended to the acquisition geometry. The CT reconstruction operation is analytically derived with respect to the acquisition geometry. This allows to propagate gradient information from a loss function on the reconstructed image into the geometry parameters. As a proof-of-concept experiment, this idea is applied to rigid motion compensation. The cost function is parameterized by a trained neural network which regresses an image quality metric from the motion-affected reconstruction alone. Since this regressed quality index and the geometry parameters are connected in a differentiable manner, optimization can be performed using standard gradient-based optimization procedures. Oppositely, all previous approaches rely on gradient-free optimization in this context. The proposed motion compensation algorithm improves the structural similarity index measure (SSIM) from 0.848 for the initial motion-affected reconstruction to 0.946 after compensation. It also generalizes to real fan-beam sinograms which are rebinned from a helical trajectory where the SSIM increases from 0.639 to 0.742. Furthermore, we can show that the number of target function evaluations is decreased by several orders of magnitude compared to gradient-free optimization. Using the proposed method, we are the first to optimize an autofocus-inspired algorithm based on analytical gradients. Next to motion compensation, we see further use cases of our differentiable method for scanner calibration or hybrid techniques employing deep models. The GPU-accelerated source code for geometry-differentiable CT backprojection in fan-beam and cone-beam geometries is publicly available at https://github.com/mareikethies/geometry_gradients_CT [1].

References

1. Thies M, Wagner F, Maul N, Folle L, Meier M, Rohleder M et al. Gradient-based geometry learning for fan-beam CT reconstruction. Phys Med Biol. 2023;68(20):205004.

Segmentation-inspired Image Registration

Saskia Neuber[1], Pia F. Schulz[1], Sven Kuckertz[2], Jan Modersitzki[1,2]

[1]Institute of Mathematics and Image Computing, University of Lübeck, Germany
[2]Fraunhofer Institute of Digital Medicine, MEVIS, Lübeck, Germany
s.neuber@uni-luebeck.de

Abstract. Artificial intelligence has been used with great success for the segmentation of anatomical structures in medical imaging. We use these achievements to improve classical registration schemes. Particularly, we derive geometrical features such as centroids and principal axes of segments and use those in a combined approach. A smart filtering of the features results in a two phase preregistration, followed in a third phase by an intensity guided registration. We also propose to use a regularization, which enables a coupling of all components of the 3D transformation in a unified framework. Finally, we show how easily our approach can be applied even to challenging 3D medical data.

1 Introduction

Image registration is one of the main tasks in daily clinical routine and is required when for example images of different times have to be compared [1].Inspired by the seminal paper of Wasserthal et. al. [2] we propose a new segmentation based registration procedure. The key idea is that based on a powerful segmentation tool, we generate a set of corresponding features, that is used to initialize the overall registration. Based on the automatically deduced features, we suggest a multi-phase approach similar to [3, 4]. In both approaches [3, 4], it is assumed that corresponding landmarks pairs are available. In a first phase, a starting value is obtained from plain landmark based preregistration. Based on this starting point, an overall energy including an image based similarity measure is minimized in a second phase. In [3] a 2D vector field (VF) regularization [5] and a simple penalty for the landmark match is used. In [4] landmarks are included as a hard constraint and a thin-plate spline (TPS) model for arbitrary dimensions is used for phase one and a curvature regularizer for phase two. In this work, we assume a segmentation, e.g., using the TotalSegmentator (TS) [2] and apply a three-phase procedure. In phase one, we generate landmarks by computing the centroids of segments and include these as a hard constraint in the preregistration. In phase two, we assume the images to be roughly aligned and derive correspondences of additional moment based features, specifically principal axes. Based on this additional information, we continue similarly to phase one. Finally, in phase three, we include an image based similarity term and replace the landmark constraint by an application specific penalty. In all phases, we use the same 3D VF regularizer [6]. To the best of our knowledge this VF regularization has not been used in 3D image registration before. Numerical results on challenging 3D thorax data are presented. Our results highlight the power of this combined approach as well as the advantages and limitations of geometrical features.

© Der/die Autor(en), exklusiv lizenziert an
Springer Fachmedien Wiesbaden GmbH, ein Teil von Springer Nature 2024
A. Maier et al. (Hrsg.), *Bildverarbeitung für die Medizin 2024*,
Informatik aktuell, https://doi.org/10.1007/978-3-658-44037-4_59

2   Material and methods

In this section we first formulate the general registration problem. Thereafter details of the landmark extraction from the segments as well as of the registration phases will be given. Next the procedure is adapted to a specific application, precisely the registration of 3D thorax data. Lastly, we present the experimental data set and the evaluation measures.

2.1   Variational formulation of the registration problem

We briefly recall the general formulation of a registration problem; for details see [1, 7]. Solving a registration problem means minimization of an overall energy J

$$J(y) = D(T[y], R) + S(y) + P(y) \quad \text{subject to} \quad C(y) = 0 \tag{1}$$

where $y : \mathbb{R}^d \to \mathbb{R}^d$ is the wanted transformation, d is the spatial dimension, template T and reference R are functions with compact support in an interval $\Omega \subset \mathbb{R}^d$ and $T[y]$ is the transformed image with $T[y](x) = T(y(x))$ for all x. Moreover D is a potential similarity measure, S is a regularizer, P is a potential penalty, and C is a potential constraint. More details are discussed in the following sections.

Although regularization is in principle arbitrary, we suggest the family

$$S(y; \gamma, W) := \int_W \gamma \|\nabla \operatorname{div} y\|^2 + (1 - \gamma)\|\nabla \operatorname{rot} y\|^2 \, dx \tag{2}$$

where either $W = \mathbb{R}^d$ or $W = \Omega$ and $\gamma \in (0, 1)$ balances divergence and curl of the field y. These regularizers perform on complete VF and not only on its components individually [5, 6]. A 2D version and the choice of an optimal parameter γ is discussed in [3]. For our 3D results we use the special case $\gamma = 0.5$, which coincides with the TPS energy as in [4]. However, we use this energy for all phases of the registration. Note, that our approach covers essentially all similarity measures, regularizers and penalty terms and is not limited to a particular setting. For our specific application, we discuss a similarity measure D and a penalty P in Section 2.4.

2.2   Segmentation-based feature extraction

We now discuss the feature generation. Basically, we derive geometrical landmarks from the segments, which we represent as characteristic functions. We assume pairs (τ_j, ρ_j), $j = 1, \ldots, L$ for the segments of the template and reference image. Our procedure is identical for all pairs (τ_j, ρ_j) and therefore we describe it only for one particular pair and omit the index j. Based on moments, we compute centroids c and principal axes v^k [1]. Note that the main axes transformation theorem gives $MV = V\Sigma$, where M is essentially the second order moment matrix, $\Sigma = \operatorname{diag}(\sigma_k^2, k = 1, \ldots, d)$ with $\sigma_j \geq \sigma_{j+1}$ an ordered diagonal matrix of eigenvalues and $V = (v^k, k = 1, \ldots, d)$ the corresponding normalized eigendirection matrix with $\det V = 1$. Besides to the centroids c, we derive potentially $2d$ additional landmarks per segment: $c \pm \sigma_k v^k$, $k = 1, \ldots, d$. However, the computation of the axes is only robust, if the segment has clear orientation, i.e. $\sigma_j \gg \sigma_{j+1}$ for all j. We therefore use the landmarks $c \pm \sigma_k v^k$ only in the latter case

(Fig. 1). For finding correspondences of the additional landmarks based on the principal axes, we assume that after the initial phase (centroids alignment), the main axes of τ and ρ are close to each other. Here we sketch the situation for $d = 2$; the 3D case is along the same lines. Without loss of generality we choose r_A as the first landmark for the principal axes of ρ. Our ordering of the additional landmark is r_A, r_B, r_C, r_D and is motivated by a right handed coordinate system. From the angles $\angle r_A c t_a$ and $\angle r_A c t_b$, we conclude that t_a and not t_b corresponds to r_A. With this ordering the list of landmarks for τ is thus t_a, t_b, t_c, t_d (Fig. 1). We extend the centroid feature list by adding these points.

2.3   Registration Scheme

Following classical landmark registration [1], in the first phase we compute y^C as the minimizer of Equation. (1) with $D = 0$, $P = 0$, $S(y) = S(y; \gamma, \mathbb{R}^d)$ and $C(y) = \sum_{j=1}^{L} \| y(r_j) - t_j \|$. Next we compute y^{LM} as minimizer of the same functional, where now the extended feature list derived from the pre-aligned images is used. Note that y^C is calculated as an intermediate step to find corresponding landmarks as described in Sec. 2.2, but is discarded as soon as y^{LM} is calculated in the second phase. The intensity based registration performed in the third phase is the minimization of Eq. (1) with $S(y) = \alpha \cdot S(y - y^{LM}; \gamma, \Omega)$ and $C = 0$. D and P are chosen application specific (Sec. 2.4). Note that the similarity measure is no longer zero and thus we need to introduce a balancing parameter α. Moreover, we only regularize the difference to the preregistration, as this difference can be interpreted as an update of y^{LM}. We restrict the regularization to Ω with Dirichlet boundary condition.

2.4   Application specific parametrization

While the general approach is clearly outlined, it remains to discuss the application depending parametrization and feature extraction. In this paper we focus on the 3D thorax data described in Section 2.5. The output of the TS contains various segments that are not usable in our registration procedure. We exclude all segments that are not fully contained in both images. For the first phase, we bypass the problem of large deformations through breathing motion inside the chest and abdomen by restricting the

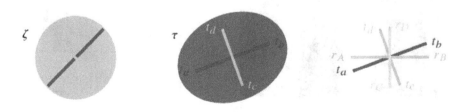

Fig. 1. Visualization of extraction and assignment of additional features. From left to right (main axis: strong, second axis: light): Segment ζ with $\sigma_1 \approx \sigma_2$ (additional features are discarded); segment τ with $\sigma_1 \gg \sigma_2$ and its principal axes; principal axes of τ, ρ after aligning the centroids.

set of centroids to those of rigid structures such as bones. Some segments are visualized in Fig. 2. For the principal axes in the second phase, we only use segments of rigid structures with clear orientation, i.e. $\log_2(\sigma_j/\sigma_{j+1}) > \text{tol}$, where tol $= 1/3$ is suggested. As similarity measure in the third phase we focus on the classical sum of squared differences restricted to a set $W \subset \Omega$

$$SSD(y;T,R,W) := 1/2 \cdot \|T[y] - R\|^2_{L^2(W)} \tag{3}$$

In particular, we define interior regions of the thorax $\Sigma_T, \Sigma_R \subset \Omega$ using the convex hull of centroids of bone structures (even if they may not be fully contained in both images). Let $\chi_{\Sigma_T}, \chi_{\Sigma_R}$ denote the characteristic functions on these. We assume that after preregistration, the exterior and interior regions roughly align, i.e $\chi_{\Sigma_T}[y^{LM}] \approx \chi_{\Sigma_R}$, but due to the lung motion not necessarily $T[y^{LM}] \approx R$ in the interior region. Therefore, we suggest the similarity measure $D(T[y], R) := SSD(y;T, R, \Sigma_R \cap y(\Sigma_T))$, to get a better alignment in the interior region. At the same time we want to keep the alignment of the exterior regions and thus use the penalty $P(y) := \beta \cdot SSD(y; \chi_{\Sigma_T}, \chi_{\Sigma_R}, \Omega)$ with $\beta \in \mathbb{R}_{\geq 0}$.

2.5 Data set

We show results for the publicly available data set [8], which consists of 3D HRCT thorax images with an inspiration and an expiration scan for each subject. We arbitrarily pick case 021 from the test data set and perform the registration between expiration (reference) and inspiration (template). The size of the data is $192 \times 192 \times 208$ voxel each. The TS is used for segmentation followed by the filtering outlined in Sec. 2.4. We obtain eleven bone segments, of which only five provide valid information about the principal axes (Fig. 2). The data set comes with two major challenges, namely large lung motion and a cropped expiration scan.

2.6 Evaluation Measures and Computational Details

The proposed method is evaluated using dice scores for corresponding segments (τ_j, ρ_j) and the energy of the difference image restricted to the thorax region in the reference

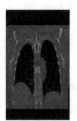 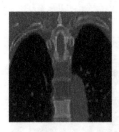 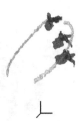 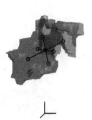

Fig. 2. Visualization of the inspriration scan [8] and bone segments from the TS. From left to right: Coronal slice overlayed with segments; details; 3D view of selected segments (blue and green indicate that only centroids or both, centroids and principal axes are used, respectively); a detailed segment with its centroid and principal axes.

Tab. 1. Mean dices of segments and distances (SSD) in the exterior ($\Gamma \setminus \Sigma_R$) and interior ($\Sigma_R$) of the thorax region ($\Gamma$) before and after registration.

	mean dice of segments in		dist [$\cdot 10^6$] in		
	$\Gamma \setminus \Sigma_R$	Σ_R	$\Gamma \setminus \Sigma_R$	Σ_R	Γ
without registration	0.24	0.51	1.2	5.6	6.9
after preregistration	0.64	0.32	2.0	4.4	6.6
after full registration	0.58	0.61	0.5	4.3	4.9

image $\Gamma \subset \Omega$ or some subset of Γ

$$\mathrm{dice}_j(y) := 2|\tau_j[y] \cap \rho_j|/(|\tau_j[y]| + |\rho_j|) \quad \mathrm{dist}(y) := SSD(y, T, R, \Gamma) \qquad (4)$$

In the implementation we use a multilevel approach similar to [4]. The data is interpolated on a 64x64x64 grid, therefore the coarsest level is $l_{\min} = 3$ and the finest level is $l_{\max} = 6$. We set the parameters $\alpha = 500$, $\beta = 10^3$. For the optimization we use a Gauss-Newton scheme and conjugate gradient as solver. All calculations are performed on MATLAB R2022b. Furthermore the FAIR package as described in [7] is used.

3 Results

Next we present numerical results for the 3D thorax data described in Sec. 2.5. Using the parameters from Sec. 2.6 the registration procedure yields transformations y^{LM} and y after preregistration and full registration, respectively. Table 1 summarizes the mean dices of the segments in the interior region $\Sigma_R \subset \Gamma$ and the exterior region $\Gamma \setminus \Sigma_R$ of the thorax region Γ. Additionally the distances in these parts are shown for the different phases of the registration. For the mean dice, we observe that after preregistration it improves considerably on the exterior, whereas it deteriorates in the interior. The latter is due to lung motion and the distribution of landmarks. Therefore, the third phase of our approach focusses on the interior region by adapting the similarity measure and adding a region specific penalty, tolerating a small degradation on the exterior region (Tab. 1). For the distances, we observe an increase on the exterior after preregistration. This is to be expected as this step does not include intensity information. However, the overall approach improves particularly the distance on the thorax region Γ (Tab. 1 and Fig. 3).

4 Discussion

We propose a new segmentation inspired registration procedure. From the automatically derived segments, we extract geometrical features such as centroids and principal axes. These features serve as input for a two-phase landmark based preregistration. Using sensible filtering, the preregistration comprises a rough alignment based on segments of bones in phase one and an extension to principal axes type features in phase two. With this approach, we overcome the difficulty of 3D landmark extraction and in addition provide an outstanding starting value for an intensity based third registration phase.

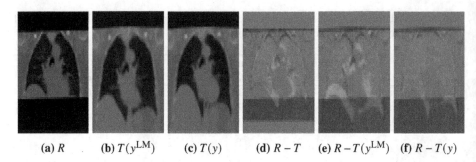

(a) R (b) $T(y^{LM})$ (c) $T(y)$ (d) $R - T$ (e) $R - T(y^{LM})$ (f) $R - T(y)$

Fig. 3. Exemplary selected coronal slices of the 3D thorax images: expiration scan (R); transformed inspiration scan landmark based $T(y^{LM})$ and final result $T(y)$; and corresponding difference images.

Similarly to [3], we use a vector field regularization energy for all phases. This energy is based on divergence and curl and enables a coupling of all components of the vector field. Note that [3] considers only 2D registration in which the curl is simply a scalar, while we extend to 3D, where the curl becomes a vector field.

A proof of concept is given for challenging 3D thorax data, which show a variety of difficulties including large lung motion and cropped images. We demonstrate that the scheme can easily be adapted to cover also this application, produces impressive results, and reveals the advantages of a hybrid, landmark and intensity based, registration.

In future work, we perform a more comprehensive evaluation on data from different applications. Moreover, we also compare the approach to state-of-the-art alternatives.

References

1. Modersitzki J. Numerical Methods for Image Registration. New York: Oxford University Press, 2004.
2. Wasserthal J, Breit HC, Meyer MT, Pradella M, Hinck D, Sauter AW et al. TotalSegmentator: Robust segmentation of 104 anatomic structures in CT images. Radiol: Artifl Intell. 2023;5(5).
3. Sorzano COS, Thévenaz P, Unser M. Elastic registration of biological images using vector-spline regularization. IEEE Trans Biomedi Engin. 2005;52(4):652–63.
4. Haber E, Heldmann S, Modersitzki J. A scale-space approach to landmark constrained image registration. Proceedings of the Second International Conference on Scale Space Methods and Variational Methods in Computer Vision (SSVM). Springer LNCS, 2009:1–12.
5. Amodei L, Benbourhim M. A vector spline approximation. J Approx Theory. 1991;67(1):51–79.
6. Dodu F, Rabut C. Vectorial interpolation using radial-basis-like functions. Comput & Math Appl. 2002;43(3-5):393–411.
7. Modersitzki J. FAIR: Flexible Algorithms for Image Registration. SIAM, 2009.
8. Hering A, Murphy K, Ginneken B. Lean2Regchallenge: CT lung registration-training data [data set]. 2020.

Exploring Epipolar Consistency Conditions

Mareike Thies[1], Fabian Wagner[1], Mingxuan Gu[1], Siyuan Mei[1], Yixing Huang[1],
Sabrina Pechmann[2], Oliver Aust[3], Daniela Weidner[3], Georgiana Neag[3],
Stefan Uderhardt[3], Georg Schett[3], Silke Christiansen[2,4], Andreas Maier[1]

[1]Pattern Recognition Lab, FAU Erlangen-Nürnberg
[2]Fraunhofer Institute for Ceramic Technologies and Systems IKTS, Forchheim
[3]Department of Rheumatology and Immunology, FAU Erlangen-Nürnberg
[4]Physics Department, Freie Universität Berlin
mareike.thies@fau.de

Abstract. Intravital X-ray microscopy (XRM) in preclinical mouse models is of vital importance for the identification of microscopic structural pathological changes in the bone which are characteristic of osteoporosis. The complexity of this method stems from the requirement for high-quality 3D reconstructions of the murine bones. However, respiratory motion and muscle relaxation lead to inconsistencies in the projection data which result in artifacts in uncompensated reconstructions. Motion compensation using epipolar consistency conditions (ECC) has previously shown good performance in clinical CT settings. Here, we explore whether such algorithms are suitable for correcting motion-corrupted XRM data. Different rigid motion patterns are simulated and the quality of the motion-compensated reconstructions is assessed. The method is able to restore microscopic features for out-of-plane motion, but artifacts remain for more realistic motion patterns including all six degrees of freedom of rigid motion. Therefore, ECC is valuable for the initial alignment of the projection data followed by further fine-tuning of motion parameters using a reconstruction-based method.

1 Introduction

Computed tomography (CT) imaging aids the reconstruction of internal structures of an object or organism by measuring X-ray projection images from multiple angles. When applied to living animals or humans, stillness of the subject is required throughout the scan as reconstruction algorithms rely on a highly accurate knowledge of the geometry between object, source, and detector pixels. This assumption cannot always be fulfilled due to inevitable motion in living organisms including cardio-respiratory motion or muscle relaxation.

The X-ray microscope (XRM) that was utilized in this study is a specialized cone-beam CT scanner with a resolution down to 500 nm. Thus far, such scanners have mainly been used to investigate static samples in materials science, geoscience, or life science [1]. Recently, X-ray microscopy has garnered interest from the biomedical research field. The scope of our work is to improve the understanding of bone remodelling diseases like osteoporosis, at a high-resolution microscopic level, with the aid of XRM imaging of living mice. Whilst it is widely accepted that osteoporosis not only affects macroscopic parameters such as bone mass but also microscopic bone geometry, the dynamics of these changes from disease onset until diagnosis remain unclear to date [2]. One central reason for this is the lack of longitudinal studies which jointly observe macroscopic and microscopic changes of bone structures in the same animal. With its non-invasive measurement procedure, high contrast between bone and soft tissue, and excellent resolution, XRM constitutes the ideal technology to enable such intravital longitudinal studies [3]. However, this requires imaging living animals and, consequently, the problem of subject motion has to be dealt with.

As demonstrated in [4], motion from the mice's respiration and muscle relaxation can severely degrade the reconstructed XRM images up to a point where they become unusable for the attempted downstream tasks. There exists a plethora of works targeting rigid motion compensation in clinical settings [5–8]. However, it is unclear how these algorithms translate to the special case of in-vivo XRM. As a first step, in this study, we investigate the applicability of epipolar consistency conditions (ECC) for motion compensation in XRM measurements of living mice. ECC are well-studied for artifact reduction in clinical cone-beam CT and have proven of great use for motion compensation in interventional C-arm head CT data [6, 9] or empirical scatter and over-exposure correction [10, 11]. Compared to such clinical use cases, the described XRM setting differs in a multitude of aspects, such as the scanner hardware, imaging protocols, geometry settings, and the structural properties of the object being scanned. We investigate the potential and limits of motion compensation with ECC for the given use case to assess whether it can pave the way toward high resolution in-vivo measurements for preclinical investigations of osteoporosis in a mouse model.

2   Materials and methods

2.1   Epipolar consistency conditions

The key idea of ECC for motion compensation is to exploit the redundancy in the projection data of a scan. As all acquired detector signals are projections of the same object under different geometries, they share common information which is related by the geometry settings. Motion introduces a mismatch in geometry and hence reduces the consistency in the data. Minimizing the inconsistency with respect to the geometry is a way to recover the mismatch introduced by subject motion. Aichert et al. [5] formally introduced ECC for transmissive radiation like X-rays and a way to apply them to cone-beam CT systems. The inconsistency between two corresponding epipolar lines l_0 and l_1 in the cone-beam case is computed via

$$\Delta M = \frac{d}{dt}\rho_{I_0}(l_0) - \frac{d}{dt}\rho_{I_1}(l_1) \tag{1}$$

where $\frac{d}{dt}\rho_I$ refers to the derivative of the 2D Radon transform of projection image I in t direction, i.e., line distance to the image origin. In the ideal, motion-free case, this inconsistency is minimal for all pairs of epipolar lines. Hence, the motion compensation target function is the sum of all pairwise inconsistencies ΔM over all projection images in a scan and over all corresponding epipolar lines per pair. We refer the reader to the work of Aichert et al. [5] for a more in-depth explanation of ECC. The ECC target function is implemented based on the openly available source code by Aichert et al. (`https://github.com/aaichert/EpipolarConsistency`), but we develop additional Python bindings for the original code base written in C++. Since Python has evolved to one of the most common coding languages for research in medical image processing, we make our bindings available to the community as a prebuilt, ready-to-use Python package at `https://github.com/mareikethies/epipolar_consistency_python`.

2.2 Motion simulation

As XRM data of living mice are not currently available, we resorted to XRM measurements of an ex-vivo murine tibia sample. The scan has $N = 1601$ projection images acquired on a short scan trajectory which we downsampled by a factor of 4 for shorter run-time resulting in a size of 409×509 pixels with a pixel size of $5.6\,\mu m$. Motion was artificially simulated by multiplying rigid transformation matrices T_i to the projection matrices P_i with $i = 1, \ldots, N$. The idea is to find rigid transformations T_i^* which recover the original, correct projection matrices from the manipulated ones (Fig. 1)

$$P_i^{\text{recovered}} = P_i^{\text{motion}} T_i^* = P_i^{\text{original}} T_i T_i^* \qquad (2)$$

Each of the rigid transformations has six degrees of freedom (3D rotation (r_x, r_y, r_z) and 3D translation (t_x, t_y, t_z)). Assuming that the motion of all projection images is independent, the problem has $6N$ degrees of freedom. Similar to prior work [9], we instead use a spline-based representation to enforce smoothness of the motion throughout the scan and reduce the dimensionality during optimization. A separate Akima-spline for each of the six motion parameters fits a smooth curve through specified nodes and reduces the number of free parameters from $6N$ to $6M$ where $M < N$ is the number of nodes for the spline. Motion simulation is performed using splines with $M = 9$ nodes and a maximum perturbation of $\pm 50\,\mu m$ and $\pm 1°$ for translation and rotation.

2.3 Optimization details

We minimize the projection-wise inconsistency quantified by ECC subject to the node values of the spline representations for the rigid transformation parameters. Three different scenarios are investigated relative to the plane spanned by the source positions during

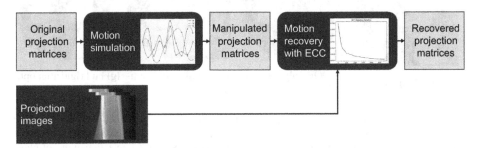

Fig. 1. The original projection matrices are first manipulated and then recovered by minimizing the inconsistency in the projection images measured by ECC.

the scan: Optimization of (1) only out-of-plane parameters (t_z, r_x, r_y), (2) only in-plane parameters (t_x, t_y, r_z), and (3) all six parameters of rigid transformations. As suggested in the seminal work [5], gradient-free optimization is performed using an adaptive Nelder-Mead downhill simplex optimizer [12] for a maximum of 1000 iterations for scenario (1) and (2) and 2000 in scenario (3). All free parameters are initialized as zero and bounds are provided according to the maximum motion added during simulation. To assess the ability of the algorithm to recover the introduced motion independent of the modelling capacity of the spline, motion recovery is performed with a spline of the same type and with identical node positions as during motion simulation.

3 Results

Reconstructions are performed by an FDK algorithm [13] using the downsampled projection images and the original, manipulated or recovered projection matrices. Figure 2 shows reconstruction results of the three investigated scenarios. The internal structure of the bone can only be recovered if just out-of-plane motion is considered (Fig. 2e). For the other two cases with in-plane motion only and full rigid transformations, artifacts remain. Nevertheless, the general shape of the bone is improved. These findings are also represented quantitatively in Table 1. Mean-squared error (MSE) and structural

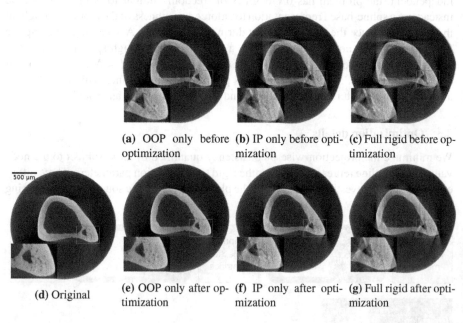

(a) OOP only before optimization (b) IP only before optimization (c) Full rigid before optimization

(d) Original (e) OOP only after optimization (f) IP only after optimization (g) Full rigid after optimization

Fig. 2. Reconstruction results before (upper row) and after motion compensation (lower row). We show an off-center slice because effects of rotation do not exhibit themselves well in the center slice. (d) is the ground truth reconstruction, (a) and (e) correspond to optimization of out-of-plane (OOP) parameters only, (b) and (f) correspond to optimization of in-plane (IP) parameters only, and (c) and (g) correspond to a full rigid optimization.

Tab. 1. The error in reconstruction domain is measured by MSE and SSIM to the ground truth reconstruction. The L_1 error quantifies the mean absolute error over all projection images for the considered transformation parameters. All values are presented as *before → after optimization.*

	out-of-plane only	in-plane only	rigid complete
# parameters	27	27	54
MSE [$*10^{-8}$]	0.59 → 0.17	3.53 → 1.49	3.64 → 1.93
SSIM	0.91 → 0.94	0.80 → 0.87	0.80 → 0.84
L1 error t_x [µm]	x	20.95 → 12.37	20.95 → 15.23
L1 error t_y [µm]	x	23.98 → 4.83	23.98 → 8.91
L1 error t_z [µm]	21.19 → 12.67	x	21.19 → 7.92
L1 error r_x [deg]	0.41 → 0.18	x	0.41 → 0.19
L1 error r_y [deg]	0.33 → 0.10	x	0.33 → 0.19
L1 error r_z [deg]	x	0.44 → 0.43	0.44 → 0.41

similarity (SSIM) are improved in each case, but very high agreement with the ground truth reconstruction can only be achieved in the simplified setup of just out-of-plane motion. The error of transformation parameters is reduced in all cases but the reduction is only marginal for rotations in z.

4 Discussion

The results imply that it is generally feasible to improve the reconstruction quality of motion-corrupted XRM scans using ECC-based optimization. The overall bone shape is improved in the motion compensated reconstructions and, for the case of just out-of-plane parameters, even the small structures inside the bone are recovered. For in-plane and full rigid motion, restoring the small-scale structures within the bone has shown to be difficult. It is apparent that the algorithm cannot compensate all six motion types with the same accuracy, especially rotation around z is only poorly recovered. This can be explained as it occurs within the epipolar planes and, therefore, does not have a large influence on the target function. Also, the considered bone is highly symmetric regarding rotation around its long axis which further complicates the formulation of a discriminative target function. Additionally, subject motion is not the only factor influencing the ECC target function. Other physical phenomena such as noise, scatter or beam hardening can also introduce mismatch between projection images and disturb the motion correction when close to the optimal solution. We further acknowledge that by using identical node positions between motion simulation and recovery, we do not mimic a realistic setup. But as the algorithm does not yield satisfactory results for all parameters in this simplified scenario, we did not include results of more complicated settings. Further, the presented algorithm will experience major performance drops as soon as the projections are laterally truncated, i.e., the object does not fully fit into the field-of-view. The ECC target function compares plane integrals through the measured object evaluated in different projection images. If projection images are truncated, the integral can only be evaluated in the non-truncated region which introduces an error and makes the ECC target function hardly usable for motion compensation. When imaging at smaller pixel sizes or larger anatomical regions of the tibia such as its proximal end (knee region), truncation might occur due to the limited field-of-view of the XRM scanner.

In conclusion, while ECC is valuable for a first alignment of motion corrupted data, reconstruction-based methods [7] seem to be more suitable for motion compensation in in-vivo XRM studies because they do not depend on non-truncated projection images and are more sensitive to changes in all six parameters of rigid motion.

Acknowledgement. The research leading to these results has received funding from the European Research Council (ERC) under the European Union's Horizon 2020 research and innovation program (ERC Grant No. 810316). The authors gratefully acknowledge the HPC resources provided by NHR@FAU. The hardware is funded by the German Research Foundation (DFG).

References

1. Jacobsen C. X-ray Microscopy. (Advances in Microscopy and Microanalysis). Cambridge University Press, 2019.
2. Mader KS, Schneider P, Müller R, Stampanoni M. A quantitative framework for the 3D characterization of the osteocyte lacunar system. Bone. 2013;57(1):142–54.
3. Wagner F, Thies M, Karolczak M, Pechmann S, Huang Y, Gu M et al. Monte Carlo dose simulation for In-vivo X-ray nanoscopy. Proc BVM. 2022:107–12.
4. Mill L, Bier B, Syben C, Kling L, Klingberg A, Christiansen S et al. Towards In-Vivo X-Ray nanoscopy: the effect of motion on image quality. Proc BVM. 2018:115–20.
5. Aichert A, Berger M, Wang J, Maass N, Doerfler A, Hornegger J et al. Epipolar consistency in transmission imaging. IEEE Trans Med Imaging. 2015;34(11):2205–19.
6. Frysch R, Rose G. Rigid motion compensation in interventional C-arm CT using consistency measure on projection data. Proc MICCAI. 2015:298–306.
7. Sisniega A, Stayman JW, Yorkston J, Siewerdsen JH, Zbijewski W. Motion compensation in extremity cone-beam CT using a penalized image sharpness criterion. Phys Med Biol. 2017;62(9):3712–34.
8. Thies M, Wagner F, Maul N, Folle L, Meier M, Rohleder M et al. Gradient-based geometry learning for fan-beam CT reconstruction. Phys Med Biol. 2023;68(20):205004.
9. Preuhs A, Ravikumar N, Manhart M, Stimpel B, Hoppe E, Syben C et al. Maximum likelihood estimation of head motion using epipolar consistency. Proc BVM. 2019:134–9.
10. Hoffmann M, Würfl T, Maaß N, Dennerlein F, Aichert A, Maier AK. Empirical scatter correction using the epipolar consistency condition. Proc CT-meeting. 2018:193–7.
11. Preuhs A, Berger M, Xia Y, Maier A, Hornegger J, Fahrig R. Over-exposure correction in CT using optimization-based multiple cylinder fitting. Proc BVM. 2015:35–40.
12. Gao F, Han L. Implementing the Nelder-Mead simplex algorithm with adaptive parameters. Comput Optim Appl. 2012;51(1):259–77.
13. Thies M, Wagner F, Huang Y, Gu M, Kling L, Pechmann S et al. Calibration by differentiation–Self-supervised calibration for X-ray microscopy using a differentiable cone-beam reconstruction operator. J Microsc. 2022;287(2):81–92.

Abstract: Enabling Geometry Aware Learning Through Differentiable Epipolar View Translation

Maximilian Rohleder[1,2], Charlotte Pradel[1], Fabian Wagner[1], Mareike Thies[1], Noah Maul[1,2], Felix Denzinger[1,2], Andreas Maier[1], Bjoern Kreher[2],

[1]Friedrich-Alexander-University, Erlangen-Nürnberg, Germany
[2]Siemens Healthineers AG, Erlangen, Germany
Maxi.Rohleder@fau.de

Epipolar geometry is exploited in several applications in the field of Cone-Beam Computed Tomography (CBCT) imaging. By leveraging consistency conditions between multiple views of the same scene, motion artifacts can be minimized, the effects of beam hardening can be reduced, and segmentation masks can be refined. So far, these conditions have been formulated as optimization criteria to be minimized in post-processing. In this work, we explore the idea of enabling deep learning models to access the known geometrical relations between views in order to improve the prediction. The implicit 3D information contained in the relative pose between views can potentially enhance various projection domain algorithms such as segmentation, detection, or inpainting. Based on this hypothesis, we introduce a differentiable feature translation operator, which uses available projection matrices to calculate and integrate over the epipolar line in a second view. After geometrically translating all channels of a layer's output feature map, we concatenate these activations to a second instance of the same architecture processing a second view of the same 3D scene. As an example application, we evaluate the effects of this operation on the task of projection domain metal segmentation. By re-sampling a stack of projections into orthogonal view pairs, we segment each projection image jointly with a second view acquired 90° apart. The comparison with an equivalent single-view segmentation model reveals an improved segmentation performance of 0.95 over 0.91 measured by the dice coefficient. By providing an implementation of this operator as an open-access differentiable layer, we seek to enable future research [1].

References

1. Rohleder M, Pradel C, Wagner F, Thies M, Maul N, Denzinger F et al. Enabling Geometry Aware Learning Through Differentiable Epipolar View Translation. Proc MICCAI. 2023:57–65.

Abstract: Realistic Collimated X-ray Image Simulation Pipeline

Benjamin El-Zein[1], Dominik Eckert[2], Thomas Weber[2], Maximilian Rohleder[1], Ludwig Ritschl[2], Steffen Kappler[2], Andreas Maier[1]

[1]Pattern Recognition Lab, Friedrich-Alexander University, Erlangen-Nuremberg, Germany
[2]Siemens Healthineers, Forchheim, Germany
benjamin.el-zein@fau.de

Collimator detection in X-ray systems has long posed a formidable challenge, particularly when information about the detector's position relative to the source is either unreliable or completely unavailable. In this paper [1], we introduce a physically motivated image processing pipeline designed to simulate the intricate characteristics of collimator shadows in X-ray images. The primary objective of this pipeline is to address the scarcity of training data for deep neural networks, which are increasingly promising for collimator detection. By applying the pipeline to deep networks initially limited by small datasets, our approach equips them with the necessary information to learn and generalize effectively. Our pipeline is a comprehensive solution that leverages several key components to generate realistic collimator images. Employing randomized labels to describe collimator shapes and their respective locations ensures diversity and representativeness. In addition, we integrate a convolution kernel based scattered radiation simulation mechanism, which is a crucial factor in real-world X-ray imaging. To complete the simulation process, we introduce Poisson noise to replicate the inherent characteristics of collimator shadows in X-ray images. Comparing the simulated data with real collimator shadows demonstrates the authenticity of our approach and its potential to bridge the gap between synthetic and real-world data. Moreover, incorporating simulated data into our deep learning framework not only serves as a valid substitute for real collimators but also significantly improves generalization in real-world applications, holding great promise for the field of collimator detection. The concepts and information presented in this paper are based on research and are not commercially available.

References

1. El-Zein B, Eckert D, Weber T, Rohleder M, Ritschl L, Kappler S et al. Realistic collimated X-ray image simulation pipeline. Proc MICCAI 2023. Springer Nature. 2023.

Abstract: RecycleNet
Latent Feature Recycling Leads to Iterative Decision Refinement

Gregor Koehler[1,2], Tassilo Wald[1,3], Constantin Ulrich[1,4], David Zimmerer[1,3],
Paul F. Jaeger[3,5], Jörg K.H. Franke[7], Simon Kohl[8], Fabian Isensee[1,3,6],
Klaus H. Maier-Hein[1,3,4,9]

[1]German Cancer Research Center (DKFZ) Heidelberg, Division of Medical Image Computing,
Germany
[2]Helmholtz Information and Data Science School for Health, Karlsruhe/Heidelberg, Germany
[3]Helmholtz Imaging, DKFZ
[4]National Center for Tumor Diseases (NCT), NCT Heidelberg, a partnership between DKFZ and
University Medical Center Heidelberg
[5]Interactive Machine Learning Group, DKFZ
[6]Applied Computer Vision Lab, DKFZ
[7]Machine Learning Lab, University of Freiburg, Freiburg, Germany
[8]Latent Labs (latentlabs.com), London, UK
[9]Pattern Analysis and Learning Group, Heidelberg University Hospital, Heidelberg, Germany
g.koehler@dkfz.de

Abstract

Despite the remarkable success of deep learning systems over the last decade, a key
difference still remains between neural network and human decision-making: As humans, we can not only form a decision on the spot, but also ponder, revisiting an initial
guess from different angles, distilling relevant information, arriving at a better decision.
Here, we propose RecycleNet, a latent feature recycling method, instilling the ponder-
ing capability for neural networks to refine initial decisions over a number of recycling
steps, where outputs are fed back into earlier network layers in an iterative fashion. This
approach makes minimal assumptions about the neural network architecture and thus
can be implemented in a wide variety of contexts. Using medical image segmentation as
the evaluation environment, we show that latent feature recycling enables the network
to iteratively refine initial predictions even beyond the iterations seen during training,
converging towards an improved decision. We evaluate this across a variety of segmentation benchmarks and show consistent improvements even compared with top-performing
segmentation methods. This allows trading increased computation time for improved
performance, which can be beneficial, especially for safety-critical applications [1].

References

1. Koehler G, Wald T, Ulrich C, Zimmerer D, Jaeger PF, Franke JKH et al. RecycleNet:
   Latent Feature Recycling Leads to Iterative Decision Refinement. 2024 Winter Conference
   on Applications of Computer Vision (WACV). 2024.

© Der/die Autor(en), exklusiv lizenziert an
Springer Fachmedien Wiesbaden GmbH, ein Teil von Springer Nature 2024
A. Maier et al. (Hrsg.), *Bildverarbeitung für die Medizin 2024*,
Informatik aktuell, https://doi.org/10.1007/978-3-658-44037-4_63

Self-supervised Vessel Segmentation from X-ray Images using Digitally Reconstructed Radiographs

Zichen Zhang[1], Baochang Zhang[1,2], Mohammad F. Azampour[1],
Shahrooz Faghihroohi[1], Agnieszka Tomczak[1,2], Heribert Schunkert[2], Nassir Navab[1]

[1]Computer Aided Medical Procedures, Technical University of Munich, Munich, Germany
[2]German Heart Center Munich, Munich, Germany
baochang.zhang@tum.de

Abstract. Coronary artery segmentation on angiograms can be beneficial in the diagnosis and treatment of coronary artery diseases. In this paper, we propose a self-supervised vessel segmentation framework that incorporates the knowledge from generated digitally reconstructed radiographs(DRRs) to perform vessel segmentation on angiographic images without manual annotations. The framework is built based on domain randomization, adversarial learning, and self-supervised learning. Domain randomization and adversarial learning are able to effectively reduce the domain gaps between DRRs and angiograms, whereas self-supervised learning enables the network to learn photometric invariant and geometric equivariant features for angiographic images. The experimental results demonstrate that we achieve a better performance compared with the state-of-the-art methods.

1 Introduction

Coronary segmentation from X-ray images is an essential yet challenging task in medical imaging due to its significance in diagnosing and treatment planning for cardiovascular diseases. This difficulty arises from the intricate and small anatomy of the coronary arteries, low contrast and noise in X-ray images, variability among patients, and the need to balance radiation exposure.

Supervised learning-based methods [1] require labor-intensive manual annotations, which are often error-prone and subjective. Besides, they face the challenge of poor generalization, as models trained on specific datasets may struggle to perform effectively on new or unseen data. In recent years, some self-supervised methods have been proposed to tackle this task [2–4]. These approaches use mathematically generated vessel-shaped fractals to synthesize angiogram-like images to perform unsupervised domain adaptation. However, there still is a large morphological gap between the generated fractals and real vascular structures, which limits the vessel segmentation performance.

In this work, the main contributions are as follows:

- To our knowledge, we are the first to introduce DRRs to achieve better vessel segmentation performance without the need for angiographic image annotations.
- A detailed ablation study is conducted to explore the effectiveness of domain randomization, adversarial learning, and self-supervised learning for vessel segmentation.

© Der/die Autor(en), exklusiv lizenziert an
Springer Fachmedien Wiesbaden GmbH, ein Teil von Springer Nature 2024
A. Maier et al. (Hrsg.), *Bildverarbeitung für die Medizin 2024*,
Informatik aktuell, https://doi.org/10.1007/978-3-658-44037-4_64

- The proposed method reasonably leverages these techniques to deliver superior segmentation results compared to other state-of-the-art approaches.

2 Materials and methods

2.1 Dataset

We regard the DRR dataset and the angiographic image dataset as the source domain and the target domain respectively.

For DRR dataset, it contains 25337 coronary DRR samples which are generated using Diff-DeepDRR [5] based on the public ASOCA dataset [6, 7]. Here, 12 standard views are referenced to generate the DRR images and corresponding masks both in a resolution of 512×512.

For the angiographic image dataset, we use the public XCAD dataset [2], which contains a training set of 1621 unannotated coronary angiography images and a testing set of 126 independent angiographic images with vessel annotations. Each image in XCAD has a resolution of 512×512 pixels with one channel.

2.2 Framework details

2.2.1 Framework overview. We propose a self-supervised end-to-end framework for vessel segmentation (Fig. 1). It involves three parts: 1) domain randomization, 2) adversarial learning, 3) self-supervised learning. Domain randomization is used to reduce the domain gaps between DRRs and angiograms. Adversarial learning is employed to encourage feature-level alignment and enable the model to learn domain-invariant features. Meanwhile, the framework enforces the network to output consistent predictions under random perturbations via self-supervised learning.

2.2.2 Domain randomization. Various image transforms are utilized for domain randomization, including rotation, flipping, cropping, Gaussian noise, color jitter, gamma transform, and Fourier-based augmentation. For Fourier-based augmentation [8], Fourier Transform is applied on both the source and target images. Then, the central regions of the source images' amplitude maps are replaced by those of the target images' amplitude maps, thus the source images have a similar style to the target images.

Taking advantage of DRR generation, DRR-based vessel supervised learning is performed using U-Net [9] as the segmentation network S with a loss function L_{seg}, which is defined as

$$L_{seg} = L_{dice} + \lambda_1 L_{bce} + \lambda_2 L_{cldice} \tag{1}$$

where L_{dice}, L_{bce} and L_{cldice} are Dice loss [10], Binary Cross Entropy loss, and clDice loss [11] respectively. We set λ_1 and λ_2 to 0.5.

2.2.3   Adversarial learning. Domain alignment is encouraged by applying adversarial learning to the features produced by the encoder S_{en} of the segmentation network S. A discriminator D with three convolutional layers, similar to the one used in PatchGAN [12], is used to distinguish the source features and the target features. Least-square loss function [13] is employed as the adversarial loss for S_{en} and is formulated as

$$L_{adv}(S_{en}) = \lambda_S E_{x_t} \left[(D(S_{en}(x_t)) - l_s)^2 \right] \tag{2}$$

where x_t are target domain images and λ_S is set to 0.001. We denote source label and target label as l_s and l_t. Meanwhile, the adversarial loss for D is formulated as

$$L_{adv}(D) = \lambda_D E_{x_t} \left[(D(S_{en}(x_t)) - l_t)^2 \right] + \lambda_D E_{x_s} \left[(D(S_{en}(x_s)) - l_s)^2 \right] \tag{3}$$

where x_s are source domain images and λ_D is set to 0.5.

2.2.4   Self-supervised learning. The network is regularized to have consistent predictions under augmentations, in which it can learn robust features for segmentation [14]. These augmentations can be regarded as perturbations, and they are basically the same as those in domain randomization except for Fourier-based augmentation (Sec. 2.2.2). The angiograms are first forwarded to the segmentation model to obtain the segmentations. Then, the angiograms and the segmentations are perturbed with the augmentations, and the perturbed angiograms are fed to the segmentation model to produce the corresponding segmentation masks. Finally, a consistency loss L_{con} based on binary cross entropy is defined between these segmentation masks and the perturbed segmentation results of the original angiograms as pseudo masks to ensure the prediction consistency.

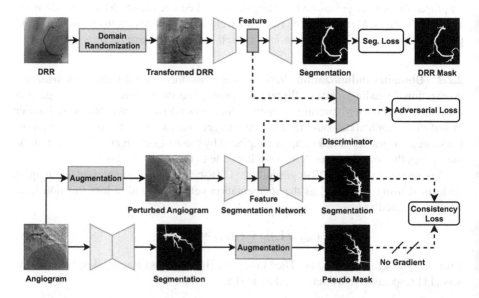

Fig. 1. An overview of the proposed method, it mainly consists of domain randomization, DRR-based supervised learning, adversarial learning, and self-supervised learning.

Tab. 1. Performance comparison between different methods on XCAD, where the subscripts of the values are the standard deviations. The SSVS results [2] are produced using the released code.

Method	Jaccard	Dice	Acc.	Sen.	Spe.	Pre.
SSVS [2]	0.401 ± 0.065	0.569 ± 0.068	0.948 ± 0.009	0.623 ± 0.092	0.968 ± 0.007	0.538 ± 0.097
DARL [3]	0.471 ± 0.076	0.636 ± 0.072	0.962 ± 0.010	0.597 ± 0.090	0.985 ± 0.007	0.701 ± 0.115
FreeCOS [4]	0.499 ± 0.083	0.661 ± 0.076	0.960 ± 0.014	0.687 ± 0.107	0.977 ± 0.014	0.625 ± 0.095
Ours	0.518 ± 0.097	0.677 ± 0.088	0.966 ± 0.010	0.675 ± 0.132	0.983 ± 0.008	0.699 ± 0.091
Ours(DR)	0.441 ± 0.083	0.607 ± 0.082	0.951 ± 0.012	0.710 ± 0.124	0.965 ± 0.013	0.550 ± 0.110
Ours(AL)	0.512 ± 0.093	0.672 ± 0.084	0.963 ± 0.011	0.699 ± 0.122	0.979 ± 0.010	0.665 ± 0.099
Ours(SSL)	0.365 ± 0.095	0.528 ± 0.105	0.945 ± 0.016	0.581 ± 0.171	0.967 ± 0.017	0.520 ± 0.121
Ours(fractal)	0.234 ± 0.113	0.366 ± 0.143	0.925 ± 0.041	0.399 ± 0.194	0.957 ± 0.047	0.432 ± 0.198

2.2.5 Implementation details. The overall objective function of our method is as

$$L_{total} = L_{seg} + L_{adv}(S_{en}) + L_{adv}(D) + 0.15L_{con} \tag{4}$$

The framework is trained on a single NVIDIA Quadro RTX 6000 GPU. For the segmentation network, the SGD optimizer is employed with an initial learning rate of 0.001, and we set the momentum and weight decay to 0.9 and 1e-4. The discriminator is trained using Adam [15] with an initial learning rate of 0.0001. The learning rates are linearly decayed to their $1/10$. We employ a batch size of 8 and train the framework for 20 epochs. We apply CLAHE histogram equalization [16, 17] to the source images and the target images, and convert their pixel values to $[-1, 1]$.

3 Results

Six metrics are employed to evaluate the performance of our proposed method, including Dice, Jaccard index (Jaccard), accuracy (Acc.), sensitivity (Sen.), specificity (Spe.), precision (Pre.). We compare our method with the state-of-the-art self-supervised approaches (Tab. 1). It can be seen that our framework surpasses these methods in these

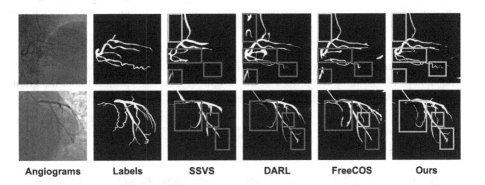

| Angiograms | Labels | SSVS | DARL | FreeCOS | Ours |

Fig. 2. The visualized results of vessel segmentation.

evaluation metrics. Besides, some of the visualized results are shown (Fig. 2). The pink boxes refer to insufficient or excessive segmentation results, whereas the green boxes are more accurate ones. The segmentation masks produced by our approach have a better preservation of local fine-grained details leading to a better overall performance.

A detailed ablation study is conducted to explore the contribution of each component in our method (Tab. 1). We denote domain randomization as DR, adversarial learning as AL, and self-supervised learning as SSL. In our experiments, domain randomization indeed is an effective technique to improve the model's generalization and performance on vessel segmentation demonstrated by the large performance drop when DR is removed. Meanwhile, there is a slight performance improvement after adding adversarial learning verifying that AL can further boost performance through an explicit domain alignment. Besides, our experiments show that the removal of the self-supervised learning component results in a substantial performance decline, where the network is deprived of the opportunity to directly access the distribution of the target domain images, which limits its performance on the target domain. To validate the contribution of DRR usage, one more experiment is conducted, where the DRR input is replaced by the fractals [4]. Notably, the segmentation performance drops significantly, which demonstrates the effectiveness of DRR utilization for angiogram vessel segmentation.

4   Conclusion

In this paper, we focus on designing a self-supervised vessel segmentation framework for angiograms. Since the angiograms are not annotated, we incorporate generated DRRs into the learning process and utilize domain randomization, adversarial learning, and self-supervised learning to reach a decent performance. We conduct experiments on a commonly used public dataset and compare our method with several state-of-the-art approaches, and the experimental results prove the effectiveness of our framework.

Domain randomization and adversarial learning are powerful tools for domain adaptation, and self-supervised learning is a crucial step to learning effective representations. This paper can serve as an inspiring starting point for applying DRRs and these techniques to X-ray image analysis, especially in cases where there are no annotations available. Because of the flexible scalability of DRR generation, using large-scale DRRs and unlabeled target domain data to perform representation learning can be a competitive proposal for medical image computing.

Acknowledgement. The project was supported by the Bavarian State Ministry of Science and Arts within the framework of the "Digitaler Herz-OP" project under the grant number 1530/891 02 and the China Scholarship Council (File No.202004910390).

References

1. Iyer K, Najarian CP, Fattah AA, Arthurs CJ, Soroushmehr SR, Subban V et al. Angionet: a convolutional neural network for vessel segmentation in X-ray angiography. Sci Rep. 2021;11(1):18066.

2. Ma Y, Hua Y, Deng H, Song T, Wang H, Xue Z et al. Self-supervised vessel segmentation via adversarial learning. Proc IEEE. 2021:7536–45.

3. Kim B, Oh Y, Ye JC. Diffusion adversarial representation learning for self-supervised vessel segmentation. The Eleventh International Conference on Learning Representations. 2023.

4. Shi T, Ding X, Zhang L, Yang X. FreeCOS: self-supervised learning from fractals and unlabeled images for curvilinear object segmentation. Proc IEEE. 2023:876–86.

5. Zhang B, Faghihroohi S, Azampour MF, Liu S, Ghotbi R, Schunkert H et al. A patient-specific self-supervised model for automatic X-ray/CT registration. Med Image Comput Comput Assist Interv. Springer. 2023:515–24.

6. Gharleghi R, Adikari D, Ellenberger K, Ooi SY, Ellis C, Chen CM et al. Automated segmentation of normal and diseased coronary arteries: the ASOCA challenge. Comput Med Imaging Graph. 2022;97:102049.

7. Gharleghi R, Adikari D, Ellenberger K, Webster M, Ellis C, Sowmya A et al. Annotated computed tomography coronary angiogram images and associated data of normal and diseased arteries. Sci Data. 2023;10(1):128.

8. Yang Y, Soatto S. Fda: fourier domain adaptation for semantic segmentation. Proc IEEE. 2020:4085–95.

9. Ronneberger O, Fischer P, Brox T. U-net: convolutional networks for biomedical image segmentation. Med Image Comput Comput Assist Interv. Springer. 2015:234–41.

10. Milletari F, Navab N, Ahmadi SA. V-net: fully convolutional neural networks for volumetric medical image segmentation. Proc Int Conf 3D Vis. Ieee. 2016:565–71.

11. Shit S, Paetzold JC, Sekuboyina A, Ezhov I, Unger A, Zhylka A et al. clDice-a novel topology-preserving loss function for tubular structure segmentation. Proc IEEE. 2021:16560–9.

12. Isola P, Zhu JY, Zhou T, Efros AA. Image-to-image translation with conditional adversarial networks. Proc IEEE. 2017:1125–34.

13. Mao X, Li Q, Xie H, Lau RY, Wang Z, Paul Smolley S. Least squares generative adversarial networks. Proc IEEE. 2017:2794–802.

14. Melas-Kyriazi L, Manrai AK. Pixmatch: unsupervised domain adaptation via pixelwise consistency training. Proc IEEE. 2021:12435–45.

15. Kingma D. Adam: a method for stochastic optimization. Int Conf Learn Represent. 2014.

16. Zuiderveld K. Contrast limited adaptive histogram equalization. Graph Gems. 1994:474–85.

17. Pizer SM, Amburn EP, Austin JD, Cromartie R, Geselowitz A, Greer T et al. Adaptive histogram equalization and its variations. Comp Vis Graph Image Proc. 1987;39(3):355–68.

Influence of imperfect annotations on deep learning segmentation models

Christopher Brückner, Chang Liu, Leonhard Rist, Andreas Maier

Pattern Recognition Lab, Department of Computer Science, Friedrich-Alexander-Universität
Erlangen-Nürnberg
chris.brueckner@fau.de

Abstract. Convolutional neural networks are the most commonly used models for multi-organ segmentation in CT volumes. Most approaches are based on supervised learning, which means that the data used for training requires expert annotations, which is time-consuming and tedious. Errors introduced during that process will inherently influence all downstream tasks and are difficult to counteract. To show the impact of such annotation errors when training deep segmentation models, we evaluate simple U-Net architectures trained on multi-organ datasets including artificially generated annotation errors. Specifically, three types of common masks are simulated, i.e. constant over- or under-segmentation error at the organ's boundary and the mixed-segmentation error. Our results show that using the ground truth data leads to mean dice score of 0.780, compared to mean dice scores of 0.761 and 0.663 for the constant over- and under-segmentation errors respectively. In contrast the mixed segmentation introduces a rather small performance decrease with a mean dice score of 0.771.

1 Introduction

In the complex landscape of medical image segmentation, deep learning plays a key role, especially in the segmentation of organs from CT scans. However, the dependency on annotated datasets, which may be error-prone, poses a challenge [1]. It is widely perceived that annotation errors have a negative impact on the model performance and several researches have been established on related topics. Eugene et al. perturbs the annotation of tumors in brain MRI using rigid transformation and analyses the impact on multiple segmentation networks [2]. Similarly, Nicholas et al. creates contour-wise perturbations to mimic the human errors in abdominal CT scans [3] and Șerban et al. creates object-wise perturbations to cell segmentation task [4]. Existing studies [1] address variability and sporadic errors, but leave a critical gap: the consistent impact of annotation errors on multi-organ segmentation models. This work fills this gap by investigating the effects of constant annotation errors, which are often overlooked in the current literature. Experimentally, we aim to determine how such errors affect multi-organ segmentation in CT images. Understanding and mitigating these effects are crucial for improving the performance of segmentation models in medical image analysis.

2 Materials and Methods

To investigate the effects of imperfect annotations, different models are trained on the original dataset as well as on datasets with artificial annotation errors, using a 3D U-Net [5]. The annotations of the training dataset are artificially adjusted to reproduce annotation errors likely to be found. In this work three annotation errors are simulated, namely over-segmentation, under-segmentation, and mixed-segmentation, i.e. the mixed over-segmentation and under-segmentation errors. Examples and sketches of the different errors are shown in Figure 1. The following section describes the dataset utilized, and explains the generation of the various errors.

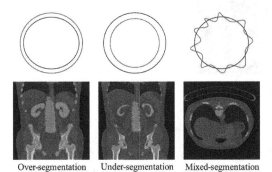

Fig. 1. Illustration of various annotation errors with corresponding examples: The ground truth is marked by a black circle, errors are shown by red lines. The best visibility for the mixed segmentation error is achieved with a coronal view.

Over-segmentation   Under-segmentation   Mixed-segmentation

2.1 Dataset

The CT-ORG dataset [6] was used as the segmentation dataset. It consists of 140 CT scans, including 3D annotations for six organs, namely liver, lungs, bones, kidneys, bladder and brain. Volumes with size smaller than $128 \times 128 \times 128$ are excluded to keep a reasonable voxel size. 89 volumes were used for training and 20 for testing. As only few volumes in the dataset contain the brain, the segmentation results are excluded in evaluation.

2.2 Annotation errors

As mentioned above, the segmentation labels of the training data are artificially manipulated to create three different kinds of annotation errors. The first two individual annotation errors represent the constant over- or under-segmentation error, mimicking annotators who tend to include the regions exceeding or shrinking the object boundaries. The third error represents mixed-segmentation, for annotators who are unsure about objects boundaries, as shown in Figure 2. Mathematical morphological operations are used for constant over-segmentation and constant under-segmentation. In particular, erosion is used for under-segmentation and dilation to create an over-segmentation error. For the mixed-segmentation error, a custom function is used to create the "wavy" boundaries. For each label instance, a certain percentage of boundary pixels are selected, at which a circular area is either added or removed from the segmentation masks, resulting in an alternating over- and under-segmentation mask.

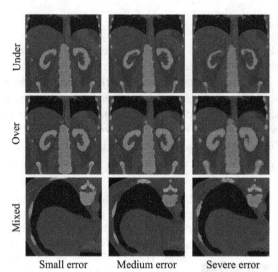

Fig. 2. Zoomed-in CT slices that clearly visualize the different artificially generated errors and their severity. "Under" refers to the constant under-segmentation error, "Over" to the constant over-segmentation error and "Mixed" to the third error, which is an alternating over- and under-segmentation error.

2.3 Level of errors

For further investigation of the influence of severity, three different error levels were defined for each annotation error, as shown in Figure 2. For the two constant errors, their magnitude is defined by the number of repetitions of the morphological operations. To be specific, for a small error around each label, one voxel is either added or removed from the segmentation, for a medium error two voxels and for a severe error five voxels. The percentage of boundary pixels determines the degree of mixed error. For a small error 0.1 %, for a medium error 1 %, and for a severe error 5 % of the boundary pixels are taken into account and a circular area with a radius of five pixels is either added or removed.

2.4 Experiments

The experiments are divided into constant and mixed error experiments to mimic the real-world scenarios with a different number of annotators when creating a segmentation dataset. The impact of each annotation error at different error levels is investigated by the average dice score (DSC) and that of each single organ. The DSC evaluates the spatial overlap of the prediction with the ground truth, which is defined as [7]

$$\text{DSC} = \frac{2\,|A \cap B|}{|A| + |B|} \tag{1}$$

where A is the ground truth mask and B is the prediction of a model. In addition, the impact of mixed error is investigated as a simulation of multiple annotators. For this purpose, equal parts of ground truth annotations and annotations containing artificially introduced medium errors are mixed into a training dataset. Finally, the impact of combining over- and under-segmentation errors are investigated to determine whether the model can adapt to these two types of errors and achieve accurate organ segmentation,

Tab. 1. Average overall dice score of constant error models and average dice score for the individual organs of constant error models.

Model	Avg.	Liver	Bladder	Lung	Kidneys	Bone
Baseline	0.780	0.909	0.279	0.977	0.645	0.880
Medium Wavy	0.771	0.853	0.253	*0.975*	*0.689*	0.868
Small Expand	0.770	0.858	0.320	0.946	0.685	0.828
Small Wavy	0.767	*0.878*	0.277	0.969	0.618	*0.870*
Medium Expand	0.761	0.859	0.439	0.915	0.628	0.746
Severe Wavy	0.757	0.817	0.326	0.954	0.625	0.833
Small Shrink	0.743	0.837	0.355	0.889	0.622	0.775
Severe Expand	0.698	0.810	*0.456*	0.834	0.564	0.566
Medium Shrink	0.663	0.781	0.188	0.797	0.538	0.692
Severe Shrink	0.494	0.659	0.230	0.487	0.250	0.37

Tab. 2. Average overall dice score of mixed error models and average dice score for the individual organs of mixed error models.

Model	Avg.	Liver	Bladder	Lung	Kidneys	Bone
Baseline	0.780	0.909	0.279	0.977	0.645	0.880
Original & Wavy	0.753	0.857	0.202	*0.976*	*0.617*	*0.873*
Original & Expand	0.750	*0.868*	*0.308*	0.963	0.535	0.843
Original & Shrink	0.693	0.846	0.202	0.873	0.483	0.768
Expand & Shrink	0.689	0.795	0.163	0.853	0.598	0.742

or whether it inherits an error. This investigation can indicate which of the two constant errors may be more problematic.

For training of these models, the volumes and associated labels are partitioned into smaller sub-volumes of size $64 \times 128 \times 128$ due to memory limitations. Each 3D U-Net model was trained for 30 epochs using the Adam optimizer with a learning rate of 10^{-3}.

3 Results

In the following section, the quantitative and qualitative results of the differently trained models are presented. All models trained with over-segmentation errors are referred to as "Expand", models trained with under-segmentation errors are referred to as "Shrink", and models trained with mixed over- and under-segmentation errors are referred to as "Wavy". Depending on the level of error, the models are named Small, Medium or Severe together with the respective error type. The models trained with errors mixed into the fine dataset are named Original & the type of error, and finally the model trained with a mixture of different errors is named Expand & Shrink.

Table 1 shows the quantitative results of the constant error models with the average total DSC in descending order as well as the average DSCs for the individual organs. The quantitative results of the mixed error experiments are shown in Table 2, which has the same structure as Table 1. The Baseline model has the overall highest average DSC of 0.780, followed by the Medium Wavy model with 0.771 and the Small Expand model with 0.770. The overall worst performing model is the Severe Shrink model with an average DSC of 0.494. With respect to each organ, models with small and medium wavy errors achieve the lowest performance decrease for liver, lung, kidneys and bone. All models show limited performance for the bladder, with Baseline DSC of only 0.279. Several example slices of the models are shown in Fig. 3.

As explained in section 2.1, the bones in the CT-ORG dataset were labeled using morphological operations, which can lead to inaccuracies. Consequently, over-segmentation is observed around the ribs and collarbone. The Baseline model, as well as the Medium Wavy model, generate segmentation masks quite similar to the ground truth. Over- and under-segmentation in the training data leads to the same errors in the test.

Table 2 shows the results of the mixed error experiments. The model mixing the error-free with the medium wavy error data achieves the least drop in average DSC, and results in a total DSC of 0.753, while the model mixing the medium expand and medium shrink data has the highest drop in DSC, achieving a total DSC of 0.689. The Expand & Shrink model shows under-segmentation for all organs, as illustrated in Figure 4, with further qualitative results from mixed error models.

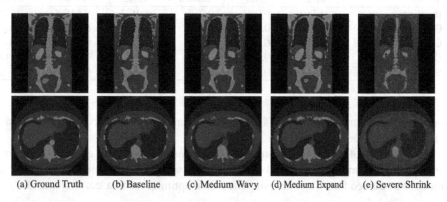

(a) Ground Truth   (b) Baseline   (c) Medium Wavy   (d) Medium Expand   (e) Severe Shrink

Fig. 3. The ground truth labels and qualitative results of selected constant error models. The different colors represent the different organs.

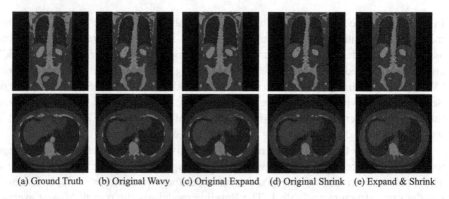

(a) Ground Truth   (b) Original Wavy   (c) Original Expand   (d) Original Shrink   (e) Expand & Shrink

Fig. 4. The ground truth labels and qualitative results of the mixed error models.

4 Discussion and Conclusion

To investigate the influence of different annotation errors and their severity on the performance of the segmentation models, artificial datasets were created. Several models were trained on these datasets and their performance compared. It can be observed in the DSC results that the original data will not always lead to highest DSC, indicating that the original dataset cannot be completely assumed as error-free. However, our experiments still show that the performance of segmentation networks is affected by annotation errors in different ways, depending on the type and the level of the error. In particular, when constant annotation errors are involved, i.e. constant over- or under-segmentation error, the segmentation performance systematically decreases and the errors are inherited by the models, which can be observed in the qualitative results. Hard-to-segment organs, like the bladder, benefit from over-segmentation, as seen in models with the highest bladder scores. Despite this, the Expand & Shrink model reveals that under-segmentation errors exert a greater impact on overall results than over-segmentation errors, leading to decreased organ recognition probability with erosion and increased probability with dilation. An interesting observation is that the segmentation network is robust to mixed-segmentation errors, where quantitative metrics are only slightly affected even with severe mixed-segmentation error. Such observations can contribute to useful suggestions to annotators of segmentation datasets, that imperfect boundary sketch is less crucial than the constant over- or under-segmentation.

Acknowledgement. The authors gratefully acknowledge the HPC resources provided by the Erlangen National High Performance Computing Center (NHR@FAU) of the Friedrich-Alexander-Universität Erlangen-Nürnberg (FAU).

References

1. Gonzalez-Jimenez A, Lionetti S, Gottfrois P, Gröger F, Pouly M, Navarini AA. Robust T-Loss for Medical Image Segmentation. MICCAI 2023. Springer. 2023.
2. Vorontsov E, Kadoury S. Label Noise in Segmentation Networks: Mitigation Must Deal with Bias. DGM4MICCAI 2021. Springer International Publishing, 2021:251–8.
3. Heller N, Dean J, Papanikolopoulos N. Imperfect Segmentation Labels: How Much Do They Matter? LABELS Workshop MICCAI 2017. Springer International Publishing, 2018:112–20.
4. Vădineanu Ş, Pelt D, Dzyubachyk O, Batenburg J. An Analysis of the Impact of Annotation Errors on the Accuracy of Deep Learning for Cell Segmentation. Medical Imaging with Deep Learning. 2022.
5. Ronneberger O, Fischer P, Brox T. U-net: Convolutional networks for biomedical image segmentation. MICCAI 2015. Springer. 2015:234–41.
6. Bilic P, Christ PF, Vorontsov E, Chlebus G, Chen H, Dou Q et al. The Liver Tumor Segmentation Benchmark (LiTS). CoRR. 2019.
7. Kaur H, Kaur N, Neeru N. Evolution of multiorgan segmentation techniques from traditional to deep learning in abdominal CT images – A systematic review. Displays. 2022.

Addressing the Bias of the Dice Coefficient

Semantic Segmentation of Peripheral Airways in Lung CT

Fenja Falta, Mattias P. Heinrich, Marian Himstedt

Institute of Medical Informatics, University of Lübeck
fenja.falta@student.uni-luebeck.de

Abstract. While self-configuring U-Net architectures excel at a vast majority of supervised medical image segmentation tasks, they strongly rely on the chosen loss function. We demonstrate that a commonly employed Dice or cross entropy loss leads to a bias of the trained network, that is critical for the clinical application of airway segmentation from CT scans. The effort to produce the most accurate segmentations is skewed towards larger anatomical structures, leaving smaller peripheral airways with poorer quality. To address this bias, we explore several different choices of amending the label definition, including morphological dilation, and find that separating the binary airway segmentations into at least two distinct structures yields substantial improvements of approximately 4 % in peripheral areas. This finding could directly benefit several clinically relevant tasks, among others virtual CT bronchoscopy.

1 Introduction

Segmentation of lung airways is a fundamental task in numerous medical applications for diagnosis and interventions. It is a key requirement for electromagnetic navigation bronchoscopy (ENB) being frequently carried out in conjunction with lung cancer biopsies. In particular, airway segmentation is conducted prior to interventions for planning paths and registration of virtual (CT-rendered) and in vivo bronchoscopy sequences for tracking a bronchoscope inside the airways primed by electromagnetic (EM) sensors [1]. Pulmonary nodules often develop in deep lung tissue. That means the segmentation of peripheral airway structures is inevitably of high importance for navigational guidance. Airway segmentation also provides benefits for lung image registration [2]. In particular, the additional anatomical features obtained can improve intra- and inter-patient (atlas) registration as well as multi-modal alignment. Besides navigation and registration tasks airway segmentation can be used to aid the treatment of chronic obstructive pulmonary disease (COPD) through automatic assessment of airway wall thicknesses and wall area percentages [3].

The recent multi-site (binary) airway segmentation challenge ATM [4] demonstrated that U-Net based network models excel in terms of Dice overlap for this task. The well-established nnU-Net framework provides a standardised and out-of-the-box method for deep learning-based semantic segmentation, that works well for a broad number of segmentation tasks [5]. By default, it employs Dice and Cross-Entropy Loss during training. For multi-label segmentation, a weighting of the losses counterbalances class imbalances, however, for binary segmentation tasks, differently sized sub-structures are

© Der/die Autor(en), exklusiv lizenziert an
Springer Fachmedien Wiesbaden GmbH, ein Teil von Springer Nature 2024
A. Maier et al. (Hrsg.), *Bildverarbeitung für die Medizin 2024*,
Informatik aktuell, https://doi.org/10.1007/978-3-658-44037-4_66

treated identically. Alternative strategies in prior work for tubular segmentation tasks included the use of dilated ground truth masks [2, 6], centreline-based losses [7] and object boundary attention [8].

Mispredictions of a segmentation network in lower branching levels of the airways, where they are more narrow, can quickly result in underestimation of bronchi lengths or disconnections in the segmentations, which is crucial for clinical application. However, since the width of the airways in these lower levels is significantly smaller, the impact of those errors on nnU-Net's loss values but also on average metrics used in prominent challenges is relatively small. This problem is in line with the assessment of many biomedical challenge organisers that noted research efforts are often focused on overfitting to the current metrics and fail to advance the solution of the imminent clinical problem [9].

Hence, there is a need to evaluate the segmentation of peripheral parts of the airway and adapt different multi-label airway segmentation setups to the clinical relevance of this aspect.

2 Materials and methods

2.1 Dataset

Since most publicly available datasets, including the ATM challenge dataset, only provide binary masks, we use the public LIDC-IDRI dataset [10] that comprises 40 CT scans with voxel-accurate airway segmentations and amend it using segmentations of singular bronchi up to tertiary bronchi depth that are obtained from [6] for the same scans to train our airway segmentation network. We use these combined annotations to create (up to) two separate labels, i.e. peripheral and non-peripheral bronchi. Later, we also employ lung lobe segmentations for further subdivisions. The dataset is split into 32 and 8 samples for training and testing respectively.

2.2 Label generation

We compare a total of four different label settings for airway segmentation. First, as a baseline, we train the network using the full binary labels provided alongside the LIDC-IDRI dataset, reaching from the trachea to peripheral bronchi. Second, we remove all parts of the airway up to tertiary bronchi from the segmentation (using the annotations provided by [6]) to obtain only segmentations of the peripheral bronchi. Third, we add the removed part of the airway back into the segmentation as a second label. For the fourth approach, we employ the Total Segmentator [11] to obtain segmentations of the five lung lobes and divide the airway segmentations into six labels based on these: one for each part of the airway located in one of the lung lobes and one for airway located outside the lung. Figure 1 displays an example of each segmentation.

2.3 Dilation

In previous works regarding semantic airway segmentation [2, 6], dilation of segmentations prior to training has shown to be beneficial in regard to anatomical structures with small sizes. We therefore compare results obtained with dilated and non-dilated labels. For the dilated approaches, 3×3×3 kernels are applied prior to training, which results in a dilation of 1 voxel in each direction. Erosions using the same kernels are subsequently applied to the predictions.

2.4 Training details

The segmentation network is trained for 250 epochs using a fixed training/test split. Since lung anatomy differs between the left and right lung, mirroring as data augmentation and nnU-Net's test time adaptation (averaging the prediction for mirrored images) is disabled. Apart from these alterations, the standard hyperparameters of the nnU-Net framework are kept.

3 Results

We evaluate the overall prediction as well as the prediction in the peripheral area for our different training setups. For that, we calculate a binary dice by binarising segmentations to obtain binary segmentations of the full airway, a peripheral dice by evaluating the score only on the peripheral labels and a peripheral sensitivity by calculating all detected peripheral voxels in the binarised segmentations. The best results are achieved when training with merged two-label segmentations (Tab. 1). It achieves a higher segmentation accuracy than using binary training labels or solely providing peripheral airway annotations. This shows, that the incorporation of non-peripheral airway in the segmentation as an additional label benefits the segmentation quality of peripheral bronchi. Since there are no edges inside the airway that indicate the location of the end and start of one label, finding the exact position of the segmentation edges poses as a difficult task.

Dilation and erosion of ground truth labels produce slightly inaccurate labels and result in segmentations with dice scores of 99.36%. When comparing results for dilated

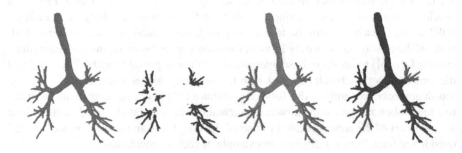

Fig. 1. The four different annotations for one image. From left to right: Full binary segmentation, segmentation of only peripheral bronchi, merged two-label segmentations and lobe-based segmentation.

Tab. 1. Quantitative results of the different training setups. Binary Dice Score for binarised segmentations, Dice Score for peripheral bronchi and the sensitivity of binarised labels for peripheral bronchi detection. Standard deviation across the 8 test cases is given in brackets.

Method	Binary Dice (%) ↑	Peripheral Dice (%) ↑	Peripheral Sensitivity (%) ↑
Without dilation			
Full binary segmentation	93.52 (1.93)	–	67.06 (6.27)
Only peripheral bronchi	–	65.8 (5.51)	57.31 (6.27)
Two-label segmentation	93.97 (1.83)	69.4 (5.86)	68.52 (5.81)
Lobe-based segmentation	93.42 (1.75)	–	63.93 (5.04)
With dilation			
Full binary segmentation	92.45 (2.99)	–	62.90 (11.66)
Only peripheral bronchi	–	64.08 (8.08)	58.11 (10.61)
Two-label segmentation	92.16 (3.34)	65.33 (8.60)	63.53 (11.67)
Lobe-based segmentation	92.04 (3.36)	–	63.17 (12.85)

Tab. 2. Dice Scores for all labels of the lobe-based segmentation. The standard deviation across the 8 test cases is given in brackets.

Label	Dice without dilation (%)	Dice with dilation (%)
Outside	97.25 (0.40)	96.76 (1.44)
Left Upper Lobe	77.21 (4.60)	73.97 (9.11)
Left Lower Lobe	75.81 (5.06)	72.94 (9.30)
Right Upper Lobe	76.51 (2.33)	72.67 (7.70)
Right Middle Lobe	67.84 (11.07)	68.99 (11.33)
Right Lower Lobe	72.19 (7.47)	69.86 (10.29)

and undilated segmentations, we see that the nnU-Net segments even small peripheral bronchi better with accurate non-dilated labels. The only advantage is seen when segmenting significantly smaller structures, i.e. the bronchi in the right middle lobe (Tab. 2), which – according to the results – also seem to be the structures that are the hardest to accurately segment.

4 Discussion

To address the task of semantic airway segmentation we explored several different setups for the nnU-Net training that incorporate a differentiation of different parts of the airway as well as a dilation of ground truth labels. We showed that dividing the ground truth labels into two sub-labels, referring to the peripheral and non-peripheral part of the airway, yields the best results in regard to segmentation accuracy. This finding provides clinical benefit for applications that involve modelling deeper inside the pulmonary anatomy. The results also suggest that a more detailed subdivision of segmentations could benefit the automatic analysis of other complex anatomical structures.

References

1. Reichl T, Luo X, Menzel M, Hautmann H, Mori K, Navab N. Hybrid electromagnetic and image-based tracking of endoscopes with guaranteed smooth output. IJCARS. 2013;8:955–65.
2. Falta F, Hansen L, Himstedt M, Heinrich MP. Learning an airway atlas from lung CT using semantic inter-patient deformable registration. Proc BVM. 2022:75–80.
3. Chauhan NS, Sood D, Takkar P, Dhadwal DS, Kapila R. Quantitative assessment of airway and parenchymal components of chronic obstructive pulmonary disease using thin-section helical computed tomography. Pol J Radiol. 2019;84:54–60.
4. Zhang M, Wu Y, Zhang H, Qin Y, Zheng H, Tang W et al. Multi-site, multi-domain airway tree modeling. Med Image Anal. 2023;90:102957.
5. Isensee F, Jaeger PF, Kohl SA, Petersen J, Maier-Hein KH. nnU-Net: a self-configuring method for deep learning-based biomedical image segmentation. Nat Methods. 2021;(2):203–11.
6. Tan Z, Feng J, Zhou J. SGNet: structure-aware graph-based network for airway semantic segmentation. Proc MICCAI. 2021:153–63.
7. Paetzold JC, Shit S, Ezhov I, Tetteh G, Ertürk A, Munich HZ et al. clDice—A novel connectivity-preserving loss function for vessel segmentation. Medical Imaging Meets NeurIPS 2019 Workshop. 2019.
8. Mishra D, Chaudhury S, Sarkar M, Soin AS. Ultrasound image segmentation: a deeply supervised network with attention to boundaries. IEEE Trans Biomed Eng. 2018;66(6):1637–48.
9. Eisenmann M, Reinke A, Weru V, Tizabi MD, Isensee F, Adler TJ et al. Why is the winner the best? Proc IEEE CVPR. 2023:19955–66.
10. Armato III SG, McLennan G, Bidaut L, McNitt-Gray MF, Meyer CR, Reeves AP et al. The lung image database consortium (LIDC) and image database resource initiative (IDRI): a completed reference database of lung nodules on CT scans. Med Phys. 2011;38(2):915–31.
11. Wasserthal J, Breit HC, Meyer MT, Pradella M, Hinck D, Sauter AW et al. Totalsegmentator: robust segmentation of 104 anatomic structures in ct images. Radiol Artif Intell. 2023;5(5).

Automated Tooth Instance Segmentation and Pathology Annotation Pipeline for Panoramic Radiographs
Mask-R-CNN Approach with Elastic Transformations

Christopher J. Hansen[1], Jonas Conrad[2], Ronald Seidel[1], Nicolai R. Krekiehn[1], Eren Yilmaz[1,3], Niklas Koser[1], Martin Goetze[1], Toni Gehrmann[2], Sebastian Lauterbach[2], Christian Graetz[2], Christof Dörfer[2], Claus C. Glüer[1]

[1] Section Biomedical Imaging, Dept. of Radiology and Neuroradiology, University Medical Center Schleswig-Holstein (UKSH), Campus Kiel
[2] Clinic of Conservative Dentistry and Periodontology, University of Kiel
[3] Dept. of Computer Science, Ostfalia University of Applied Sciences, Wolfenbüttel, Germany
christopher.hansen@rad.uni-kiel.de

Abstract. Caries detection in dental radiographs is a challenging and time consuming task even for experts in the field. Recent studies have shown the potential of tooth instance segmentation and caries detection with neural networks. We present a tooth level pathology annotation pipeline, based on automated tooth instance segmentation and numbering with a Mask-R-CNN architecture followed by the extraction of the bounding boxes of individual teeth as patches, that can be reassembled to the original image. 5-fold cross validation resulted in mean average precision (mAP) of 0.898 ± 0.02 for tooth instance segmentation. Augmentation focusing on elastic transformation increased the mAP by 0.053 to 0.951 ± 0.014 and enhanced robustness across folds. At performance levels at least similar to published data our approach provides flexibility for patch-based pathology diagnosis combined with the option to reassemble annotated patches to the original image. This will permit combining tooth-number-specific, neighborhood-based and entire image based features in future modeling along with tooth-centric review and diagnoses by clinical needs of dentists.

1 Introduction

In 2019, approximately 335 million people of the European Region's population (33.6%) suffered from caries of permanent teeth [1]. Modern clinical devices allow for rapid acquisition of full dental X-rays suitable for the visualization of dental pathologies, but dentists are more and more challenged in evaluating the increasing amount of image data. As a growing body of studies suggests, artificial intelligence (AI) and neural networks can support radiologists and dentist in tooth detection, segmentation and numbering with different approaches on panoramic dental X-ray images [2–6]. Furthermore, neural networks can also assist in caries detection [7] predominantly on bitewing X-ray [8] and panoramic dental X-ray images [9] or making caries classifications on single teeth [10]. The latter is similar to the manual approach, as the dental pathology diagnosis is usually made at the tooth level. A current hurdle in the application of artificial intelligence in dentistry for pathology detection on tooth level, however, is the lack of an end-to-end

© Der/die Autor(en), exklusiv lizenziert an
Springer Fachmedien Wiesbaden GmbH, ein Teil von Springer Nature 2024
A. Maier et al. (Hrsg.), *Bildverarbeitung für die Medizin 2024*,
Informatik aktuell, https://doi.org/10.1007/978-3-658-44037-4_67

workflow, with high functionality and adaptability in the daily routine. We addressed this problem in the present study and suggest an innovative strategy for tooth instance segmentation, which facilitates further tooth level pathology annotation. The annotations on those tooth patches can seamlessly be patched back to the original full dental X-ray images, which allows simple and reliable integration into the majority of existing clinical workflows. Several different approaches on tooth detection, instance segmentation and tooth numbering exist, including the use of Faster R-CNN [4], or DetectNet with Grad-Cam [5]. The Mask-R-CNN architecture [11] is a state-of-the-art framework for instance segmentation, excelling in tasks like tooth detection with bounding boxes, encompassing both segmentation and classification [3]. For comparisons of model performance, for example, of Mask-R-CNN with PANet see Silva et al. [2]. Leite et al. [6] presented a different approach, with a two step AI model, based on a detector and a fine-tuner segmenting and numbering individual teeth. In this study, we chose the Mask-R-CNN architecture as our framework, because it showed satisfying results across different studies and data sets while outputting tooth detection, segmentation and classification [2, 3]. As previous studies suggested we also investigated the applicability of data augmentation techniques with tooth X-ray images [2], because there is only very limited experience with advanced augmentation techniques suited for dental AI modelling [4, 5]. Several augmentation types were tested with a specific focus on elastic augmentation.

2 Materials and methods

Our workflow (Fig. 1) is a novel approach to tooth segmentation, providing a pipeline for pathology annotation on tooth level. During inference the panoramic dental X-ray is input into the Mask-R-CNN model (A). The model will perform an automated instance segmentation of each single tooth, including numbering according to the Fédération Dentaire Internationale (B). After segmentation the tooth bounding boxes are exported as individual images for further diagnostics on tooth level (e.g. caries) (C). Each segmented tooth can be assigned back to the original image and has all relevant metadata stored, specifically the diagnostic outcome (D). This allows subsequent data usage for e.g. pathology detection on both, the single tooth instances, a limited neighbourhood of multiple teeth and the full dental X-ray. Our model was initialized with pre-trained weights from imagenet [12].

2.1 Augmentations

We investigated different data augmentation techniques. All augmentations have been applied together in a fixed range of magnitude, with a probability of 0.5 for each image to have all augmentations applied to the image. We are intentionally excluding augmentations that are clinically nonsensical. We used a common image augmentation pipeline consisting of Gaussian Blur, Gaussian Noise, Brightness, CoarseDropout and CropAndPad. While elastic transformations [13] usually deform the image slightly we took a different approach and chose a small and fixed σ value of 0.25 creating a distorted field and giving a small range of magnitude of (0.0, 5.0) for the image smoothing α value. This generalizes the morphology of the teeth, while making it possible to still clearly distinguish the single teeth. To give the model the chance to learn the core of what a tooth is, the mask was, left unchanged for the elastic transformation.

2.2   Patching and re-patching

When using images for training in a Mask-R-CNN the original images (Fig. 2 A) can be of different size, but they are resized by the model and output in a uniform size during training (Fig. 2 B). The same is true for the detected tooth patches (Fig. 2 C, D). This in total leads to 4 different image sizes (Fig. 2). To patch and re-patch each annotation the metadata is stored in a table. The re-sizing of the annotations is calculated from that metadata. This allows further data usage without having to compromise on data accessibility or immense time loss for re-annotating. Annotations made on a single tooth can be moved to the full dental X-ray and vice versa.

Fig. 1. Pipeline for tooth level pathology annotation from the input radiograph (A), tooth instance segmentation (B), extraction of single tooth image patches for pathology annotation (C), to the re-patched annotation (D).

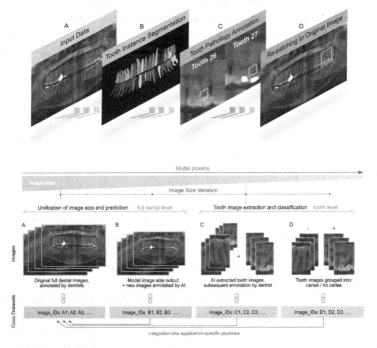

Fig. 2. Patching and Re-Patching workflow of annotations between single tooth images and full dental X-rays. The annotations can be moved from the single tooth image to the full X-ray and vice versa.

2.3 Metrics

For the evaluation of the model we use the mean-Average-Precision (mAP) to compare our work with previous studies [2]. mAP is a commonly used metric in Object Detection to evaluate the true positives (TP), false positives (FP) and false negatives (FN). It is calculated by $mAP = 1/n * \Sigma_{k=1}^{k} AP_k$ where AP_k is the average precision of the current class and n is the number of classes. The metric itself is not sensitive to single classes, as it averages over all classes. We use a further metric, as suggested by [14], which is the Normalized-Surface-Distance (NSD), a boundary based metric, for each tooth. The NSD is a commonly used metric in medical imaging to compare two shapes and quantify how similar they are. The distance between the GT_{Mask} circumference and the $Pred_{Mask}$ circumference for each point is calculated and then normalized with the circumference of the GT_{Mask}. The NSD from GT_{Mask} to $Pred_{Mask}$ and vice versa is not equal, so we average over both.

2.4 Data and annotations

For this study we used the publicly available dataset from Universidade Federal da Bahia, Brasil [2] which consists of 1321 panoramic radiographs in 10 categories. Dentists from the University Hospital Schleswig-Holstein, Kiel, Germany, annotated tooth segmentations on 276 images with CVAT (Computer Vision Annotation Tool) [15]. The data were split in a 5-fold-cross-validation for training. In each fold, 220 images were used for training and 56 images for validation.

3 Results

After training we used the two aforementioned metrics to evaluate the model performance on detecting, segmenting and numbering the teeth. Tab. 1 shows the mAP results for each fold and each augmentation pipeline. Training without any augmentations resulted in a mAP between 0.883 and 0.911, across the 5-folds for all tooth classes. Training with the standard augmentation pipeline resulted in mAP between 0.878 and 0.955. Adding the elastic transformation to the augmentation pipeline we achieved mAP levels of 0.939 to 0.958, improving the results by 0.003 to 0.061. On average the training without augmentation was 0.898, with augmentation but without elastic transformation was 0.930 and with the elastic transformation at 0.951. The latter increased the performance on average by 5.3% compared to unaugmented training. With elastic transformation, the deviation between the folds is the lowest with 1.9%, highest without elastic transformation at 7.7% and 2.8% without any augmentation. Hence elastic transformation not only increases performance, but also reduces the inter fold variability, i.e. it increases the robustness of the model performance. Fig. 3 shows the results for the NSD with elastic transformation. The results are split by tooth class and averaged over all folds. The NSD shows a difference in the performance of the single tooth instances across tooth classes. The '8s' on each quadrant have the largest distance (bad), while the '6s' and '7s' on average have the smallest distance (good). Outliers can be found for all teeth and do not show a particular pattern.

Tab. 1. mAP at 50% overlap threshold over all teeth for all folds with different augmentation techniques. The best result for each augmentation method is marked in bold.

	no augmentations	w/o elastic	w/ elastic
Fold1	0.897	0.940	0.948
Fold2	0.883	0.878	0.939
Fold3	0.910	*0.955*	*0.958*
Fold4	*0.911*	0.945	*0.958*
Fold5	0.890	0.933	0.954
Mean	0.898	0.930	0.951

4 Discussion

The selected augmentation techniques have shown, by using elastic transformations, that we can achieve results comparable to other publications even with a smaller subset of the same dataset used for training and validation compared to [2]. It reduces the need for time consuming annotation work from experts and, more importantly also improves robustness of the model performance across folds. This supports our hypothesis of elastic transformations helping in generalizing the tooth features for the model. With the NSD metric we could identify a difference in detectability of the different tooth classes, showing that the '8s' (wisdom teeth) are the hardest to segment. This is plausible, as the '8s' do look different in different patients, whereas the shape of the '6s' (first molar) and '7s' (second molar) is rather uniform and defined. Our approach provided a novel workflow that automates tooth segmentation as single instances which enables pathology diagnostics on the tooth level. The tooth level diagnostics maintain compatibility with the original dental X-ray and providing dentist-oriented methodology typical for the effective current clinical workflow, as confirmed by the dentists involved in this project. The approach holds potential for flexible further model training, providing a variety of modeling options e.g.: single tooth-focused models, class-group based models (e.g. all '4s' (first premolar)), and annotated full dental X-rays. Our study has some limitations as incomplete dentures or dentures with implants have been excluded and it requires testing in independent datasets. In conclusion our model shows state-of-the-art performance for

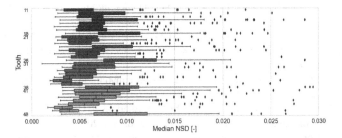

Fig. 3. NSD for all tooth classes over all folds combined. The color indicates the quadrant 1-4 from top to bottom. The bar shows the interquartile range with the whiskers noting the min. and max. value. Single dots show outliers. Less than 4% of data being above the threshold.

tooth instance segmentation, and highlights potential of elastic transformation, as a data augmentation technique suited for panoramic radiographs. Our workflow enables development of diagnostic models, i.e. pathology detection on tooth level, with the ability to investigate tooth class separately or in combination.

Acknowledgement. Our work was supported by funds of the Molecular Imaging North Competence Center and the Section Biomedical Imaging, Kiel.

References

1. World Health Organization (WHO) Europe. WHO Europe calls for urgent action on oral disease as highest rates globally are recorded in European Region. WHO Media Release. Accessed November 2023.
2. Silva B, Pinheiro L, Oliveira L, Pithon M. A study on tooth segmentation and numbering using end-to-end deep neural networks. Conf Graph Images (SIBGRAPI). IEEE. 2020.
3. Jader G, Fontineli J, Ruiz M, Lima K, Pithon M, Oliveira L. Deep instance segmentation of teeth in panoramic X-ray images. 2018:400–7.
4. Tuzoff DV, Tuzova LN, Bornstein MM, Krasnov AS, Kharchenko MA, Nikolenko SI et al. Tooth detection and numbering in panoramic radiographs using convolutional neural networks. Dentomaxillofacial Radiol. 2019;48(4). PMID: 30835551:20180051.
5. Muramatsu C, Morishita T, Takahashi R, Hayashi T, Nishiyama W, Ariji Y et al. Tooth detection and classification on panoramic radiographs for automatic dental chart filing: improved classification by multi-sized input data. Oral Radiol. 2021.
6. Leite AF, Gerven AV, Willems H, Beznik T, Lahoud P, Gaêta-Araujo H et al. Artificial intelligence-driven novel tool for tooth detection and segmentation on panoramic radiographs. Clin Oral Investig. 2021;25(4):2257–67.
7. Schwendicke F, Tzschoppe M, Paris S. Radiographic caries detection: a systematic review and meta-analysis. J Dent. 2015;43(8). Epub 2015 Feb 24. Erratum in: J Dent. 2021 Nov;114:103783. PMID: 25724114.:924–33.
8. Mertens S, Krois J, Cantu AG, Arsiwala LT, Schwendicke F. Artificial intelligence for caries detection: randomized trial. J Dent. 2021;115:103849.
9. Geetha V, Aprameya KS, Hinduja DM. Dental caries diagnosis in digital radiographs using back-propagation neural network. Health Inf Sci Syst.
10. Oliveira J, Proença H. Caries detection in panoramic dental X-ray images. Comput Vis Med Image Proc. Ed. by Tavares JMRS, Jorge RMN. Dordrecht: Springer Netherlands, 2011:175–90.
11. He K, Gkioxari G, Dollár P, Girshick R. Mask r-cnn. Proc IEEE. 2017:2961–9.
12. Deng J, Dong W, Socher R, Li LJ, Li K, Li FF. ImageNet: a large-scale hierarchical image database. 2009:248–55.
13. Simard P, Steinkraus D, Platt J. Best practices for convolutional neural networks applied to visual document analysis. Proc IEEE. 2003:958–63.
14. Maier-Hein L, Reinke A, Godau P, Tizabi MD, Buettner F, Christodoulou E et al. Metrics reloaded: recommendations for image analysis validation. 2023.
15. OpenCV. Computer vision annotation tool. https://github.com/opencv/cvat. Accessed November 2023.

Multi-task Learning to Improve Semantic Segmentation of CBCT Scans using Image Reconstruction

Maximilian E. Tschuchnig[1], Julia Coste-Marin[2], Philipp Steininger[2], Michael Gadermayr[1]

[1]Salzburg University of Applied Sciences
[2]MedPhoton GmbH
maximilian.tschuchnig@fh-salzburg.ac.at

Abstract. Semantic segmentation is a crucial task in medical image processing, essential for segmenting organs or lesions such as tumors. In this study we aim to improve automated segmentation in CBCTs through multi-task learning. To evaluate effects on different volume qualities, a CBCT dataset is synthesised from the CT Liver Tumor Segmentation Benchmark (LiTS) dataset. To improve segmentation, two approaches are investigated. First, we perform multi-task learning to add morphology based regularization through a volume reconstruction task. Second, we use this reconstruction task to reconstruct the best quality CBCT (most similar to the original CT), facilitating denoising effects. We explore both holistic and patch-based approaches. Our findings reveal that, especially using a patch-based approach, multi-task learning improves segmentation in most cases and that these results can further be improved by our denoising approach.

1 Introduction

Segmentation is a crucial field of automated medical image analysis, for a multitude of applications, from segmenting low-level (e.g., nuclei) to high-level tissue structure (differentiation between cancer, stroma, and necrosis). Classical segmentation methods (thresholding, region-based, watershed), though useful for both 2D and 3D segmentation, often struggle with the complexity of pathological and anatomical structures, particularly high-level structures observed in medical imaging. Deep learning methods exhibit the state-of-the-art for semantic segmentation, commonly employing encoder-decoder models [1–3]. These models are trained to encode latent information in a bottleneck and then use this information to reconstruct a mask (segmentation) or the original volume (image reconstruction). Fully-convolutional networks, exemplified by Unet [4], utilize this encoder-decoder structure to generate segmentation masks. Models like nn-unet [1] extend Unet's architecture to 3D and demonstrate state-of-the-art performance on various computed tomography (CT) segmentation tasks [5]. UnetR [2] and SegFormer [3] adapt nn-unet by incorporating transformer blocks like multihead attention.

Multi-task learning (MTL) aims to share knowledge over multiple tasks of a common model for knowledge transfer, regularization and data efficiency. E.g. MTL approaches have previously been investigated by Weninger et al. [6] to reduce the amount of needed labelled training data by adding a reconstruction to a segmentation task. Similarly, Mlynarski et al. [7] include a task of 2D tumor detection score estimation. Both approaches

© Der/die Autor(en), exklusiv lizenziert an
Springer Fachmedien Wiesbaden GmbH, ein Teil von Springer Nature 2024
A. Maier et al. (Hrsg.), *Bildverarbeitung für die Medizin 2024*,
Informatik aktuell, https://doi.org/10.1007/978-3-658-44037-4_68

use encoder-decoder structures. Therefore, the addition of multiple tasks increase the amount of data that can be used to train their encoder.

We propose a novel, model agnostic, extension to semantic segmentation. By formulating model optimisation through MTL of segmentation and image reconstruction we facilitate morphology based regularisation. For experimental validation, we select the state-of-the-art for automated semantic segmentation, 3D nn-unet [1, 5]. The evaluation is conducted using the Liver Tumor Segmentation Benchmark (LiTS) [5]. To assess our proposed adaptation at different data quality, we synthesise cone-beam CT (CBCT) from the original LiTS, with varying numbers of projections employed for CBCT reconstruction. We further evaluate the effect of using CBCT corresponding to the highest quality volumes as the reconstruction target, facilitating a denoising effect.

2   Method

Our model agnostic approach, shown applied to a 3D nn-unet in Fig. 1, is to 1) add a regularisation term to semantic segmentation through MTL with the additional task of image reconstruction and 2) add denoising effects to the reconstructions of 1) by always reconstructing the highest quality volume.

In detail, the proposed multi-task method describes a generic adaptation of the training stage of semantic segmentation approaches. Additionally to performing segmentation the multi-task model mt-c is trained to reconstruct the current volume for regularisation. Assuming binary cross-entropy (BCE) as the segmentation and L2 as the reconstruction loss, a combined loss can be formulated as $Loss = BCE(\hat{s}, s) + l2(\hat{v}, v)$. With s as the real and $\hat{s}$ as the predicted segmentation as well as v denoting the current and $\hat{v}$ the reconstructed image. The intuition is to explicitly regularise the learned segmentation using morphology. By synthesizing CBCTs from LiTS using different amounts of used projections, different quality CBCT volumes are generated. By replacing v with the highest quality volume v_o, the model is further trained to denoise lower visual quality volumes. We refer to this method as mt-b (best quality).

As shown in Fig. 1, a 3d nn-unet [1, 4] is chosen as the baseline (red path). This unet consists of an encoder with 3 double convolution layers and $3 \times 3 \times 3$ convolutional kernels, connected by 3d max pooling. The latent space consists of one double convolution block leading into the unet decoder which mirrors the encoder. As is typicall for unet, each double convolutional output in the encoder is also connected to the decoder double convolutional block of the same order. Additionally, one 3d convolutional layer is added to the decoder with a filter size of $1 \times 1 \times 1$ and the number of filters set to the amount of segmentation classes. The rest of the convolutional layers are set to $\{32, 64, 128, 256\}$ filters along the stream direction in the encoder. Batch norm is applied after each layer in the double convolutional blocks. The model is trained utilizing a sum ($Loss_1$) of BCE and Dice $Loss_1 = BCE(\hat{s}, s) + Dice(\hat{s}, s)$.

We apply the multi-task adaptation, shown in Fig. 1 (combining both the red and blue path), on the introduced baseline. The last double convolutional layer output is used multistream, with one stream feeding into the baseline segmentation layer and the other stream feeding into a 3d convolutional layer with filter size $1 \times 1 \times 1$ and a linear activation function to facilitate reconstruction. The baseline loss is adapted by adding the l2 $Loss_2 = \alpha \cdot (BCE(\hat{s}, s) + Dice(\hat{s}, s)) + (1 - \alpha) \cdot l_2(\hat{v} - v)$ with $\alpha = 0.8$. Depending on the setup, the optimal v_o is used instead of v in training.

2.1 Dataset

Evaluation is performed using the LiTS dataset. LiTS consists of 131 abdominal CT scans in the training set and 70 test volumes. The 131 train volumes include segmentations of 1) the liver and 2) liver tumors. The dataset contains data from 7 different institutions with a diverse set of liver tumor diseases. For further information we refer to Bilic et al. [5]. To evaluate effects on vastly different volume qualities, the LiTS dataset was converted into synthetic CBCT scans. Corresponding projections were simulated per CT volume, with the number of projections $n_p \in \{490, 256, 128, 64, 32\}$. 490 projections was chosen as the default configuration to show a visual quality similar to the original CT and 32 as the lowest configuration, showing little information and many artifacts.

2.2 Experimental setup

We evaluate the introduced methods holistically and patch based on liver and liver tumor segmentation [5, 8–10]. Segmentation are evaluated using the Dice score. A threshold of 0.5 is applied to the model output before Dice calculation to establish binary labels. To fit the holistic data on an NVIDIA RTX A6000 grafics card the volumes are downscaled by the factor 2. For patched segmentation, patches of the size $192 \times 192 \times 192$ are extracted from the CBCT data. On inference, the patch segmentations are re-agregated before calculating a holistic Dice. Models and setups are evaluated using the different

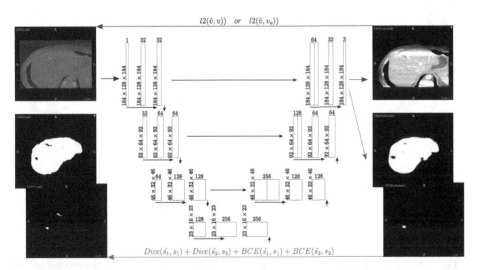

Fig. 1. Segmentation unet (red path) and the reconstruction task (blue), facilitating MTL. The volumes are used in patches and holistically (downscaled by 2). The multi-task trained model performs segmentation and reconstruction at once (red and blue paths). The final loss includes Dice, BCE and L2 to facilitate training both segmentation and reconstruction.

quality CBCT datasets with the quality depending on the amount of used projections for simulation $n_p \in \{490, 256, 128, 64, 32\}$. A further investigated parameter is the reconstruction target with the two investigate setups, mt-c and mt-b. The setup mc-c uses the input volume of the current quality as its reconstruction target while mt-b always uses the best possible quality input volume (v_o). Therefore, in the case $n_p = 490$ both mt-b and mt-c lead to the same results. All setups are trained and evaluated 4 times to facilitate stable results with the same random splits for results comparability. Since annotations are not available for the LiTS test dataset, the test dataset was disregarded for this publication and the original train set was separated into training-validation-testing data [8, 9]. The separation was performed with the ratio 0.7, 0.2 and 0.1 (training:0.7, validation:0.2, testing:0.1).

3   Results

The segmentation results of the holistic approach are shown in Fig. 2. It shows boxplots of segmentation results using different quality levels based on the amount of projections. The 3 upper boxplots show the results of our baseline (nn-unet), mt-c and mt-b with the highest quality reconstruction target ($n_p = 490$). The top row shows Dice results based on liver segmentation. The bottom row shows liver tumor Dice. Fig. 3 follows the same structure for patch based liver and liver tumor segmentation. Holistic segmentation was most successful using the baseline nn-unet with the best scores for liver segmentation with a Dice of 0.88 for 490 and 256 projections and 0.78 for 32 projections. The mt-c

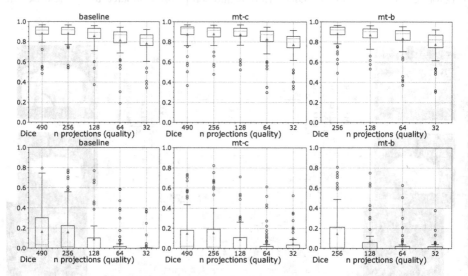

Fig. 2. Holistic segmentation results using different quality levels based on the amount of projections (boxplot x-axis). The 3 upper boxplots show the results of baseline (nn-unet), mt-c and mt-b. The top row shows Dice scores based on liver segmentation. The bottom row shows liver tumor Dice scores. The orange lines show the median and green triangles the mean.

approach lead to a minor improvement of 0.01 in the case of 128 projections and mt-b lead to an improvement of 0.02 from 0.82 to 0.84 with 64 projections. Regarding liver tumor segmentation, the baseline nn-unet performed best in all cases except 32 projections, where mt-c proposed regularisation lead to an improvement of 0.02. For patch based segmentation, mt-c and mt-b show dominance. mt-c displays best values for 490 and 128 projections with an increase in performance to the baseline by 0.04 and 0.02 respectively. For 256 and 64 projections, mt-b led to best Dice scores with an increase of 0.02 and 0.03 over the baseline. The effect regarding liver tumor segmentation is similarly positive.

4 Discussion

Our investigation of MTL for image segmentation shows a notable distinction between holistic approaches, characterized by holistic volume understanding, and patched approaches, emphasizing high-frequency information with smaller receptive fields (in terms of real tissue). The holistic approaches generally show superior results, but the impact of MTL is more pronounced in our patched approaches. We assume that the increased effect of mt-c in the patched approaches is due to the retention of high-frequency information. This high frequency information proves valuable for segmenting complex structures such as liver tumors. Additionally, mt-b further improves patched, full-scale approaches, suggesting that the denoising effects are more useful when high-frequency information is preserved. These findings lead to two key insights. Firstly, the results affirm that MTL improves segmentation accuracy. Adding an image reconstruction tasks,

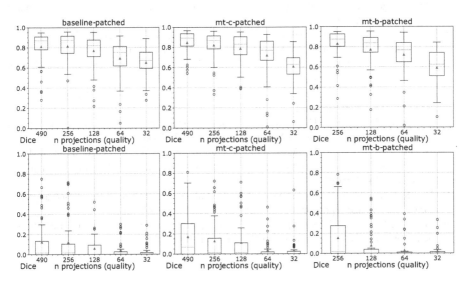

Fig. 3. Patch-based segmentation results using different quality levels based on the amount of projections (boxplot x-axis). The 3 upper boxplots show the results of our baseline (nn-unet), mt-c and mt-b. The top row shows Dice scores based on liver segmentation. The bottom row shows liver tumor Dice scores. The orange lines show the median and green triangles the mean.

especially if there is important morphological, high-frequency information, enhances the model's ability to segment complex structures. Secondly, the downscaling needed for holistic approaches might hinder the model's capacity to leverage MTL fully. To further validate these findings, we propose a future investigation of full-resolution, holistic approaches to remove the possible confounding factor of volume resolution.

In conclusion, we evaluate MTL to improve 3D semantic segmentation through the addition of image reconstruction. We evaluate multiple different volume qualities and setups and show that MTL can improve segmentation performance, especially in a high resolution, patched setup.

Acknowledgement. This project was partly funded by the Austrian Research Promotion Agency (FFG) under the bridge project "CIRCUIT: Towards Comprehensive CBCT Imaging Pipelines for Real-time Acquisition, Analysis, Interaction and Visualization" (CIRCUIT), no. 41545455 and by the county of Salzburg under the project AIBIA.

References

1. Isensee F, Petersen J, Klein A, Zimmerer D, Jaeger PF, Kohl S et al. nnU-Net: self-adapting framework for U-net-based medical image segmentation. Proc BVM. 2019:22–2.
2. Hatamizadeh A, Tang Y, Nath V, Yang D, Myronenko A, Landman B et al. Unetr: transformers for 3d medical image segmentation. Proc IEEE. 2022:574–84.
3. Xie E, Wang W, Yu Z, Anandkumar A, Alvarez JM, Luo P. SegFormer: simple and efficient design for semantic segmentation with transformers. Proc IEEE. 2021;34:12077–90.
4. Ronneberger O, Fischer P, Brox T. U-net: convolutional networks for biomedical image segmentation. Proc IEEE. 2015:234–41.
5. Bilic P, Christ P, Li HB, Vorontsov E, Ben-Cohen A, Kaissis G et al. The liver tumor segmentation benchmark (lits). Med Image Anal. 2023;84:102680.
6. Weninger L, Liu Q, Merhof D. Multi-task learning for brain tumor segmentation. Brainlesion: Glioma, Multiple Sclerosis, Stroke and Traumatic Brain Injuries: 5th International Workshop, BrainLes 2019, Held in Conjunction with MICCAI 2019, Shenzhen, China, October 17, 2019, Revised Selected Papers, Part I 5. 2020:327–37.
7. Mlynarski P, Delingette H, Criminisi A, Ayache N. Deep learning with mixed supervision for brain tumor segmentation. J Med Imaging. 2019;6(3):34002–2.
8. Araújo JDL, Cruz LB da, Diniz JOB, Ferreira JL, Silva AC, Paiva AC de et al. Liver segmentation from computed tomography images using cascade deep learning. Comput Biol Med. 2022;140:105095.
9. Han K, Liu L, Song Y, Liu Y, Qiu C, Tang Y et al. An effective semi-supervised approach for liver CT image segmentation. Proc IEEE. 2022;26(8):3999–4007.
10. Wang J, Zhang X, Lv P, Wang H, Cheng Y. Automatic liver segmentation using EfficientNet and attention-based residual U-net in CT. J Digit Imaging. 2022:1–15.

Non-specialist Versus Neural Network
An Example of Gender Classification from Abdominal CT Data

Stephan Prettner, Tatyana Ivanovska

Technical University of Applied Sciences OTH Amberg-Weiden
s.prettner@oth-aw.de

Abstract. The general paradigm is the following: more input information for a system leads to a better performance. Our assumption is that the information must be rather appropriate than excessive, especially, when the training data is limited. Moreover, the requirements of a machine learning system might differ from the ones of a human observer. In this work, we analyze and compare the performance of several neural network architectures and human readers, who had only basic common knowledge on the subject. The example task is gender classification using abdominal computerized tomography (CT) data. It has been demonstrated by our study that training of a neural network purely on pelvic bone segmentation masks is the most efficient and produces highly accurate results, whereas for human observers this information is not sufficient. The study confirms our original assumptions and emphasizes the importance of the appropriate input feature selection for a better performance of a specific task.

1 Introduction

Recently, artificial neural networks have become extremely successful in many computer vision tasks, even outperforming human experts in some cases [1, 2]. In the medical field, artificial intelligence (AI) systems are as well increasingly adopted for such applications as computer-aided diagnosis and image-based screening. However, it has been recently demonstrated by Larrazabal et al. [3] that the performance of a neural network on a specific task can be significantly decreased, if there is, for instance, a gender imbalance in the dataset. This raises an important issue, namely, what information is important for a training of a neural network to produce highly accurate results. In our opinion, there are two main interrelated components, namely, the model itself (i. e., the corresponding model complexity [4]) and the appropriate input data. The latter is especially relevant, when the amount of available training data is limited, which is usually the case in the medical domain.

In this work, we consider the gender identification as an example task and run a study to compare the performance of a neural network and non-specialists dependent on the input data. The goal of the study is to find answers to the following questions. What information is relevant for a neural network to correctly determine the gender? How is it comparable to a human observer? This task has been selected due to several reasons. First, the gender information is usually given in the metadata such as DICOM tags of a 3D scan. Therefore, the groundtruth of such a classification task is already provided. Second, different input variants are possible in this case. We assume that even a non-specialist can easily determine the patient's gender using a 3D view of an abdominal

© Der/die Autor(en), exklusiv lizenziert an
Springer Fachmedien Wiesbaden GmbH, ein Teil von Springer Nature 2024
A. Maier et al. (Hrsg.), *Bildverarbeitung für die Medizin 2024*,
Informatik aktuell, https://doi.org/10.1007/978-3-658-44037-4_69

CT scan. On the other hand, the task becomes rather challenging, if a layman without a specific knowledge about the human anatomy is required to determine the gender using the pelvic bones only. The performance of a neural network on the gender classification task can be also evaluated using the whole abdominal CT scan and the pelvic bones only as input data. We also analyze the performance of a non-expert human observer with and without the special training on the gender-specific differences of pelvic bone anatomy. Third, it is known that the detection of gender from CT data is useful for forensic and bioarchaelogical applications. For instance, bones of the pelvis and skull parts have been used for post-mortem gender identification [5]. These applications are relevant, but not our primary target though.

The paper is organized as follows. In Section 2, we describe the input data and the neural network architectures that have been utilized. In Section 3, we present the results of our experiments. The findings as well as the outlook are discussed in Section 4.

2   Materials and methods

2.1   Materials

In this work, a subset of a large-scale pelvic bone dataset, namely, the CTPelvic1K was utilized. The CT data originated from different open-source datasets, and the segmentation masks of the pelvic bones were provided by the team of Liu et al. [6]. In our work, a subset from five open-source datasets was utilized. We selected only the subjects with a segmentation mask for the pelvic bones. The sacrum part was excluded from the segmentation mask. The datasets with severe artifacts, like major pelvic fractures or external fixtures, were excluded. For about 40% of the samples, the gender was provided in the DICOM tags. The remaining samples were manually annotated by two observers with experience in medical imaging. If the annotations were not consistent, the subject was excluded from the dataset. The details of the final dataset are summarized in Table 1.

The final 955 samples were converted to a common spacing $(0.78, 0.78, 0.8)$ and randomly split into training and validation (80%, 767 subjects) and test (20%, 188 subjects) sets. The training and validation part was used for 5-fold cross-validation during the training of the neural networks. The average distribution of gender in five folds was 46% males and 54% females. The test set consisted of 73 males and 115 females. Three different groups of input data representations were generated:

- the whole abdominal CT scan (3D volume),
- the abdominal CT cropped to the location of the pelvis (3D volume),
- the pelvic bones only (3D volume).

To analyze the performance of non-expert human observers, 50 samples from the test set (25 male and 25 female subjects, respectively) were randomly selected. The example views from two subjects (one male, one female) from the reduced test set are given in Figure 1.

Tab. 1. A summary of the subset of the CTPelvic1K dataset.

Dataset	Samples	M / F	Spacing mm	Resolution
COLONOG [7]	700	326 / 374	(0.75, 0.75, 0.81)	(512, 512, 323)
KITS19 [8]	32	12 / 20	(0.82, 0.82, 1.25)	(512, 512, 240)
ABDOMEN [9]	35	15 / 20	(0.76, 0.76, 3.80)	(512, 512, 73)
CERVIX [9]	41	0 / 41	(1.02, 1.02, 2.50)	(512, 512, 102)
MSD_T10 [10]	147	72 / 75	(0.77, 0.77, 4.55)	(512, 512, 63)
Total	955	425 / 530	(0.78,0.78,0.8)	

2.2 Methods

2.2.1 Manual analysis. The human observers were selected to be non-experts in the field of medical imaging, radiology, or surgery, i. e., they had only basic common knowledge about the pelvic bone anatomy.

The samples from each group were presented to each observer in a random order using a 3D volume rendering viewer in MeVisLab software [11]. The manual analysis was conducted in four rounds for each human reader. Each round took approximately 20 minutes. First, the pelvic bones only group was presented and analyzed. Second, the whole abdominal CT scan was evaluated. Third, the observer was given a short explanation on the gender dimorphism of pelvic bones, and several examples of male and female pelvic bones from the training and validation part were demonstrated. Thereafter, the evaluation on the bone group was repeated. Finally, the gender was identified on the cropped abdominal CT scan group. Each group was shown separately, i. e., the observer was not allowed to switch between the groups during each evaluation round.

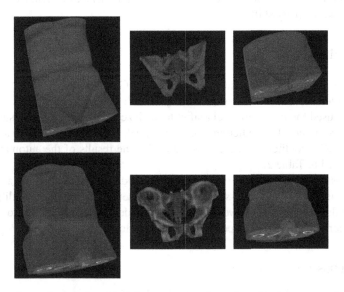

Fig. 1. Three views of a female subject (upper row) and a male subject (lower row). Left: a full CT scan; Middle: pelvic bones only; Right: cropped CT scan.

Tab. 2. Validation and test AUC_ROC metrics for each fold of the 5-fold cross-validation and the ensemble consisting of five models.

Model	Validation Folds					Ensemble (Test set)
	Fold 1	Fold 2	Fold 3	Fold4	Fold 5	
DenseNet264$_{\text{FullCT}}$	0.9475	0.9426	0.9730	0.9671	0.9391	0.9533
DenseNet121$_{\text{FullCT}}$	0.9493	0.9509	0.9773	0.9664	0.9402	0.9512
DenseNet264$_{\text{CropCT}}$	0.9595	0.9521	0.9712	0.9725	0.9711	0.9602
DenseNet121$_{\text{CropCT}}$	0.9571	0.9514	0.9500	0.9709	0.9744	0.9602
DenseNet264$_{\text{Bones}}$	0.9975	0.9730	0.9945	0.9984	0.9699	0.9741
DenseNet121$_{\text{Bones}}$	0.9972	0.9774	0.9983	0.9987	0.9777	0.9736

2.2.2 Automated analysis with neural network classification. For automated gender classification, a 3D version of the well known dense architecture, namely, DenseNet [12] was utilized. The pooling operations and convolutions are configured and used for the three-dimensional space. The aim of the DenseNet is to achieve a high flow of information from the original image to the classification using the so called dense blocks and transition layers. At the end of the network, a pooling layer, a fully connected layer and the softmax activation function are utilized to carry out the class prediction. Two model sizes, namely, DenseNet264 (40.25 Mln parameters) and DenseNet121 (11.24 Mln parameters) were trained for each input data group. The 3D implementation was provided by MONAI Framework [13]. The models were trained for maximally 300 epochs with early stopping parameters $\delta = 0$, patience $= 10$ using Adam optimizer and static learning rate $lr = 0.34391$. The other hyperparameters are Batch_Size $= 2$, Patch_Size $= 96 \times 96 \times 96$, Dropout_Rate $= 0.2$, and Cross Entropy Loss function. The decision threshold was selected 0.5. The data augmentation included random flips, rotation, and intensity shifts.

3 Results

Area Under the Receiver Operating Characteristic Curve (ROC AUC) [14] was used as the evaluation metric of the automated analysis both for validation and test sets. The five folds were used for an ensemble classifier to analyze the full test set (188 subjects). The ensemble computes the predictions for each model, then these values are averaged and the AUC_ROC coefficients are computed on it. The results of the automated analysis are presented in Table 2.

The results of the manual evaluation of the reduced, completely balanced test set (50 subjects) from three non-specialists are presented in Table 3. Additionally, the correspondent Ensembles of five DenseNet264 models were also applied to this reduced test set. Here, the sensitivity, specificity, and F1 values were computed.

4 Discussion

As it can be observed in Table 2, both full and cropped CT data are more confusing for the networks than the pelvic bones only. We assume that with more training data,

Tab. 3. Evaluation metrics for the reduced completely balanced test set from human observers and the best Ensembles.

Reader	Sensitivity	Specificity	F1 Score
Bones, No explanations for human observers			
Observer$_1$	44%	52%	45.83%
Observer$_2$	32%	36%	32.65%
Observer$_3$	64%	44%	58.18%
Full CT scan			
Observer$_1$	96%	100%	97.96%
Observer$_2$	80%	92%	85.1%
Observer$_3$	76%	88%	80.85%
EnsembleDenseNet_264	88%	92%	89.8%
Bones, After explanation for human observers			
Observer$_1$	88%	92%	89.8%
Observer$_2$	84%	84%	84%
Observer$_3$	60%	84%	68.18%
EnsembleDenseNet_264	96%	92%	94.11%
Cropped CT scan			
Observer$_1$	84%	80%	82.35%
Observer$_2$	72%	92%	80%
Observer$_3$	68%	80%	74%
EnsembleDenseNet_264	92%	96%	93.88%

a neural network could learn to detect the required features from a complete CT scan with similar results. The bone information only, obviously, represents strong features for classification, which can be learned by a neural network from a moderately large training set. Both DenseNet models performed quite similar. The larger model resulted with slightly higher AUC scores for most of the folds. The results on the full test set confirmed our observations, as shown in Table 2.

In contrast, the observations for a non-trained human observer were significantly easier on the full CT scans, where the gender specific features were mainly recognizable. This is demonstrated in Table 3. After the short explanation on gender dimorphism, all human observers improved their results, but they did not outperform the results for the full CT scan. The cropped CT scan allowed the users to classify the gender groups less accurately than using the full scans, which is well understandable, since less information is given, and the observers had to concentrate on the lower body only. The ensemble model performed the best on the pelvic bone data. However, due to the small size of the reduced test set, the differences with the results of the models trained on cropped CT data is not that distinct.

These findings demonstrate the importance of the appropriate input for an artificial intelligence model and the excessive information, which might be crucial for a human observer, is not always helpful to obtain better results from a neural network.

In this work, we analyzed the performance of several neural network models and non-specifically educated human observers for the task of gender classification from abdominal CT data. It was demonstrated that pelvic bones only represented the most informative features for a neural network, whereas human observers required more information. Even after explanations on gender-specific differences, the human readers could not outperform the models using the bone data as training input. In future work, we will investigate the question of the appropriate input features for other imaging modalities, such as MRI, and organ areas, for instance, human respiratory system.

Acknowledgement. The authors would like to thank the MONAI team for the excellent framework and the non-specialist human observers, who participated in the manual analysis.

References

1. Esteva A, Chou K, Yeung S, Naik N, Madani A, Mottaghi A et al. Deep learning-enabled medical computer vision. NPJ Digit Med. 2021;4(1):5.
2. Voulodimos A, Doulamis N, Doulamis A, Protopapadakis E et al. Deep learning for computer vision: a brief review. Comput Intell Neurosci. 2018;2018.
3. Larrazabal AJ, Nieto N, Peterson V, Milone DH, Ferrante E. Gender imbalance in medical imaging datasets produces biased classifiers for computer-aided diagnosis. Proc Natl Acad Sci. 2020;117(23):12592–4.
4. Hu X, Chu L, Pei J, Liu W, Bian J. Model complexity of deep learning: a survey. Knowl Inf Syst. 2021;63:2585–619.
5. Inskip S, Scheib CL, Wohns AW, Ge X, Kivisild T, Robb J. Evaluating macroscopic sex estimation methods using genetically sexed archaeological material: the medieval skeletal collection from St John's Divinity School. Am J Phys Anthropol. 2019;168(2):340–51.
6. Liu P, Han H, Du Y, Zhu H, Li Y, Gu F et al. Deep learning to segment pelvic bones: large-scale CT datasets and baseline models. Int J Comput Assist Radiol Surg. 2021;16:749–56.
7. Johnson CD, Chen MH, Toledano AY, Heiken JP, Dachman A, Kuo MD et al. Accuracy of CT colonography for detection of large adenomas and cancers. N Engl J Med. 2008;359(12):1207–17.
8. Heller N, Sathianathen N, Kalapara A, Walczak E, Moore K, Kaluzniak H et al. The kits19 challenge data: 300 kidney tumor cases with clinical context, ct semantic segmentations, and surgical outcomes. arXiv preprint arXiv:1904.00445. 2019.
9. Landman B, Xu Z, Igelsias J, Styner M, Langerak T, Klein A. Miccai multi-atlas labeling beyond the cranial vault-workshop and challenge. Proc MICCAI. Vol. 5. 2015:12.
10. Antonelli M, Reinke A, Bakas S, Farahani K, Kopp-Schneider A, Landman BA et al. The medical segmentation decathlon. Nat Commun. 2022;13(1):4128.
11. Ritter F, Boskamp T, Homeyer A, Laue H, Schwier M, Link F et al. Medical image analysis. IEEE Pulse. 2011;2(6):60–70.
12. Huang G, Liu Z, Van Der Maaten L, Weinberger KQ. Densely connected convolutional networks. Proc IEEE Conf Comput Vis Pattern Recognit. 2017:4700–8.
13. Cardoso MJ, Li W, Brown R, Ma N, Kerfoot E, Wang Y et al. Monai: an open-source framework for deep learning in healthcare. arXiv preprint arXiv:2211.02701. 2022.
14. Fawcett T. An introduction to ROC analysis. Pattern Recognit Lett. 2006;27(8):861–74.

Automatic Segmentation of Lymphatic Perfusion in Patients with Congenital Single Ventricle Defects

Marietta Stegmaier[1], Johanna P. Müller[1], Christian Schröder[2], Thomas Day[3],
Michela Cuomo[2], Oliver Dewald[2], Sven Dittrich[2], Bernhard Kainz[1,4]

[1]FAU Erlangen-Nürnberg, Germany
[2]University Hospital Erlangen, Germany
[3]King's College London, United Kingdom
[4]Imperial College London, United Kingdom
johanna.paula.mueller@fau.de

Abstract. The Fontan circulation is the surgical end-point for a variety of single-ventricle congenital heart lesions. While recent decades have witnessed substantial improvements in survival rates, the associated physiology remains susceptible to severe complications such as protein-losing enteropathy and plastic bronchitis. These complications are often indicative of abnormal congestion in the lymphatic system, underscoring their significance as harbingers of impending co-morbidities. An accurate assessment of congestion severity requires the detailed annotation of lymphatic perfusion patterns in each volumetric scan slice. The manual labelling of such intricate data is time-consuming and demands a high level of expertise, rendering it unfeasible within the confines of standard clinical protocols. We use a curated database consisting of manually annotated T2-weighted magnetic resonance imaging (MRI) scans from 71 Fontan patients post-surgery. Following the current state-of-the-art method for biomedical image segmentation, we evaluate its performance on multiple independent test sets regarding the degree of severity and imaging quality. Incorporating the best-performing model, we have developed a user-friendly interface for the automatic segmentation of lymphatic malformations, which will be published before the conference starts.

1 Introduction

Single ventricle malformations are relatively rare diagnoses ($\sim 1.25\%$ of infants) manifesting a genetic component [1], and when left untreated, they can be fatal in the neonatal period. To address this, the majority of univentricular abnormalities undergo a multi-stage surgical protocol, ultimately resulting in the establishment of the Fontan circulation. While there have been significant improvements in the long-term survival rates for Fontan patients over recent decades, their unique hemodynamics can lead to severe complications, such as protein-losing enteropathy and plastic bronchitis. Detecting early signs of these comorbidities is crucial. They are often manifested as abnormalities in lymphatic perfusion patterns, resulting from congestion in the venous system. To facilitate the recognition of these complications, early diagnosis, and the categorisation of lymphatic malformations into different degrees of severity is imperative. T2-weighted MRI of the thorax and abdomen has proven to be a valuable tool in this classification process, as it portrays lymphatic fluid with high intensity [2]. We established a curated

© Der/die Autor(en), exklusiv lizenziert an
Springer Fachmedien Wiesbaden GmbH, ein Teil von Springer Nature 2024
A. Maier et al. (Hrsg.), *Bildverarbeitung für die Medizin 2024*,
Informatik aktuell, https://doi.org/10.1007/978-3-658-44037-4_70

dataset comprising Fontan patients who received treatment at the Erlangen University Hospital between the years 2007 and 2020. As part of their routine follow-up examinations, conducted six months after Fontan Completion, these patients underwent a standard MRI protocol. At the time of our study, our database encompassed records from 71 patients. Collaborating with a pediatric cardiologist, we manually annotated lymphatic perfusion patterns using MRI-specific labelling software. Manual labelling introduces fuzzy labels into the learning pipeline, e.g., induced by different levels of annotator expertise, specific ambiguity inherited in the data, varying granularity and complexity of annotations, and annotator bias, represented by specific uncertainty and ambiguity. In our specific case, semantic annotation required a pixel-wise binary classification of lymphatic and non-lymphatic structures. Given the complexity of lymphatic perfusion patterns, we had to consider several factors to distinguish between foreground and background. The defining characteristic of lymphatic fluid is its heightened intensity in T2-weighted MR images, which proves insufficient due to the presence of numerous structures exhibiting similar brightness. Thus, anatomical expertise played a pivotal role in excluding gastrointestinal areas and blood vessels. We utilised quality ratings assigned by the pediatric cardiologist and focused on developing models capable of making accurate predictions with a limited amount of labelled data through data augmentation, cross-validation, and distinctions based on image quality, severity levels, and anatomical regions. So far, the authors could only identify one similar study [3] with fewer patients (n=48) for measuring lymphatic burden, and a related one [4] with fewer patients (n=22) for quantifying thoracic lymphatic flow patterns using dynamic contrast-enhanced MR lymphangiography.

1.1 Contributions

1. We manually annotated lymphatic perfusion abnormalities in T2-weighted MRI samples of Fontan patients six months after surgery completion. We curated the collection of annotated samples to a novel database consisting of 71 samples.
2. We test and evaluate the performance of state-of-the-art segmentation models on ill-defined labels in few-shot scenarios. Through 5-fold cross-validation and ensemble prediction, we show the generalisability of our trained models in challenging cases.
3. To complete our contributions, we offer a user-friendly interface that facilitates the automatic prediction of lymphatic perfusion patterns in input data, also with probability maps for prediction.

2 Materials and methods

Timely classification of patients into different severity types based on lymphatic malformations is crucial due to potential complications. Manual annotation, while time-consuming and impractical for routine clinical use, can be significantly streamlined by automated segmentation tools, taking advantage of recent deep learning advancements. To facilitate supervised learning, a dataset of T2-weighted MR images from Fontan patients with lymphatic malformations has been annotated.

Tab. 1. Data folds for model training.

	Model	1	2	3	4	5	6	7.1	7.2	7.3	Dataset
	Samples	81	81	81	60	45	80	12	46	20	105
	Abdominal	28	28	28	19	17	27	3	17	8	36
Region	Whole-body	25	25	25	22	11	26	6	12	4	33
	Thoracic	28	28	28	19	17	27	3	17	8	36
	0	3	3	3	3	1	3	0	0	0	4
	1	12	12	12	12	6	14	12	0	0	18
Quality (n)	2	46	46	46	32	20	42	0	46	0	52
	3	20	20	20	12	14	20	0	0	18	26
	4	0	0	0	1	4	1	0	0	2	5
	1	2	2	2	0	7	5	1	1	0	7
Severity (n)	2	28	28	28	0	38	29	3	15	10	38
	3	50	50	50	58	0	45	8	29	10	58
	4	1	1	1	2	0	1	0	1	0	2

2.1 Dataset curation

In Erlangen University Hospital, all patients with univentricular heart defects undergo a standardised protocol which was first introduced in 2007. Apart from numerous other steps, the plan includes a retrospective analysis of T2-weighted MR images with fat saturation six months after the Fontan Completion to assess potential lymphatic malformations. In the years 2007-2020, a total of 71 children received this scan creating the basis for a dataset that can be extended in the future. The dataset properties and patient distribution are presented in the underlying medical study [2], which compiles abnormal abdominal lymphatic perfusion patterns and investigates their impact on serum protein readings. Reference annotations were created for all patients with the assistance of a specialised pediatric cardiologist. The semantic annotation involved a binary pixel-wise classification into lymphatic and non-lymphatic structures. Due to the complexity of the perfusion patterns, several aspects had to be considered to differentiate between the fore- and background. Considering only the high intensity of lymphatic fluid in T2-weighted MR images, this criterion is not sufficient because multiple other structures are depicted in a similar brightness. Hence, anatomical knowledge was vital to rule out gastrointestinal areas or blood vessels. Apart from that, previous research about common locations of lymphatic abnormalities was considered during the decision-making process [2, 5]. To factor these disparities into the evaluation, the scans were rated concerning their quality by the pediatric cardiologist. Given the large differences in intensity between *BLADE* and *SPACE* MRI sequences, the latter were exempt from the general quality assessment. The remaining images were assigned ranks from one to four, with one representing the best and four representing the worst quality, see quality distribution in Table 1. Reasons for low quality were large slice thickness, motion artefacts and imaging resolution. As a final step of the data curation, the cases were assigned a severity type describing the degree of lymphatic malformations. All patients in the database had been previously classified by two independent experts according to the system introduced by [2, 5]. The para-aortic, portal-venous, and thoracic regions are considered separately for this evaluation, resulting in three ranks per patient. For thoracic-only scans, the thoracic ranks by both raters were averaged (Fig. 1); abdominal-only images were assigned the mean of the para-aortic and portal-venous ratings by both raters. The severity types mapped to whole-body scans comprised the ranks of all three regions.

2.2 Segmentation framework

To create a standardised and robust segmentation tool, we chose to use the nnU-Net [6] as a state-of-the-art segmentation model. This self-configuring model preserves the overall structure of conventional U-Nets, yet systematizes the re-design of the pipeline for individual tasks. One key advantage of the network is its ability to learn efficiently from minimal training data, which is particularly important in our project since the available training cases of Fontan patients with lymphatic malformations are very limited. Another benefit of the nnU-Net is its accessibility without demanding expert knowledge or advanced computing resources to provide fast and accurate results, especially, for future clinical deployment.

3 Results

In Table 2, the 2D-, 3D- and Ensemble U-Nets yield similar results. A more detailed evaluation reveals that the superiority of specific configurations depends on the anatomical region of the scans. Abdominal-only images perform better with the 2D network, while thoracic-only scans tend to favour the 3D U-Net, and no clear preference between configurations is observed for whole-body cases. Concerning the different training schemes for the models, one can note that the performance of the networks improves substantially the more data augmentation functions are included. This observation also applies to mirroring, comparing Model 3 with the default augmentation and Model 2 without mirroring. Independent of the specific configurations and data folds, the anatomical

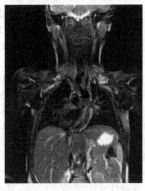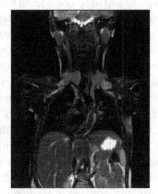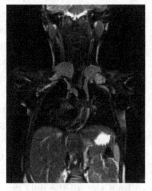

(a) Original Scan   (b) Predicted Segmentation   (c) Ground Truth Label

Fig. 1. Example of a high-performing MRI scan with characteristics: Region "Thoracic-only", Severity type "2", Quality rank "2".

Tab. 2. Evaluation scores for predictions with the best checkpoint (best scores of each configuration shown in bold) (DSC: dice similarity coefficient; IoU: Intersection over Union).

		2D Configuration		3D Configuration		Ensemble of 2 D and 3 D	
		DSC	IoU	DSC	IoU	DSC	IoU
	1	0.39 ± 0.21	0.24 ± 0.16	0.38 ± 0.22	0.23 ± 0.18	0.39 ± 0.22	0.24 ± 0.18
	2	0.43 ± 0.20	0.27 ± 0.16	0.43 ± 0.19	0.27 ± 0.16	0.43 ± 0.20	0.27 ± 0.17
	3	0.45 ± 0.20	0.29 ± 0.17	0.44 ± 0.20	0.28 ± 0.19	0.45 ± 0.22	0.29 ± 0.20
Model	4	0.41 ± 0.18	0.26 ± 0.14	0.38 ± 0.16	0.23 ± 0.12	0.40 ± 0.17	0.25 ± 0.14
	5	0.40 ± 0.19	0.25 ± 0.15	0.37 ± 0.18	0.23 ± 0.14	0.38 ± 0.19	0.23 ± 0.15
	6	$\mathbf{0.45 \pm 0.17}$	$\mathbf{0.29 \pm 0.16}$	$\mathbf{0.46 \pm 0.17}$	$\mathbf{0.30 \pm 0.15}$	$\mathbf{0.46 \pm 0.18}$	$\mathbf{0.30 \pm 0.17}$
	7	0.38 ± 0.23	0.23 ± 0.20	0.39 ± 0.22	0.24 ± 0.21	0.40 ± 0.24	0.25 ± 0.22

Tab. 3. Average scores for anatomical regions, qualities, and severities (best scores of each category shown in bold) (DSC: dice similarity coefficient; IoU: intersection over union; NSD: normalized surface distance).

		DSC	IoU	Box-IoU	NSD
	Abdominal	0.42 ± 0.19	0.27 ± 0.16	0.29 ± 0.10	0.70 ± 0.13
Region	Whole-body	0.26 ± 0.16	0.15 ± 0.11	0.22 ± 0.08	0.60 ± 0.23
	Thoracic	$\mathbf{0.49 \pm 0.18}$	$\mathbf{0.32 \pm 0.18}$	$\mathbf{0.34 \pm 0.12}$	$\mathbf{0.74 \pm 0.26}$
	0	0.19 ± 0.17	0.10 ± 0.12	0.18 ± 0.11	0.55 ± 0.25
	1	0.33 ± 0.19	0.20 ± 0.14	0.27 ± 0.10	0.69 ± 0.22
Quality (n)	2	0.41 ± 0.18	0.26 ± 0.15	0.29 ± 0.13	0.71 ± 0.28
	3	0.41 ± 0.17	0.26 ± 0.13	$\mathbf{0.30 \pm 0.11}$	$\mathbf{0.78 \pm 0.20}$
	4	$\mathbf{0.44 \pm 0.30}$	$\mathbf{0.28 \pm 0.29}$	0.30 ± 0.15	0.39 ± 0.28
	1	0.26 ± 0.14	0.15 ± 0.10	0.20 ± 0.09	0.59 ± 0.26
Severity (n)	2	0.39 ± 0.19	0.24 ± 0.16	0.28 ± 0.11	0.67 ± 0.29
	3	$\mathbf{0.43 \pm 0.21}$	$\mathbf{0.27 \pm 0.19}$	$\mathbf{0.31 \pm 0.13}$	0.71 ± 0.28
	4	0.39 ± 0.13	0.24 ± 0.08	0.29 ± 0.07	$\mathbf{0.76 \pm 0.12}$

region of a scan largely dictates the results of the segmentation as depicted in Table 3. Thoracic-only images are predicted most accurately, followed by abdominal-only- and, lastly, whole-body cases. Apart from the anatomical region, the severity ranks assigned to the scans seem to have a noticeable impact on the scores, with types 3 and 4 outperforming groups 1 and 2. In contrast to severity ranks, image qualities have a minor impact on the results except from the SPACE sequence (quality 0) with poor performance due to its contrast characteristics.

4 Discussion

The choice of model configuration is crucial for optimising segmentation results in the context of lymphatic abnormalities, particularly when considering different anatomical regions. The 2D and 3D U-Net models and their ensemble do not show a significant trend in performance. While the 2D model works well for abdominal-only scans, the 3D model excels in segmenting thoracic-only images due to the need for three-dimensional context. The ensemble model does not consistently outperform the others. The comparison of quality distributions reveals that the quality of training images does not significantly impact segmentation performance. In the context of lymphatic perfusion patterns, the rarity of positive foreground pixels in scans can lead to high precision but low sensitivity, which is problematic for clinical diagnosis. Comparing different models with varying foreground-to-background ratios in training sets, it is evident that the size of the training set has a more significant impact on performance than the fore-to-background ratio, highlighting the importance of having a substantial number of training cases in the dataset. For challenging scans with reduced intensity contrast between lymphatic abnormalities and surrounding structures, e.g., where the gastrointestinal tract's similar intensity and texture further complicate the task, the models tend to under-segment the portal-venous region instead of over-segmenting the gastrointestinal tract, as the latter is a larger structure, and the models favour not assigning a foreground label when uncertain. Although the current model performance may benefit from more extensive training data, the efforts to enhance the database of Fontan patients at Erlangen University Hospital are ongoing. To aid clinical professionals in the annotation process, a user interface has been developed that provides predicted segmentation masks and probability maps.

Acknowledgement. The authors gratefully acknowledge the scientific support and HPC resources provided by the Erlangen National High Performance Computing Center (NHR@FAU) under the NHR projects b143dc and b180dc. NHR funding is provided by federal and Bavarian state authorities. NHR@FAU hardware is partially funded by the German Research Foundation (DFG) – 440719683. Additional support was also received by the ERC - project MIA-NORMAL 101083647, DFG KA 5801/2-1, INST 90/1351-1 and by the state of Bavaria.

References

1. Marin-Garcia J. Post-genomic Cardiology. Academic Press, 2011.
2. Schroeder C, Moosmann J, Cesnjevar R, Purbojo A, Rompel O, Dittrich S. A classification of abdominal lymphatic perfusion patterns after Fontan surgery. J Cardio-Thorac Surg. 2022;62(4):ezac103.
3. Vaikom House A, David D, Aguet J, Dipchand AI, Honjo O, Jean-St-Michel E et al. Quantification of lymphatic burden in patients with Fontan circulation by T2 MR lymphangiography and associations with adverse Fontan status. Heart J-Cardiovasc Imaging. 2023;24(2):241–9.
4. Zheng Q, Itkin M, Fan Y. Quantification of thoracic lymphatic flow patterns using dynamic contrast-enhanced MR lymphangiography. Radiol. 2020;296(1):202–7.
5. Biko DM, DeWitt AG, Pinto EM, Morrison RE, Johnstone JA, Griffis H et al. MRI evaluation of lymphatic abnormalities in the neck and thorax after Fontan surgery: relationship with outcome. Radiol. 2019;291(3):774–80.
6. Isensee F, Jaeger PF, Kohl SA, Petersen J, Maier-Hein KH. nnU-Net: a self-configuring method for deep learning-based biomedical image segmentation. Nat Methods. 2021;18(2):203–11.

Data Augmentation for Images of Chronic Foot Wounds

Max Gutbrod[1,2], Benedikt Geisler[1,2], David Rauber[1], Christoph Palm[1]

[1]Regensburg Medical Image Computing (ReMIC), Ostbayerische Technische Hochschule Regensburg (OTH Regensburg)
[2]equal contribution
max.gutbrod@oth-regensburg.de

Abstract. Training data for Neural Networks is often scarce in the medical domain, which often results in models that struggle to generalize and consequently show poor performance on unseen datasets. Generally, adding augmentation methods to the training pipeline considerably enhances a model's performance. Using the dataset of the Foot Ulcer Segmentation Challenge, we analyze two additional augmentation methods in the domain of chronic foot wounds - local warping of wound edges along with projection and blurring of shapes inside wounds. Our experiments show that improvements in the Dice similarity coefficient and Normalized Surface Distance metrics depend on a sensible selection of those augmentation methods.

1 Introduction

Reliable and accurate segmentation results of chronic foot wounds (CFW) help in subsequent analyses such as wound assessment or measuring. As data in the medical field is often scarce, domain-specific augmentation methods play a crucial role in the training of Neural Networks. Thus, we analyze the viability of two existing works [1, 2] in the context of CFWs. The original aim of [1] is to augment chest X-ray images by emulating artifacts generated by X-ray machines. We hypothesize that this technique also proves useful for wound segmentation tasks. This is because blurred areas within the wound may resemble artifacts originating from the image-capturing process or represent realistic variations within the wound itself. Wound boundaries are of special interest to experts as they can indicate whether the CFW is healing or deteriorating. Therefore, the second augmentation method [2] focuses specifically on these segmentation boundaries by locally warping the edges to the inside or outside of the wound, simulating its healing or deterioration process.

Since the segmentation quality of wound boundaries is not represented by the overlap-based DSC metric, we follow the recommendation of [3] and complement our evaluation with a boundary-based metric, namely the Normalized Surface Distance (NSD), which is described in Section 2.7.

2 Materials and methods

This chapter comprises a description of the dataset, the employed augmentation methods, the model architecture, the training process, and evaluation metrics.

© Der/die Autor(en), exklusiv lizenziert an
Springer Fachmedien Wiesbaden GmbH, ein Teil von Springer Nature 2024
A. Maier et al. (Hrsg.), *Bildverarbeitung für die Medizin 2024*,
Informatik aktuell, https://doi.org/10.1007/978-3-658-44037-4_71

2.1 Dataset

The Foot Ulcer Segmentation Challenge [4] from 2021 is a wound image dataset containing foot ulcer images from 889 patients, annotated by domain experts. The image size is 512×512 pixel with zero padding if necessary. The train and validation data consist of 1010 and 200 images and are publicly available. As the test set is held out, we create our own using the method described below. We do not rely on the validation images as test set because there are multiple occurrences of very similar images being contained in both the train and validation set, leading to extremely well performing models when tested against the validation set. To mitigate this, we first combine both the train and validation split into one common pool. Next, we identify and remove 25 duplicate images and then cluster all images containing wounds from the same patient to prevent test set leakage by having images of the same patient in both the train and test data. We do this in an automated fashion by making use of the pretrained CLIP model [5]. This model projects the images into a semantic space and thus allows to cluster images based on their similarity score. We set the similarity threshold to 0.999 for duplicates and between 0.7 and 0.999 for similar images. Using this approach, we identify 49 patients for which 292 similar images are present. Based on the aforementioned similarity assessment, the remaining 893 images are considered to belong to different patients.

Data augmentation was demonstrated to be most effective when applied in environments with limited training data. Hence, we trim the dataset down to 140 images. To this end, for each patient with multiple images we choose one, resulting in 49 samples. Then, 91 images are randomly sampled from the remaining image pool. We split the resulting dataset, stemming from unique patients, into 100 training, 20 validation, and 20 test images.

2.2 Network architecture

To evaluate the proposed augmentation techniques, we use the U-net architecture [6] for medical image segmentation with four symmetrical encoder and decoder layers to receive the same input and output dimensions. In contrast to the original implementation, each convolutional layer is extended with a batch normalization layer. We do not further refine the architecture and use the default PyTorch initialization for the weights and biases.

2.3 Shape projection and blurring

In [1], random geometric shapes are projected onto the object to select regions where Gaussian blurring should be applied. We extend this notion by employing resized versions of an object's corresponding segmentation mask. Ablation studies are carried out, examining the number of projected random shapes, the scaling factor of the resized segmentation mask, and the σ value of the Gaussian blur filter. As default, we set σ to 2.5, the number of random shapes to 3 and the rescale factor to 0.2.

2.4 Warping

To further increase the variance of wound edges we include the Stoachastic Evolution augmentation algorithm proposed by [2]. This algorithm aims to emulate the deterioration and healing process of medical conditions seen in different modalities. The authors have already shown segmentation improvements due to this method for breast mass, prostate, brain tumor, and lung nodule datasets. Applied to our data, warping areas are located at the wound edges and warped to the outside (deterioration) or to the inside (healing). The warping intensity is determined by the area and radius of the wound. For further details, we refer to [2]. The only necessary parameter for this method is the number of local warpings N, which are distributed around the border of the wound in a circular fashion. Figure 1 shows the result of an outside warping with $N = 8$ and the corresponding displacement field. We perform ablation studies on N for inside and outside warping separately.

2.5 Baseline

We establish the baseline by training two additional models. The first does not use any augmentation technique at all, whereas the second one uses a combination of rescaling, rotation, and horizontal flip of the whole image, which we refer to as "traditional augmentation". The scaling factor s is uniformly sampled from the interval [0.8, 1.2], the rotation angle r is sampled within the range [-90°, +90°].

2.6 Training

We train each ablation model for 350 epochs with a batch size of 20 and select the model with the best validation loss to evaluate the test set. In each epoch, we randomly

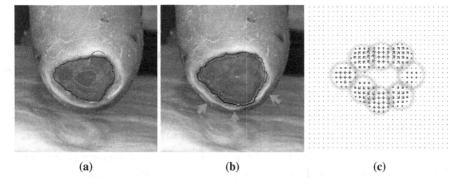

| (a) | (b) | (c) |

Fig. 1. (a) Blur augmentation with two random shapes (pink) and a resized segmentation mask (green). Inside overlapping areas (gray overlay) between the ground truth mask (black border) and the shapes, a Gaussian blur is applied. (b) Outside warping augmentation with old (gray border) and new (black border) mask. Green arrows indicate notable wound edges, induced by the warping augmentation with $N = 8$. (c) Displacement field corresponding to (b) and applied to (a). Each circled area contains one local warping area with a randomized warping strength: each located at the border of the segmentation mask.

Tab. 1. Ablation on hyperparameters of the blur augmentation method described in Section 2.3. σ corresponds to the standard deviation used in the Gaussian blur kernel, n to the number of random geometric shapes, and s to the scaling factor of the resized segmentation mask.

	random shapes			random shapes			segm. shape	
σ	DSC	NSD	n	DSC	NSD	s	DSC	NSD
0.5	59.3 ± 1.9	**41.8 ± 2.6**	1	56.9 ± 3.1	37.8 ± 3.3	0.2	**60.0 ± 2.2**	**41.2 ± 3.8**
1.0	58.7 ± 3.4	38.7 ± 4.5	2	60.5 ± 3.5	39.2 ± 3.7	0.4	59.6 ± 2.4	39.7 ± 2.7
2.0	60.2 ± 2.1	37.8 ± 4.0	3	**60.5 ± 1.8**	**41.1 ± 2.8**	0.6	59.3 ± 3.0	37.0 ± 2.4
2.5	**61.0 ± 3.2**	41.8 ± 4.0	5	59.4 ± 1.4	38.2 ± 3.7			
3.0	60.6 ± 2.8	39.5 ± 4.0						

augment 30 % of the training images. We keep this rate for the combined ablations, always use traditional augmentation, and choose additional augmentations based on a uniform Bernoulli distribution. We use SGD with momentum $\beta = 0.9$ and a OneCycle learning rate scheduler [7] with a maximum learning rate of 0.01 reached after 35 epochs. To enable the training process, the Dice similarity coefficient (DSC) between the ground truth segmentation mask and predictions is calculated and subsequently transformed into the DSC loss, denoted as $DSC_L(y, \hat{y}) = 1 - DSC(y, \hat{y})$.

2.7 Evaluation metric

Following the recommendation of [3], we complement the overlap-based DSC metric used in the loss function with a boundary-based metric, namely the NSD, to make up for the shape unawareness of the overlap-based metric. The NSD measures the overlap between two boundaries $\beta_{A|B}$ within a tolerated deviation distance τ in relation to the boundary length of both shapes

$$\text{NSD}(\beta_A, \beta_B, \tau) = \frac{|\beta_A \cap \beta_B(\tau)| + |\beta_B \cap \beta_A(\tau)|}{|\beta_A| + |\beta_B|} \tag{1}$$

Using the NSD, we hope to identify if and which augmentation technique is best suited to improve segmentations in the challenging area around wound edges. For our experiments, we set τ to two pixels, denoting the radius around the annotation border.

3   Results

In tables 1 and 2, we present the ablation results for isolated augmentation methods. Table 3 shows the results of the two baselines and the combined ablations. Means and standards deviation are calculated on repeated experiments with ten different random seeds. Our results shows the performance boost of traditional augmentation from 56.4 % (DSC) and 37.5 % (NSD) to 62.7 % (DSC) and 46.5 % (NSD). However, these results were further enhanced by additionally applying outside warping, reaching a maximum of 64.2 % (DSC) and 46.8 % (NSD). All other examined augmentation methods achieve 60.0 % – 61.0 % on DSC, and 40.5 % – 41.8 % on NSD. Thus, they perform better than no augmentation but fail to surpass the traditional augmentation. Combining the traditional

Tab. 2. Ablation on the hyperparameter of the warping augmentation described in Section 2.4. N is the number of local warpings.

	inside warp.		outside warp.	
N	DSC	NSD	DSC	NSD
6	59.4 ± 2.1	38.7 ± 4.3	**62.7 ± 3.0**	**42.4 ± 2.3**
8	58.5 ± 2.4	40.1 ± 1.9	62.0 ± 2.1	41.6 ± 2.5
10	**60.2 ± 1.9**	**40.5 ± 2.2**	61.2 ± 2.0	42.0 ± 3.2
12	58.8 ± 2.8	39.4 ± 3.1	61.5 ± 2.4	41.7 ± 1.9
16	59.7 ± 2.2	39.3 ± 3.0	61.1 ± 3.3	40.2 ± 2.9

Tab. 3. Baseline results for no augmentations and for the traditional augmentations (Tra). Additionally, the DSC and NSD results are given for combinations of augmentation methods. Augmentations in brackets are treated as one, since they cannot be used independently.

Augmentations	DSC	NSD
None	56.4 ± 0.0	37.5 ± 0.0
Tra	62.7 ± 2.9	46.5 ± 2.3
Tra + (random shapes)	63.6 ± 3.0	45.7 ± 2.1
Tra + (segm. shape)	62.6 ± 2.0	45.6 ± 2.9
Tra + (random shapes) + (segm. shape)	62.6 ± 3.2	42.5 ± 4.1
Tra + inside warp.	61.5 ± 1.7	45.6 ± 3.8
Tra + outside warp.	**64.2 ± 2.1**	**46.8 ± 2.8**
Tra + inside warp. + outside warp.	63.1 ± 3.2	44.4 ± 5.4
Tra + (random shapes) + (segm. shape) + inside warp. + outside warp.	62.8 ± 2.6	45.4 ± 4.0

method with more than one of our proposed augmentations does not improve the result but rather , at least for NSD. The augmentations inside warping and resized segmentation mask with blurring yield inferior results when combined with the traditional method. Combining all augmentations performs only slightly better than the traditional method alone.

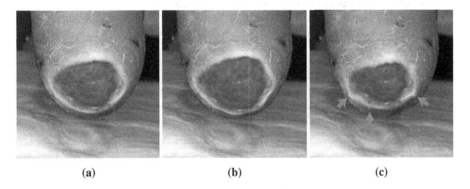

(a)   **(b)**   **(c)**

Fig. 2. (a) Original image. (b) Outside warping with $N = 8$. (c) Inside warping with $N = 8$. Compared to outside warping, clearly visible discontinuities are indicated by green arrows.

4 Discussion

Having established literature in mind, we hypothesized that all proposed methods outperform the augmentation-free baseline while ensuring none degrade performance below this level. However, in the domain of CFWs, stacking augmentations can be disadvantageous when not done carefully. Combining the traditional augmentation method with outside or inside warping, yield both the best and worst result. One reason for this might be the clearly visible discontinuities caused by inside warping, as shown in Figure 2. Further, we cannot exclude the possibility of a bias in the test set in favor of outside and to the detriment of inside warping. As outside warping is on par with the traditional method but executes 43 % faster, it might be a sensible default choice in the domain of CFWs. Both methods combined yield the best result with 1.5 percentage points more on the DSC than the traditional method alone and raise the training time by only 29 %. In terms of NSD, none of the proposed methods significantly outperforms the traditional approach, contrary to our expectations, given that they introduce variance at the wound edges. Future work might focus on the performance difference between inside and outside warping. To this end, a linear interpolation between the N warping fields could help to reduce discontinuities. Further, experiments could be carried out on a more comprehensive dataset to potentially reduce the effect of biases. Implementing a combined loss for the training process, incorporating DSC and NSD characteristics, provides another promising opportunity for future developments.

References

1. Alam MS, Wang D, Sowmya A. Image data augmentation for improving performance of deep learning-based model in pathological lung segmentation. DICTA. IEEE. 2021:1–5.
2. Liu H, Cao H, Song E, Ma G, Xu X, Jin R et al. A new data augmentation method based on local image warping for medical image segmentation. Med Phys. 2021;48(4):1685–96.
3. Maier-Hein L, Menze B et al. Metrics reloaded: pitfalls and recommendations for image analysis validation. arXiv.org. 2022;(2206.01653).
4. Wang C, Mahbod A, Ellinger I, Galdran A, Gopalakrishnan S, Niezgoda J et al. FUSeg: the foot ulcer segmentation challenge. arXiv.org. 2022;(2201.00414).
5. Radford A, Kim JW, Hallacy C, Ramesh A, Goh G, Agarwal S et al. Learning transferable visual models from natural language supervision. Proc Int Conf Mach Learn. Proc PMLR. 2021:8748–63.
6. Ronneberger O, Fischer P, Brox T. U-net: convolutional networks for biomedical image segmentation. Proc MICCAI. 2015:234–41.
7. Smith LN, Topin N. Super-convergence: very fast training of neural networks using large learning rates. Artificial Intelligence and Machine Learning for Multi-domain Operations Applications. Vol. 11006. Proc SPIE. 2019:369–86.

Segmentation of Acute Ischemic Stroke in Native and Enhanced CT using Uncertainty-aware Labels

Linda Vorberg[1,2], Oliver Taubmann[2], Hendrik Ditt[2], Andreas Maier[1]

[1]Pattern Recognition Lab, Friedrich-Alexander-Universität, Erlangen-Nürnberg, Germany
[2]Computed Tomography, Siemens Healthineers AG, Forchheim, Germany
linda.vorberg@fau.de

Abstract. In stroke diagnosis, a non-contrast CT (NCCT) is the first scan acquired and bears the possibility to identify ischemic changes in the brain. Their identification and segmentation are subject to high inter-rater variability. We develop and evaluate models based on labels that reflect the uncertainty in segmentation hypotheses by annotation of minimum ("inner") and maximum ("outer") contours of perceived presence of infarct core and hypoperfused tissue. These labels are used for training nnU-Net to segment both from NCCT and CT angiography (CTA) scans of 167 patients. The predicted output is post-processed to obtain delineations of the tissue of interest at varying distances between inner and outer contours. Compared to the ground truth, infarcts of medium size (10 to 70 ml) could be segmented in the NCCT scans with a median error of 3.7 ml (6.2 ml for CTA) of excess predicted volume, missing 6.4 ml (3.5 ml) of the infarct.

1 Introduction

Stroke is one of the leading causes of death world-wide, with ischemic stroke, which is caused by a lack of blood supply to the brain, accounting for 62.4% of all global stroke incidents [1]. In clinical practice, a non-contrast CT (NCCT) scan is acquired as a first-line imaging tool to exclude hemorrhage and decide on further treatment. In a subsequent CT angiography (CTA) scan, discontinuation of contrast agent can reveal the presence of vessel occlusions causing the stroke. Changes in gray-white matter differentiation or hypoattenuation due to water uptake can be visible in the NCCT scan but may be very subtle and hard to detect due to e. g. low signal-to-noise ratio [2, 3]. CT perfusion (CTP) can more reliably detect stroke core, tissue that is irreversibly damaged, as well as tissue at risk that is still salvageable, the so-called penumbra [4]. However, it might not always be available and is more complex to perform [5]. Prior work reports on a high inter-reader variability and uncertainty in the labels and tries to incorporate this during training of infarct segmentation in NCCT [3, 6]. In our approach, we rely on uncertainty-aware labels in which stroke core and hypo-perfused tissue (consisting in core and penumbra) were both annotated with an inner and outer contour based on CTP result maps, representing boundaries of minimum and and maximum perceived extent of the respective class instead of having one fixed delineation. We train nnU-Net models [7] to predict these annotations with either the NCCT or the CTA scans as model input and provide a meaningful evaluation scheme for the results.

2 Materials and methods

2.1 Data

The dataset used for this study consists of NCCT, CTA and CTP scans of 167 patients. All scans were acquired at a single site with a Somatom Definition AS+ scanner (Siemens Healthineers, Forchheim, Germany). The NCCT voxel spacing is $0.43 \times 0.43 \times 0.8$ mm^3 ($0.64 \times 0.64 \times 0.53$ mm^3 for CTA) on average and all slices have a size of 512×512 pixels. From CTP (voxel spacing $0.43 \times 0.43 \times 1.0$ mm^3), perfusion maps encoding the Cerebral Blood Flow (CBF), Cerebral Blood Volume (CBV) and Time to Maximum Enhancement (TMAX) were calculated to support annotation. For some patients, no appearance of acute stroke could be identified from the perfusion scans. 24 scans lacked signs of infarct core, out of which 9 also did not exhibit signs of penumbra. Additionally, 40 out of 167 patients presented with a prior infarct. The mean infarct size amongst the patients identified with acute ischemic stroke is 34.5 ± 37.3 ml (mean $\pm$ std).

2.2 Uncertainty-aware labels

In medical image classification and segmentation tasks, there is typically a difference between annotations of expert raters which hints at an underlying inherent uncertainty [8]. In stroke lesion segmentation in particular, perfusion maps from CTP, which are predominantly used in clinical routine to determine the extent of penumbra and infarct core tissue prior to treatment, often leave ample room for interpretation. Furthermore, common thresholding-derived core and penumbra masks are prone to artifacts that render them unreliable as reference labels. In this work, we therefore rely on labels that aim to describe this uncertainty pragmatically using an inner and an outer contour of the tissue to be segmented. Both boundaries are annotated for the infarct core as well as the hypoperfused tissue, which is understood as the union of the core and the surrounding penumbra. The outer contour represents the furthest presumed extent of the class, i. e. no part is expected outside of this region. The inner contour delimits the minimum extent, i. e. the actual object is expected to cover this region completely. The inner contour is enforced to lie within the outer contour, with the resulting tube-like structure between both representing an "uncertain" region. Exemplary ground truth labels of both classes can be seen in Fig. 1a. Prior infarcts are additionally annotated using only a single contour as they can be demarcated with higher confidence and only serve as an auxiliary training target to help the model distinguish prior from acute infarctions. Annotations are performed on the baseline time step of CTP, to which the NCCT and CTA data are rigidly registered to ensure alignment of inputs and targets.

2.3 Segmentation model training

We employ the 3D full-resolution U-Net configuration of nnU-Net [7], a state-of-the-art medical segmentation method, to jointly learn segmentation of the inner and outer contours for infarct core and hypoperfused volume, as well as prior infarcts as an auxiliary target, from NCCT or CTA scans as inputs. The framework additionally offers a region-based training that allows to merge individual labels for learning areas comprised of different hierarchical classes, e. g. penumbra enclosing the infarct core. The model is trained in a five fold cross-validation scheme—distinct from the nnU-Net internal cross validation of which only a single train/validation split is run in our setup—to obtain micro-averaged test statistics over all samples.

2.4 Evaluation

2.4.1 Post-processing of predicted label maps. For evaluation, a set of potential boundary realizations between the inner and outer predicted contour is created similar to a threshold sweep in ROC analysis, but based purely on geometric considerations. To this end, for every voxel location $\vec{x}$ within the "tube" between the inner and outer predicted boundaries, the Euclidean Distance Transform (EDT) [9] is computed as

$$d_k(\vec{x}) = \min_{\vec{y} \in \Omega_k} (\|\vec{x} - \vec{y}\|_2) \tag{1}$$

The distance d_k, where $k \in \{O, I\}$, is computed for the inner ($k = I$) and outer ($k = O$) contour, where $\vec{y}$ must lie inside the inner contour when $k = I$ and outside the outer contour when $k = O$, with Ω_k denoting the respective set of voxels. To convert the distances (Eq. 1) into relative distances between 0 and 1, we calculate

$$d_r(\vec{x}) = \frac{d_O(\vec{x})}{d_O(\vec{x}) + d_I(\vec{x})} \tag{2}$$

with $d_r(x) \in [0, 1]$. An example of a resulting relative distance map can be seen in Figure 1b. This map can then be thresholded at different levels, yielding isocontours corresponding to different lesion extents.

2.4.2 Evaluation metrics. To demonstrate the concept but at the same time keep the results concise, we report metrics only at relative distances of 0.0, 0.5 and 1.0 below. For

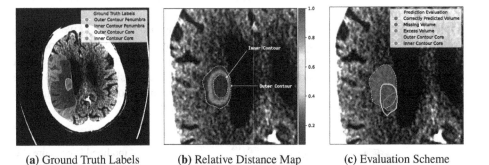

(a) Ground Truth Labels   (b) Relative Distance Map   (c) Evaluation Scheme

Fig. 1. 1a: Visualization of the ground truth labels of both core and penumbra with inner and outer boundary overlayed over the NCCT scan. 1b: Result of the post-processed prediction of core tissue resulting in the relative distance (Eq. 2). 1c: Prediction shown in 1b is thresholded at 0.0 and compared to the ground truth labels of infarct core (same contours as in 1a). Correctly predicted region is overlayed in green, missing region in red and excess volume in blue.

each, the resulting binary mask is compared to the ground truth label of the respective tissue which consists of inner and outer boundary. We assess missing volume, i. e. the region that is not part of the prediction but contained within the inner ground truth contour, and conversely excess volume, i. e. regions of the prediction outside the outer contour. Please note that this is a stricter approach than what is often done in infarct volumetry which only considers the total volume regardless of extent; in our setup, missing and excess volume can never "cancel out".

The correctly predicted region is the intersection of the predicted mask with the region enclosed by the inner and outer contour. In this way, areas outside of the inner contour but still within the outer contour are not penalized. The described measures are visualized in Figure 1c. Based on this concept, a modified Dice coefficient is

$$D(A, B_I, B_O) = \frac{2 \cdot |A \cap B_O|}{|A| + |B_I| + |A \cap (B_O \setminus B_I)|} \tag{3}$$

where A corresponds to the prediction and B_I and B_O to the regions enclosed by the inner and outer ground truth contour, respectively. This modified Dice score has the disadvantage of a variable ground truth, slightly overrating larger predictions as long as they are within the outer contour. However, it is sufficiently close to the original (which is already known to favor larger objects by design) that it still allows for a supplementary, intuitive measure of quality in a single number. It should be understood as a complement to the volumetric approach which provides more exact and nuanced, but less commonly read measurements.

3 Results

We divide our samples into four subgroups based on the mean ground truth infarct core volume (<1 ml, 1-10 ml, 10-70 ml, >70 ml). Following [6], patients with an infarct volume <1 ml are not considered relevant and are therefore excluded from the results. This leads to 142 patients remaining with 44, 77, and 21 patients in the respective subgroups (1-10 ml, 10-70 ml, >70 ml). Figure 2 shows the modified dice scores for the prediction of both hypoperfused and core tissue, averaged over the relative distances of 0.0, 0.5 and 1.0. The dice score is higher for the segmentation of the hypoperfused tissue and rises with increasing infarct size for both tissue types. The median dice score for infarct core is best for infarcts of large size (>70 ml). The left side of Figure 3 shows the minimum and maximum ground truth infarct volume, based on the inner and outer

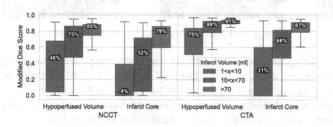

Fig. 2. Results for the modified Dice Score (Eq. 3) for hypoperfused and core region, split up by the size of the ground truth infarct for experiments with NCCT and CTA scans.

contours of the label. To compare, the three plots in each row on the right show excess and missing volume resulting from the predicted segmentation. Both measures are evaluated for the different volume subgroups and relative distances. With higher distances, leading to a smaller segmented region, the excess predicted volume is decreasing and missing volume is increasing. In general, the difference in volume is lower for the smallest infarct volume group (1-10 ml) with a median missing volume of 1.7 ml and excess volume of 0.7 ml with a relative distance of 0.5 in the NCCT scans. An exemplary case with both input images, predictions and CTP for comparison is shown in Figure 4.

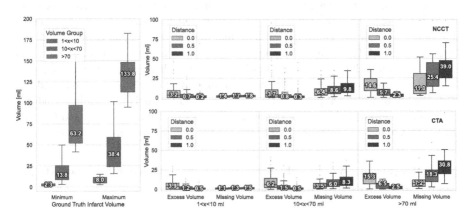

Fig. 3. Volumetric assessment for stroke core: Left plot shows minimum and maximum infarct core volume coming from inner and outer label boundaries. Three plots in each row on the right show excess predicted and missing volume per relative distance threshold. Each plot shows the results for a separate ground truth infarct volume (group). NCCT in upper row, CTA below.

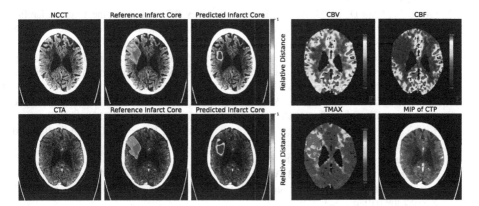

Fig. 4. Example: First column shows the original scan (NCCT/CTA). Columns two and three show the ground truth annotation and predicted label overlayed on the original scan. Right side shows perfusion maps and a Maximum Intensity Projection (MIP) of the CTP scan.

4   Discussion

This work presented an approach to develop and comprehensively evaluate models for ischemic lesion segmentation in both native and enhanced CT based on uncertainty-aware labels. Label uncertainty is of particular relevance in ischemic stroke due to the intrinsic difficulty of determining the precise extent of the infarction based on the reference standard predominantly available as initial diagnostic imaging in clinical routine, namely CT perfusion. Results for CTA were superior to NCCT, which is in line with expectation as the distribution of contrast medium gives a clearer indication of hypoperfusion, whereas early ischemic changes in the NCCT are more subtle. Therefore, for NCCT, core volume also tends to be underestimated across all volume subgroups and thresholds. Overall, we could demonstrate that the core infarct can be identified from both NCCT and CTA scans in the proposed setup, with median volumetric errors well below the volume difference due to label uncertainty. Altering the relative distance of the final contour varies the trade-off between under- and overestimating infarcted core tissue.In future work, we plan to investigate the use of models that explicitly address epistemic uncertainty (e. g., Bayesian neural networks) within this setup and look into the benefits of jointly evaluating NCCT and CTA to utilize complementary information.

Acknowledgement. We sincerely thank the Universitätsklinikum Schleswig-Holstein for providing the data used in this study.

References

1. Tsao CW, Aday AW, Almarzooq ZI, Anderson CA, Arora P, Avery CL et al. Heart disease and stroke statistics—2023 update: a report from the American Heart Association. Circ. 2023;147(8):e93–e621.
2. Grotta JC, Chiu D, Lu M, Patel S, Levine SR, Tilley BC et al. Agreement and variability in the interpretation of early CT changes in stroke patients qualifying for intravenous rtPA therapy. Stroke. 1999;30(8):1528–33.
3. Lin SY, Chiang PL, Chen PW, Cheng LH, Chen MH, Chang PC et al. Toward automated segmentation for acute ischemic stroke using non-contrast computed tomography. Int J Comput Assist Radiol Surg. 2022;17(4):661–71.
4. Mayer TE, Hamann GF, Baranczyk J, Rosengarten B, Klotz E, Wiesmann M et al. Dynamic CT perfusion imaging of acute stroke. AJNR Am J Neuroradiol. 2000;21(8):1441–9.
5. Kim Y, Lee S, Abdelkhaleq R, Lopez-Rivera V, Navi B, Kamel H et al. Utilization and availability of advanced imaging in patients with acute ischemic stroke. Circ Cardiovasc Qual Outcomes. 2021;14(4):e006989.
6. Ostmeier S, Axelrod B, Pulli B, Verhaaren BF, Mahammedi A, Liu Y et al. Random expert sampling for deep learning segmentation of acute ischemic stroke on non-contrast CT. arXiv:2309.03930. 2023.
7. Isensee F, Jaeger PF, Kohl SA, Petersen J, Maier-Hein KH. nnU-net: self-configuring deep learning-based biomedical image segmentation. Nat Methods. 2021;18(2):203–11.
8. Joskowicz L, Cohen D, Caplan N, Sosna J. Inter-observer variability of manual contour delineation of structures in CT. Eur Radiol. 2019;29:1391–9.
9. Strutz T. The distance transform and its computation. arXiv:2106.03503. 2021.

Preprocessing Evaluation and Benchmark for Multi-structure Segmentation of the Male Pelvis in MRI on the Gold Atlas Dataset

Francesca De Benetti[1], Smaranda Bogoi[1], Nassir Navab[1], Thomas Wendler[1,2,3]

[1]Chair for Computer Aided Medical Procedures and Augmented Reality, Technische Universität München, Garching, Germany
[2]Clinical Computational Medical Imaging Research, Department of Interventional and Diagnostic Radiology and Neuroradiology, University Hospital Augsburg, Augsburg, Germany
[3]Institute of Digital Health, University Hospital Augsburg, Neusaess, Germany
francesca.de-benetti@tum.de

Abstract. In radiation therapy (RTx), an accurate delineation of the regions of interest and organs at risk allows for a more targeted irradiation with reduced side effects. In the case of prostate cancer treatments, RTx planning requires the delineation of many pelvic structures. This is a time-consuming task and clinicians would greatly benefit from using robust automatic multi-structure segmentation tools. With the final purpose of introducing an automatic segmentation algorithm in clinical practice, we first address the problem of multi-structure segmentation in pelvic MR using a publicly available dataset. Moreover, we evaluate three types of preprocessing approaches to enable training and inference using different MR sequences. Despite a limited number of training samples, we report an average Dice score of 84.7 ± 10.2% in the segmentation of 8 pelvic structures. The code and the trained models are available at: https://github.com/FrancescaDB/multi_structure_segmentation_gold_atlas

1 Introduction

Recent technological developments have enabled the construction of integrated magnetic resonance (MR) linear accelerators (MR-Linacs). An accurate delineation of the regions of interest and organs at risk is used during online adaptive radiation therapy (RTx) to optimize the irradiation plan with the goal of a more targeted irradiation with reduced side effects [1], but this is a very time-consuming task. Therefore, clinicians would greatly benefit from robust automatic multi-structure segmentation approaches.

Multi-structure segmentation is an established task in the medical imaging community with a number of approaches yielding good results in different tasks (e.g., [2]). However, most of them are developed for computed tomography (CT) volumes, and only a minority address MR imaging, which is the preferred imaging modality in RTx planning because of its superior soft tissue contrast when compared to CT [3].

RTx planning for prostate cancer patients involves conventionally the delineation of many structures in the pelvic region in MR. With the final purpose of introducing a robust automatic segmentation algorithm in clinical practice, we first address the problem of multi-structure segmentation in MR using publicly available datasets. Specifically, the contributions of this work are:

© Der/die Autor(en), exklusiv lizenziert an
Springer Fachmedien Wiesbaden GmbH, ein Teil von Springer Nature 2024
A. Maier et al. (Hrsg.), *Bildverarbeitung für die Medizin 2024*,
Informatik aktuell, https://doi.org/10.1007/978-3-658-44037-4_73

- We perform an extensive literature research on MR segmentation of the pelvic region, as well as on the available public datasets.
- We evaluate three types of preprocessing approaches to enable training and inference using different MR sequences.
- We report the performance of an established Neural Network on the Gold Atlas dataset [4], addressing the lack of a benchmark for multi-structure pelvic MR segmentation on a public dataset.

1.1 Related work

The problem of multi-structure segmentation in MR of the male pelvic region is scarcely addressed in the literature. Between 2018 and 2023, 37 papers focused on the segmentation of anatomical structures in the pelvic region: four of them used synthetic MR data, 12 on CT, and 21 on MR. Among the latter, only six addressed the problem of multi-structure segmentation of three or more structures in the male pelvis.

Chen et al. [5], Elguindi et al. [6], and Savenije et al. [7] used existing architectures to segment some structures among rectum, bladder, prostate, penile bulb, seminal vesicles, rectal spacer, urethra, femoral heads and neurovascular bundles. Li et al. [8] and Nie et al. [9] proposed a few-shot segmentation approach (for the segmentation of eight structures) and a newly designed network called STRAINet (for the segmentation of prostate, bladder, and rectum), respectively. The majority of the papers used T2-weighted MR volumes [6, 8–10], whereas Savenije et al. worked on T1-weighted MR volumes [7] and Sanders et al. used a dataset of T1/T2-weighted MR and T2-weighted MR [11]. With the exception of Savenije et al. [7], the details of the normalization approaches applied to the dataset are omitted or not reported in a way to ensure reproducibility.

Concerning the data availability, six datasets of male pelvic MR are publicly available. Three[1] of them provide the segmentation of the prostate only. The AMOS dataset[2] includes the annotations of prostate, bladder, and some abdominal organs. Two datasets, namely the PROSTATE DIAGNOSIS dataset[3] and the Gold Atlas [4], contain the segmentation of more than seven pelvic structures.

2   Materials and methods

2.1   Dataset

The goal of this paper is to perform multi-structure segmentation of the male pelvis. Specifically, this a preliminary work in the direction of multi-structure segmentation in an in-house MR-Linac dataset. For this reason, we used only the T2-weighted MR volumes of the Gold Atlas dataset, because (a) it includes a high number of annotations (prostate, rectum, seminal vesicles, neurovascular bundles, penile bulb, bladder, anal canal, and femoral heads), and (b) the sequence and field-of-view are similar to the ones of our clinical use case. Therefore, the used dataset is composed of 19 T2-weighted MR

---

[1] pi-cai.grand-challenge.org; medicaldecathlon.com; liuquande.github.io/SAML/
[2] amos22.grand-challenge.org
[3] wiki.cancerimagingarchive.net/display/Public/PROSTATE-DIAGNOSIS

Tab. 1. Details of the portion of the Gold Atlas [4] data used in this work.

Site	Number of volumes	Manufacturer	Sequence	Voxel size [mm^3]
Dataset 1 # 1, # 3	12 (8+4)	GE	T2w-FRFSE	2.5 × 0.875 × 0.875
Dataset 2 # 2	7	Siemens	T2w-TSE	2.5 × 0.875 × 0.875-1.1

volumes. Twelve of them are fast recovery fast spin echo (T2w-FRFSE). The remaining seven are turbo spin echo (T2w-TSE) (Tab. 1). In the following, we will refer to them as "Dataset 1" (D1) and "Dataset 2" (D2), respectively.

2.2 Preprocessing

The two different MR sequences used within the dataset have an impact on the appearance of the volumes (Fig. 1). For this reason, we evaluated several preprocessing approaches. First, we resized the volumes to 384 × 384 in the x and y direction, while keeping the original number of slices. Second, we merged the femoral heads, which are originally segmented separately, into one label. Afterwards, we normalized the data to have a more uniform distribution. Following the consensus in the literature [12–14], we used the min-Max scaling (mM-Scale), which consists in rescaling the original MR values to the [0, 1] interval. Before the scaling, we applied three types of percentile-based clipping at the dataset level: (1) no clipping, (2) 99.5-percentile clipping, and (3) dataset-dependent clipping with 99.9-percentile clipping in D1 and no clipping in D2 (Fig. 2). The different clipping thresholds were empirically chosen in order to include all (#1), few (#3) or none of the outliers (#2) in the distribution of the intensities of the MRI voxels values.

2.3 Segmentation network set-up

We used DeepLabv3 [10] as implemented in the `segmentation-models-pytorch` package. DeepLabv3 is lightweight model and therefore its training and inference phases are faster than state-of-the-art models (such as nn-UNet), which is valuable in clinical

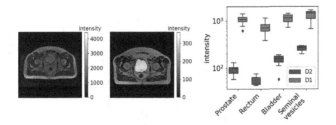

(a) Example of MR slices from D1 (left) and D2 (right).

(b) Boxplots of the original intensities of four selected organs.

Fig. 1. Visual representation of the differences between D1 and D2.

practice. The network takes as input 2D axial slices and was trained for a maximum of 300 epochs, with a learning rate of 10^{-3} and the Adam optimizer. As loss function, we combined Dice loss and weighted cross entropy (WCE) loss with equal weighting between the two. The weights of the WCE were computed based on the volumes of the structures in the training set in order to reduce class imbalance. We used the dice score (DSC) as the evaluation metric.

The two datasets were split at a patient level with 8/2/2 patients for training, validation, and testing in D1, respectively, and 4/1/2 in D2. To cope with the small size of the dataset, we applied data augmentation techniques during the training phase. Specifically, we used the torchio RandomMotion and RandomBiasField transformations (both with probability 0.1), as well as random rotation ($\in [0, 10]°$) and random affine transform (translation $\in [-38, 38]$ voxel and scale $\in [-20, 20]$ %), both with probability 0.5.

2.4 Postprocessing

To limit the number of false positives predicted by the network, we applied the largest connected component (LCC) filter, as implemented in the monai package, to the predictions. In the case of the femoral heads, seminal vesicles, and neurovascular bundle, the number of connected components was set to 2.

3 Results

The overall best performing approach ($\star$) is the mM-scale with dataset-dependent percentile clipping (#3) with LCC, with an average DSC of 84.7 ± 10.2 % (Tab. 2).

Without postprocessing, the best preprocessing type was mM-scale with dataset-dependent percentile clipping (#3), with an average DSC over the 8 structures of 79.2 ± 10.6 %, whereas the worst preprocessing was mM-scale with no clipping (#1).

Interestingly, preprocessing #1 resulted in the best performance at a structure level (penile bulb, DSC = 89.3 ± 2.2 %), as well as the worst (prostate, DSC = 47.2 ± 10.2 %).

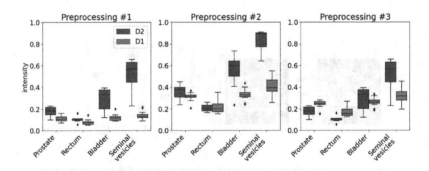

Fig. 2. Boxplots of the intensities of four selected organs for D1 and D2 after preprocessing.

Tab. 2. Dice score (mean ± std - in %) of the trained models with/without postprocessing.

Approach	#1	#2	#3	#1 + LCC	#2 + LCC	#3 + LCC
Anal canal	53.6 ± 6.7	82.8 ± 7.7	87.2 ± 4.8	73.3 ± 7.9	89.0 ± 5.1	89.2 ± 3.1
Femoral heads	85.1 ± 4.6	84.2 ± 2.4	85.2 ± 1.9	91.8 ± 3.9	92.2 ± 3.2	92.0 ± 2.0
Neurovasc. bundle	47.9 ± 6.7	58.2 ± 13.3	67.3 ± 4.4	52.4 ± 5.6	60.3 ± 11.7	73.3 ± 4.6
Penile bulb	89.3 ± 2.2	84.6 ± 8.4	80.8 ± 3.3	89.9 ± 1.2	88.2 ± 3.2	87.4 ± 2.4
Prostate	47.2 ± 10.2	71.6 ± 4.9	77.5 ± 8.5	62.2 ± 6.3	79.0 ± 5.0	84.5 ± 5.5
Rectum	69.8 ± 3.5	70.9 ± 4.7	76.0 ± 5.2	85.3 ± 4.5	84.1± 7.1	83.3 ± 6.5
Seminal vescicles	66.4 ± 7.3	70.2 ± 8.5	60.9 ± 7.7	69.7 ± 5.0	73.6 ± 7.0	63.0 ± 8.2
Bladder	51.0 ± 6.3	72.3 ± 8.6	77.9 ± 6.5	71.5 ± 11.5	86.7 ± 8.5	89.9 ± 4.0
Average	67.0 ± 18.5	77.2 ± 11.2	79.2 ± 10.6	77.3 ± 14.4	83.7 ± 10.8	84.7 ± 10.2★

When using LCC as postprocessing, the best performing structure was the femoral heads (preprocessing #2, DSC = 92.2 ± 3.2 %), and the worst-performing one is the neurovascular bundle (preprocessing #1, DSC = 52.4 ± 5.6 %).

The mM-scale with no clipping (#1) was the best for penile bulb segmentation without LCC, whereas it was the best for penile bulb and rectum after LCC. Similarly, mM-scale with 99.5-percentile clipping (#2) was the best only for seminal vesicles before LCC, but for seminal vesicles and femoral heads after LCC.

The overall high standard deviation (> 10%) shows a high variability in the performance of the network, which improved only slightly after the postprocessing.

4 Discussion

We presented the first benchmark on multi-structure segmentation of the male pelvic region in T2-weighted MR volumes. Despite the limited amount of data, we reported satisfactory performance after the LCC postprocessing (DSC ∈ [63, 89.9] %). Moreover, we evaluated the results of different normalization techniques to cope with T2-weighted MR volumes with different sequences. This is particularly important because this problem for the pelvic MR is not as widely studied as for brain MR [14].

Another challenge was represented by the different sizes of the structures to segment. Larger structures, such as the bladder (DSC = 89.9 ± 4.1 %, preprocessing #3 + LCC) and the rectum (DSC = 83.3 ± 6.5 %), are in general easier to segment than smaller structures, such as neurovascular bundle (DSC = 73.3 ± 4.6 %) and seminal vescicles (DSC = 63.0 ± 8.2 %). Interestingly, the penile bulb results in a very good segmentation (DSC = 87.4 ± 2.4 %), even though it is the smallest structure.

A comparison with the literature is not trivial, as none of the previous work address exactly our problem, and all used private datasets. Moreover, publicly available pre-trained models only focus on the prostate. In general, the performance of the best approach★ is just below the average for the bladder (DSC ∈ [90, 97] % in [5, 6, 9, 11]), within the average for the femoral heads (DSC ∈ [92, 96] % in [5, 7]), and above the average for the penile bulb (DSC = 74 % in [6]). In the case of the rectum, there is good agreement between our results and those of Chen et al. [5], Elguindi et al. [6] and Savenije et al. [7] (DSC ∈ [81, 85] %), however Sanders et al. [11] reported a higher

DSC of 91%. For the seminal vesicles and the prostate, our results are below the average (DSC = 75 % in [11] and DSC ∈ [89, 91] % in [9, 11], respectively).

Overall, this paper is a good starting point for developing robust automatic multi-structure segmentation pipelines for more reliable and less labor-intensive RTx planning.

Acknowledgement. This work was partially funded by the DFG grant NA 620/51–1.

References

1. Kawula M, Vagni M, Cusumano D, Boldrini L, Placidi L, Corradini S et al. Prior knowledge based deep learning auto-segmentation in magnetic resonance imaging-guided radiotherapy of prostate cancer. Phys Imaging Radiat Oncol. 2023.
2. Fu Y, Lei Y, Wang T, Curran WJ, Liu T, Yang X. A review of deep learning based methods for medical image multi-organ segmentation. Physica Medica. 2021.
3. Heinke MY, Holloway L, Rai R, Vinod SK. Repeatability of MRI for radiotherapy planning for pelvic, brain, and head and neck malignancies. 2022.
4. Nyholm T, Svensson S, Andersson S, Jonsson J, Sohlin M, Gustafsson C et al. MR and CT data with multiobserver delineations of organs in the pelvic area: part of the gold atlas project. Med Phys. 2018.
5. Chen X, Ma X, Yan X, Luo F, Yang S, Wang Z et al. Personalized auto-segmentation for magnetic resonance imaging-guided adaptive radiotherapy of prostate cancer. Med Phys. 2022.
6. Elguindi S, Zelefsky MJ, Jiang J, Veeraraghavan H, Deasy JO, Hunt MA et al. Deep learning-based auto-segmentation of targets and organs-at-risk for magnetic resonance imaging only planning of prostate radiotherapy. Phys Imaging Radiat Oncol. 2019.
7. Savenije MH, Maspero M, Sikkes GG, Voort van Zyp JR van der, TJ Kotte AN, Bol GH et al. Clinical implementation of MRI-based organs-at-risk auto-segmentation with convolutional networks for prostate radiotherapy. Radiat Oncol. 2020.
8. Li Y, Fu Y, Yang Q, Min Z, Yan W, Huisman H et al. Few-shot image segmentation for cross-institution male pelvic organs using registration-assisted prototypical learning. Proc IEEE ISBI. 2022.
9. Nie D, Wang L, Gao Y, Lian J, Shen D. STRAINet: spatially varying sTochastic residual AdversarIal networks for MRI pelvic organ segmentation. Trans Neur Netw Learn Syst. 2018.
10. Chen LC, Papandreou G, Schroff F, Adam H. Rethinking atrous convolution for semantic image segmentation. arXiv:1706.05587. 2017.
11. Sanders JW, Lewis GD, Thames HD, Kudchadker RJ, Venkatesan AM, Bruno TL et al. Machine segmentation of pelvic anatomy in MRI-assisted radiosurgery (MARS) for prostate cancer brachytherapy. Int J Radiat Oncol Biol Phys. 2020.
12. Isaksson LJ, Raimondi S, Botta F, Pepa M, Gugliandolo SG, De Angelis SP et al. Effects of MRI image normalization techniques in prostate cancer radiomics. Phys. Med. 2020.
13. Panic J, Defeudis A, Balestra G, Giannini V, Rosati S. Normalization strategies in multi-center radiomics abdominal MRI: systematic review and meta-analyses. IEEE Open J Eng Med Biol. 2023.
14. Scalco E, Belfatto A, Mastropietro A, Rancati T, Avuzzi B, Messina A et al. T2w-MRI signal normalization affects radiomics features reproducibility. Med Phys. 2020.

Evaluation of Semi-automatic Segmentation of Liver Tumors for Intra-procedural Planning

Dominik Pysch[1,2], Maja Schlereth[1], Mihai Pomohaci[2], Peter Fischer[2], Katharina Breininger[1]

[1]Department Artificial Intelligence in Biomedical Engineering, FAU Erlangen-Nürnberg, Erlangen, Germany
[2]Siemens Healthcare GmbH, Forchheim, Germany
dominik.pysch@fau.de

Abstract. Transarterial chemoembolization (TACE) is a common procedure for the treatment of intermediate-stage primary liver cancer, in which the blood supply of the tumor is suppressed by occluding the supplying vessels. In this procedure, contrast-enhanced cone-beam computed tomography (CBCT) scans are used to localize the tumor lesions and identify their feeding vessels, potentially aided by segmentation software. With the help of semi-automatic segmentation algorithms, a high-quality segmentation of a tumor can be achieved with minimal user input, such as drawing a line approximating the tumor's longest axis. In this paper, we conduct a user study for evaluating human tendencies when annotating tumors in this manner, build a simulator based on our findings and design a semi-automatic segmentation method based on DeepGrow, trained on simulated inputs. We compare it to the random walker algorithm, acting as an established baseline measure, on the task of liver tumor segmentation using a dataset of CBCT scans along with simulated user inputs. We discover that human users tend to overestimate tumors with an average distance of 2.8 voxels to the tumor's boundary. Our customized network outperforms the random walker with an average Dice score of 0.89 and an average symmetric surface distance (ASSD) of 1.16 voxels compared to a Dice score of 0.69 and an ASSD of 2.95 voxels. This shows the potential of learning-based methods to speed up the intraprocedural segmentation workflow.

1 Introduction

Hepatocellular carcinoma (HCC) is a primary malignant tumor of the liver, ranked as the fifth most common cause of cancer worldwide. Around 830.000 people died from liver cancer globally in 2020 and an increase of over 50% is predicted by the year 2040 [1]. Transarterial chemoembolization (TACE) is a common procedure for the treatment of intermediate-stage HCC [2], in which feeding vessels of the tumor are occluded and chemotherapeutic agents are delivered locally [3]. 3D cone-beam computed tomography (CBCT) images are acquired during the procedure to locate the tumor and its feeding vessels as accurately as possible and guide the intraoperative devices to the correct location [4]. Precisely defining the edges of the tumor to perform accurate treatment and prevent harming healthy tissue requires a robust segmentation of the tumor area. However, a complete manual segmentation of the tissue in a volumetric image is not feasible for clinical practice. Instead, a semi-automatic segmentation can be applied

© Der/die Autor(en), exklusiv lizenziert an
Springer Fachmedien Wiesbaden GmbH, ein Teil von Springer Nature 2024
A. Maier et al. (Hrsg.), *Bildverarbeitung für die Medizin 2024*,
Informatik aktuell, https://doi.org/10.1007/978-3-658-44037-4_74

which enables fast and reliable delineation of the tissue of interest. To perform semi-automatic segmentation many algorithms are applicable. Grady introduced the random walker algorithm, which converts an image into a graph representation and applies labels to the vertices (representing pixels) by computing the probabilities of a random walk stopping at pre-labeled seed vertices [5]. Amrehn et al. propose a deep learning approach for interactive human-in-the-loop segmentation using fully convolutional neural networks (CNNs), allowing the user to iteratively adjust the segmentation. They showcase that a learning-based approach can outperform classical, non-learning-based algorithms [6]. DeepGrow by Sakinis et al. [7] is another deep learning approach to interactive segmentation, providing user input as heatmaps to the network.

In order to minimize user interaction and accelerate the process, semi-automatic algorithms can be used for quicker segmentation during time-critical interventions such as TACE. In this paper, we develop a learning-based semi-automatic segmentation algorithm for liver tumors. Therefore, we modify DeepGrow to use only one single lightweight user input at the beginning (in the form of a single line along the tumor's longest axis) instead of an additional iterative sequence of corrections. We conduct a user study to investigate human interaction with the annotation tool and the accuracy and variability between users. We use our findings from these experiments for our network setup. On a dataset of liver CBCT scans with simulated user input, we evaluate two trained models compared to the random walker as a baseline.

2 Materials and methods

2.1 Dataset

An internal dataset of 98 CBCT volumes from 98 different patients is used in this study. All volumes depict the liver in the arterial phase of an intra-arterial injection of contrast agent. The volumes have been acquired in multiple hospitals and cover the liver for planning liver-directed endovascular therapy such as TACE or selective internal radiation therapy (SIRT) on fixed C-arms (Siemens Healthineers, Forchheim, Germany). Tumor lesions are annotated by a radiologist with 5 years of experience. Only non-rim arterially hyperenhancing lesions (APHE), as defined by the LIRADS lexicon with a diameter above 1 cm are included. The dataset is split by volume into 82 volumes (135 lesions) for training and validation and into 16 volumes (19 lesions) for testing. After splitting, each lesion is treated as an independent sample.

2.2 User input

In the interventional setting, it is important to select the treatment target with minimal user input. In our work, we select a line along the longest axis of the tumor as user input because radiologists are used to this form of annotation from tumor measurements. In a user study, we asked 15 medical students to annotate tumors of the LiTS training set with this method, resulting in 510 tumor annotations on a total of 56 tumors. After searching a suitable view for placing the line, the line is drawn by placing two clicks for the line's endpoints. The ratio between the longest possible line segment within the tumor visible in the selected view and the longest possible line segment in the tumor overall averages at 0.91, showing that the user is reliably able to find a suitable view for placing the line. When comparing the users' clicks with the ground truth segmentations, we find that 59.6% of the clicks lie outside of the tumor, 29.7% of the clicks lie inside of it and 10.7% of the clicks perfectly hit the tumor's boundary. Thus we conclude a tendency to overestimate tumors when annotating them by this given method. Furthermore, we find that on average, the users' clicks were off the boundary by 2.8 (±0.6) voxels, when measuring the minimal Manhattan distance between a click and the boundary.

In this work, we simulate the user input based on the ground truth segmentation of the lesion. The simulation method used in this paper is visualized in Figure 1. We first compute the three principal components of the tumor. We construct a line parallel to the primary component passing through the tumor's center of mass (dotted red line in Fig. 1a). This estimation should emulate the users ability to find a view of the tumor containing its longest axis. On each side, we select the tumor voxel that is closest to an arbitrary point on the line far outside of the tumor, delivering the outermost voxels along the primary component (green voxels in Fig. 1a). In an optional last step, the line's endpoints can get moved along the line by a random or fixed amount to account for the observed human error. In the example in Figure 1b, the two endpoints are randomly moved within the red area.

As described in Section 2.3, DeepGrow requires foreground and background seeds as user input to segment the lesion, meaning that our inputs have to be pre-processed before feeding them into the DeepGrow algorithm. We uniformly distribute two foreground seeds along the line segment between its endpoints c_1 and c_2, as well as four background seeds along the line beyond c_1 and c_2, respectively.

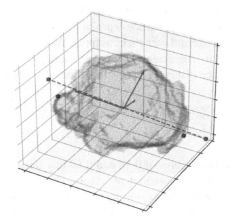 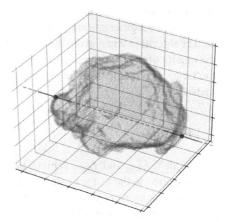

(a) Line approximating the tumor's longest axis. Resulting endpoints in green.

(b) Shifting the line's endpoints by a random amount, mimicking the average human error.

Fig. 1. Visualizing our method for simulating user input.

2.3   Deepgrow

Sakinis et al. introduced a learning-based algorithm for interactive semi-automatic segmentation called DeepGrow [7]. It uses a U-Net with three 3D input channels: the image itself and two guidance signal maps for foreground and background seeds, respectively. The user input gets stored in a binary mask of the same size as the image. A Gaussian filter is applied to the mask in order to smooth the input, producing the guidance signal map which is finally used as the network input. In Sakinis' DeepGrow, the user is able to refine the computed segmentation by iteratively adding foreground or background seeds in a human-in-the-loop process. We modified this approach such that only one initial input (formed as described in 2.2) is required. Finally, our CNN uses (32, 64, 128, 256, 512) feature maps. The image has a size of $64 \times 64 \times 64$ pixel. Intensity values of the images are normalized, mapping the range $[-120, 240]$ to $[-1, +1]$ without clipping. The Adam optimization algorithm and the Tversky loss ($\alpha = 0.4$, $\beta = 0.6$) are used. We apply a learning rate of 0.0001 and a dropout of 0.3, training for 500 epochs, whilst applying geometrical as well as intensity augmentation. The method is implemented in MONAI and pytorch.

2.4   Experiment

We train our network on the described dataset using simulated user inputs two times. The first model f_{clean} is trained with simulated input without any added errors. When training the second model f_{noisy}, we include the optional step described in section 2.2, moving the simulated endpoints of the line by an amount chosen uniformly at random out of the interval $[-6, +6]$, leading to an absolute deviation similar to the previously determined average human error of 2.8 voxels. We then apply both models to the test set, again using simulated user inputs with and without added errors. We compare the quality of the segmentation results to masks produced by the non-learning-based random walker algorithm when given the exact same image and user clicks as input. We measure the quality of the results using the Dice similarity coefficient (Dice) as an overlap-based metric as well as the average symmetric surface distance (ASSD) as a distance-based metric [8].

3   Results

Our models f_{clean} and f_{noisy} achieve average Dice scores of 0.88 and 0.89 respectively when applied to the test set using simulated user input without any errors. The random walker scores an average Dice score of 0.69. When randomly shifting the simulated clicks by an amount chosen uniformly at random out of the interval $[-6, 6]$ (comparable to the average human error) we do not see huge differences. When we increase the magnitude of the error, we measure a drop of the average Dice score of model f_{clean} down to 0.79 and a drop to 0.64 of the random walker, while still measuring a stable average Dice score of 0.88 of model f_{noisy}. The ASSD reveals the same tendency. The box plots in Figure 2 provide a summary of the segmentation results by all three algorithms across the whole test set in three cases: applying the algorithms using simulated input without any errors added, with a randomized shift of the clicks of an extent chosen uniformly at random (u.a.r) in $[-6, 6]$ and with a randomized shift of the clicks of an extent chosen u.a.r in $[-18, 18]$. Both the Dice score and the ASSD show that our network delivers consistently very good results. The random walker algorithm performs well in the majority of cases, though never as good as our model when comparing single cases. When the user input is subject to above-average errors, we can observe that the model f_{noisy}, which was already trained with erroneous inputs, delivers better results than the model f_{clean}.

Figure 3 shows a qualitative example of segmentations computed with user-input without any errors added. One sample slice out of a sample lesion of the test set together with the segmentation results of our model f_{noisy} as well as the random walker approach is displayed.

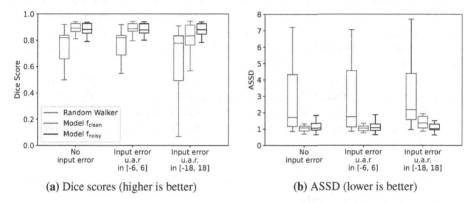

(a) Dice scores (higher is better)   (b) ASSD (lower is better)

Fig. 2. Results of applying DeepGrow models f_{clean} and f_{noisy} and the random walker on the test set using simulated user input, varying applied errors. Whisker lengths are set to 1.5 times the interquartile range.

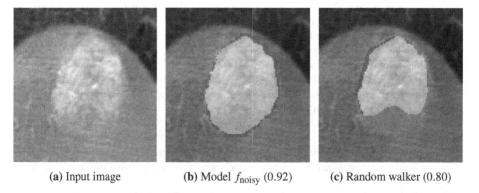

(a) Input image   (b) Model f_{noisy} (0.92)   (c) Random walker (0.80)

Fig. 3. Qualitative examples of the test set. True positives in yellow, oversegmented areas in blue, undersegmented areas in green, Dice score in parentheses.

4 Discussion

We observe that the learning-based approach for semi-automatic segmentation of liver tumors clearly delivers better results than the classical random walker algorithm when trained and applied to the described interventional CBCT dataset. This shows the potential of learning-based methods to improve the intraprocedural segmentation workflow compared to classical heuristical segmentation algorithms. We also observe that artificially adding errors to user inputs during training of such a model is advantageous, since it becomes more robust to above-average user input errors during inference. There are several limitations to the presented study. Interventional imaging data is not as widely available as diagnostic imaging data like CT or MRI. Thus, the CBCT dataset collected and annotated for this study is relatively small. We had to use a non-public dataset because the available public datasets are designed for fully automatic segmentation. Since test labels are hidden in such datasets, the generation of simulated user inputs is not possible and our method not applicable. This hampers comparison with results from other methods. The dataset is limited to a subgroup of liver lesions that could be treated with embolization. The performance of the method on hypoenhancing or rim-enhancing lesions is unclear.

In future work, one should collect real human user input and again apply the model to the test set with the collected instead of simulated input. Since we already train with the average human error included, we expect a comparable performance to the simulated user input. Furthermore, a larger dataset is required for a thorough evaluation of the method.

Disclaimer. The concepts and information presented in this paper are based on research and are not commercially available.

References

1. Rumgay H, Arnold M, Ferlay J, Lesi O, Cabasag CJ, Vignat J et al. Global burden of primary liver cancer in 2020 and predictions to 2040. J Hepatol. 2022.
2. Asafo-Agyei KO, Samant H. Hepatocellular Carcinoma. StatPearls [Internet]. 2022.
3. Lewandowski RJ, Geschwind JF, Liapi E, Salem R. Transcatheter intraarterial therapies: rationale and overview. Radiol. 2011;259(3):641–57.
4. Cui Z, Shukla P, Habibollahi P, Park HS, Fischman A, Kolber M. A systematic review of automated feeder detection software for locoregional treatment of hepatic tumors. Diagn Interv Imaging. 2020;101(7-8). Elsevier:439–49.
5. Grady L. Random walks for image segmentation. IEEE Trans Pattern Anal Mach Intell. 2006;28(11):1768–83.
6. Amrehn M, Gaube S, Unberath M, Schebesch F, Horz T, Strumia M et al. UI-Net: interactive artificial neural networks for iterative image segmentation based on a user model. Proc EG VCBM. 2017:143–7.
7. Sakinis T, Milletari F, Roth H, Korfiatis P, Kostandy P, Philbrick K et al. Interactive segmentation of medical images through fully convolutional neural networks. 2019.
8. Reinke A, Tizabi MD, Sudre CH, Eisenmann M, Rädsch T, Baumgartner M et al. Common limitations of image processing metrics: a picture story. 2021.

Generalizable Kidney Segmentation for Total Volume Estimation

Anish Raj[1,2], Laura Hansen[1], Fabian Tollens[3], Dominik Nörenberg[3], Giulia Villa[4], Anna Caroli[4], Frank G. Zöllner[1,2]

[1]Computer Assisted Clinical Medicine, Medical Faculty Mannheim, Heidelberg University, Mannheim, Germany
[2]Mannheim Institute for Intelligent Systems in Medicine, Medical Faculty Mannheim, Heidelberg University, Mannheim, Germany
[3]Department of Clinical Radiology and Nuclear Medicine, Medical University Center Mannheim, Medical Faculty Mannheim, Heidelberg University, Mannheim, Germany
[4]Bioengineering Department, Istituto di Ricerche Farmacologiche Mario Negri IRCCS, Ranica (BG), Italy
anish.raj@medma.uni-heidelberg.de

Abstract. We introduce a deep learning approach for automated kidney segmentation in autosomal dominant polycystic kidney disease (ADPKD). Our method combines Nyul normalization, resampling, and attention mechanisms to create a generalizable network. We evaluated our approach on two distinct datasets and found that our proposed model outperforms the baseline method with an average improvement of 9.45 % in Dice and 79.90 % in mean surface symmetric distance scores across both the datasets, demonstrating its potential for robust and accurate total kidney volume calculation from T1-w MRI images in ADPKD patients.

1 Introduction

Autosomal dominant polycystic kidney disease (ADPKD) is a common cause of chronic kidney disease, ultimately leading to end-stage renal disease and kidney failure in most cases [1]. The total kidney volume (TKV) can be used to monitor ADPKD progression and is also recognized as a relevant prognostic marker [2–4]. TKV calculation requires accurate delineation of kidney volumes which is usually performed manually by an expert and is time-consuming. Therefore, automated segmentation is warranted [5, 6]. However, deep learning approaches should generalize well to unseen external datasets to become clinical applicable. Hence, in this work, we develop an approach by combining Nyul normalization [7], resampling, and attention mechanisms to create a generalizable neural network for ADPKD kidney segmentation.

2 Materials and methods

2.1 Patient data

The patient T1-w MRI data were obtained from two different sources. The first dataset was obtained from the National Institute of Diabetes and Digestive and Kidney Disease

A. Maier et al. (Hrsg.), *Bildverarbeitung für die Medizin 2024*,
Informatik aktuell, https://doi.org/10.1007/978-3-658-44037-4_75

Tab. 1. Descriptive statistics from both ADPKD datasets.

Characteristic	Dataset A	Dataset B
Patient count	93	41
Male:female ratio	50:50	46:54
Average age (years)	30 ± 10	44 ± 11
Image size	256 × 256 × [30-80]	512 × 512 × [40-66]
In-plane resolution (mm^2)	1.41 × 1.41 (±0.13)	0.73 × 0.73 (±0.03)
Slice thickness (mm)	3.06 ± 0.29	4 ± 0.00
TKV (ml)	1311 ± 977	1582 ± 970

(NIDDK), National Institutes of Health, USA, and was collected in the Consortium for Radiologic Imaging Studies of Polycystic Kidney Disease (CRISP) study [1]. The second dataset was collected in the context of the EuroCYST Initiative (ClinicalTrials.gov Identifier: NCT02187432). From here on, we call the first and second Datasets A and B, respectively. Both MRI datasets were acquired in coronal orientation from ADPKD patients with CKD stages 1 to 3. Tab. 1 depicts the characteristics of each dataset.

2.2 Image annotation

Dataset A was annotated by two physicians with experience of 1 and 3 years, respectively [8]. The mean inter-user agreement for Dataset A was 0.91±0.06 (Dice) with a coefficient of variation of 0.07. Dataset B was annotated by a single expert with 4 years of experience in manual tracing of renal ADPKD.

2.3 Image pre-processing

We first resampled both datasets to a uniform resolution of 1.4×1.4×3.0 mm^3. We further resized Dataset B's image size to 256×256 voxels to keep it in line with Dataset A. Furthermore, to create similar histogram distribution between the two datasets, we trained Nyul normalizer [7] on Dataset A. Then we transformed Dataset B using the trained normalizer to align the image intensity distributions of both datasets. Next, we normalized intensities using volume-wise z-score normalization. These steps bring the distributions of both the datasets closer and help in network generalizability.

2.4 Network architecture

We implemented two U-Net [9] based architectures for kidney segmentation. The first is nnUNet [10], which we used as a baseline model. The second is based on a combination of Convolution Block Attention Module (CBAM) [11] and Attention U-Net [12]. The attention mechanisms help in extracting relevant image regions from spatial and channel dimensions of the feature maps. The CBAM and Attention modules were combined to form CBAM-Attention U-Net as described in [8]. Fig. 1 depicts the network architecture of CBAM-Attention U-Net.

2.5 Training

We trained both baseline (nnUNet) and CBAM-Attention U-Net for 100 epochs with 5-fold cross-validation on Dataset A and then make prediction on Dataset B and vice versa for testing model generalizability on unseen datasets as a function of training size. The nnUNet was trained with its standard settings [10]. The CBAM-Attention U-Net was trained with a patch size of 128×128 with a combination of cross-entropy and dice loss and the image preprocessing as described in sub-section 2.3. The training:validation:test split for Dataset A for each fold consisted of 73:2:18 patients. For Dataset B the split was 31:2:8, respectively. Further training details can be found in [8].

2.6 Evaluation

We employed two metrics to compare the network predictions to the ground-truth; the dice (DSC) score for assessing the overlap and the mean surface symmetric distance (MSSD) (in mm) which is more perceptive to alignment and shape.

3 Results

Histograms of pre- and post-Nyul normalization are shown in Fig. 2. The quantitative segmentation results are given in Tab. 2.

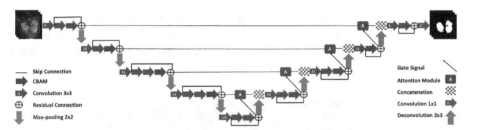

Fig. 1. CBAM-Attention U-Net with Convolution Block Attention Modules in encoder path and attention gates in decoder path of a U-Net architecture.

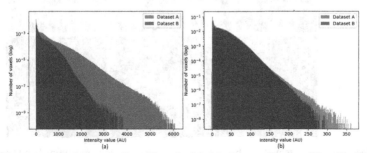

Fig. 2. Histograms of datasets before (a) and after Nyul normalization (b), with Wasserstein distances of 227.5 and 2.4, respectively.

Tab. 2. Quantitative results comparing the baseline nnUNet to our CBAM-Attention U-Net. All the scores are obtained by combining results from each test fold in 5-fold cross validation so that whole dataset is covered in testing. The best results are highlighted in italics. The up and down arrows indicate that higher and lower values denote better performance.

Network	Training dataset	DSC ↑ Dataset A	Dataset B	MSSD (mm) ↓ Dataset A	Dataset B	Volume difference (%) Dataset A	Dataset B
Baseline	A	*0.914±0.057*	0.896±0.098	2.89±4.39	8.64±14.21	1.95±11.77	-0.41±5.21
	B	0.521±0.255	0.885±0.122	17.00±15.01	8.95±14.76	40.72±36.70	*-0.24±5.66*
CBAM	A	0.910±0.054	0.898±0.052	*1.21±1.45*	1.64±1.38	*1.06±13.76*	-0.35±11.85
U-net	B	0.800±0.160	*0.915±0.044*	3.33±6.90	*1.35±1.30*	18.77±22.73	2.86±7.98

For Dataset A, CBAM-Attention U-Net attains the best MSSD (1.21±1.45 mm) and volume difference (1.06±13.76%), while the baseline attains the best DSC (0.914±0.057) when trained on Dataset A. For Dataset B, the best DSC (0.915±0.044) and MSSD (1.35±1.30 mm) are obtained by the CBAM-Attention U-Net, however, the baseline provides the best volume difference of -0.24±5.66 % (here, both trained on Dataset B). Moreover, the CBAM-Attention U-Net attains a DSC of 0.898±0.052 on Dataset B when trained exclusively on Dataset A. Finally, qualitative results from the best and worst predictions are visualized in Figs. 3 and 4.

4 Discussion

This study aimed at creating a generalizable kidney segmentation algorithm for T1-w MRI images of patients with ADPKD. Similarity of data distribution is important to create a robust algorithm that can generalize to data from multiple sources. To achieve

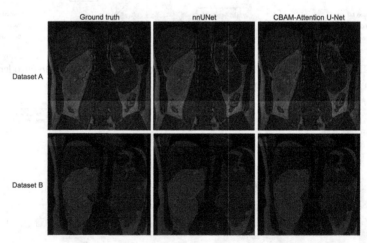

Fig. 3. Qualitative results with the best predictions from both networks trained on Dataset A and B, repectively. For Dataset A DSCs are 0.966 and 0.963 for nnUNet and CBAM-Attention U-Net and for Dataset B 0.931 and 0.959, respectively.

this, we made intensity distributions of the datasets similar by using resampling and Nyul normalization and then training CBAM-Attention U-Net. The CBAM-Attention U-Net outperformed nnUNet [10] (4/6 metric values), a common medical segmentation baseline. It exhibited generalization when trained on Dataset A, performing well on both sets (DSC ≈ 0.90). However, training on Dataset B (41 patients) showed reduced generalizability on Dataset A, indicating a likely dependence on training dataset size. Compared to other works [13, 14] (2000 and 400 cases, respectively), our approach attains lower DSC (v/s >0.97). However, they used a significantly larger training data than our study. To explore the impact of training dataset size on generalizability, additional external datasets would be necessary. In conclusion, we demonstrated that with enough data, we can create a generalizable ADPKD kidney segmentation algorithm. This approach can be helpful in reliably and automatically calculating TKV for ADPKD patients.

Disclaimer. The authors declare that they have no conflict of interest.

Acknowledgement. The Consortium for Radiologic Imaging Studies of Polycystic Kidney Disease (CRISP) was conducted by the CRISP Investigators and supported by the National Institute of Diabetes and Digestive and Kidney Diseases (NIDDK). The data from the CRISP study reported here were supplied by the NIDDK Central Repository. This manuscript was not prepared in collaboration with investigators of the CRISP study and does not necessarily reflect the opinions or views of the CRISP study, the NIDDK Central Repository, or the NIDDK. Data collection in the context of the EuroCYST Initiative was funded by ERA – EDTA. This study was supported in part by the German Federal Ministry of Education and Research (BMBF) under the funding code 01KU2102, and the Italian Ministry of Health, under the frame of ERA PerMed

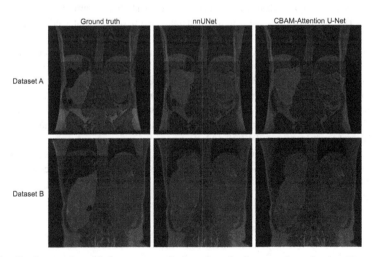

Fig. 4. Qualitative results with the worst predictions from both networks trained on Dataset A and B, respectively. The bad performance of networks is due to the presence of cysts in the liver.

(ERAPERMED2020-326 - RESPECT). We also acknowledge a grant from the Italian Association for Polycystic Kidney (Associazione Italiana Rene Policistico - AIRP).

References

1. Chapman AB, Guay-Woodford LM, Grantham JJ, Torres VE, Bae KT, Baumgarten DA et al. Renal structure in early autosomal-dominant polycystic kidney disease (ADPKD): the consortium for radiologic imaging studies of polycystic kidney disease (CRISP) cohort. Kidney Int. 2003;64(3):1035–45.

2. Irazabal MV, Rangel LJ, Bergstralh EJ, Osborn SL, Harmon AJ, Sundsbak JL et al. Imaging classification of autosomal dominant polycystic kidney disease: a simple model for selecting patients for clinical trials. J Am Soc Nephrol. 2015;26(1):160.

3. Grantham JJ, Torres VE, Chapman AB, Guay-Woodford LM, Bae KT, King Jr BF et al. Volume progression in polycystic kidney disease. N Engl J Med. 2006;354(20):2122–30.

4. Raj A, Tollens F, Caroli A, Nörenberg D, Zöllner FG. Automated prognosis of renal function decline in ADPKD patients using deep learning. Z Med Phy. 2023.

5. Zöllner FG, Kociński M, Hansen L, Golla AK, Trbalić AŠ, Lundervold A et al. Kidney segmentation in renal magnetic resonance imaging-current status and prospects. IEEE Access. 2021;9:71577–605.

6. Zöllner FG, Svarstad E, Munthe-Kaas AZ, Schad LR, Lundervold A, Rørvik J. Assessment of kidney volumes from MRI: acquisition and segmentation techniques. AJR Am J Roentgenol. 2012;199(5):1060–9.

7. Nyúl LG, Udupa JK. On standardizing the MR image intensity scale. Magn Reson Med. 1999;42(6):1072–81.

8. Raj A, Tollens F, Hansen L, Golla AK, Schad LR, Nörenberg D et al. Deep learning-based total kidney volume segmentation in autosomal dominant polycystic kidney disease using attention, cosine loss, and sharpness aware minimization. Diagnostics. 2022;12(5):1159.

9. Ronneberger O, Fischer P, Brox T. U-net: convolutional networks for biomedical image segmentation. Proc MICCAI. Springer. 2015:234–41.

10. Isensee F, Jaeger PF, Kohl SA, Petersen J, Maier-Hein KH. nnU-net: a self-configuring method for deep learning-based biomedical image segmentation. Nat Methods. 2021;18(2):203–11.

11. Woo S, Park J, Lee JY, Kweon IS. Cbam: convolutional block attention module. Proc ECCV. 2018:3–19.

12. Oktay O, Schlemper J, Le Folgoc L, Lee M, Heinrich M, Misawa K et al. Attention U-net: learning where to look for the pancreas. Proc MIDL. 2022.

13. Kline TL, Korfiatis P, Edwards ME, Blais JD, Czerwiec FS, Harris PC et al. Performance of an artificial multi-observer deep neural network for fully automated segmentation of polycystic kidneys. J Digit Imaging. 2017;30:442–8.

14. He X, Hu Z, Dev H, Romano DJ, Sharbatdaran A, Raza SI et al. Test retest reproducibility of organ volume measurements in ADPKD using 3D multimodality deep learning. Acad Radiol. 2023.

Multi-organ Segmentation in CT from Partially Annotated Datasets using Disentangled Learning

Tianyi Wang, Chang Liu, Leonhard Rist, Andreas Maier

Pattern Recognition Lab, Department of Computer Science, Friedrich-Alexander-Universität Erlangen-Nürnberg
tianyi.wang@fau.de

Abstract. While deep learning models are known to be able to solve the task of multi-organ segmentation, the scarcity of fully annotated multi-organ datasets poses a significant obstacle during training. The 3D volume annotation of such datasets is expensive, time-consuming and varies greatly in the variety of labeled structures. To this end, we propose a solution that leverages multiple partially annotated datasets using disentangled learning for a single segmentation model. Dataset-specific encoder and decoder networks are trained, while a joint decoder network gathers the encoders' features to generate a complete segmentation mask. We evaluated our method using two simulated partially annotated datasets: one including the liver, lungs and kidneys, the other bones and bladder. Our method is trained to segment all five organs achieving a dice score of 0.78 and an IoU of 0.67. Notably, this performance is close to a model trained on the fully annotated dataset, scoring 0.80 in dice score and 0.70 in IoU respectively.

1 Introduction

The emergence of deep learning (DL) has had a huge impact on the development of various fields, including biomedical imaging[1, 2]. In the field of multi-organ segmentation, DL has become a powerful tool[3, 4]. Accurate and automated multi-organ segmentation has great potential in a wide range of medical applications from diagnosis to therapy.

Despite its huge potential, the practical application of DL-based multi-organ segmentation comes with challenges. Chief among them is the quantity and quality of data. DL-based segmentation models are mostly trained in a supervised fashion, requiring a large number of paired images and annotations for a successful training. However, due to the difficulty of manual organ segmentation, such datasets are seriously downgrading model performance. Many public segmentation dataset are public available but can also be freely used because of unmatched annotations. For example, the CT-ORG[5] dataset contains annotations of bones but no abdominal organs, while the AMOS[6] dataset contains annotations of abdominal organs without bones. Both datasets cannot be used to train a network for both bones and abdominal organs segmentation because they are both partially annotated.

Several studies have attempted to solve this problem using semi-supervised learning[7], transfer learning[8] and weakly-supervised learning[9]. However, these methods usually require large amounts of unannotated data, specialised network architectures or complex training procedures. In contrast, disentangled learning is proposed to split

© Der/die Autor(en), exklusiv lizenziert an
Springer Fachmedien Wiesbaden GmbH, ein Teil von Springer Nature 2024
A. Maier et al. (Hrsg.), *Bildverarbeitung für die Medizin 2024*,
Informatik aktuell, https://doi.org/10.1007/978-3-658-44037-4_76

the network training into multiple sub-tasks, improving the training of the individual network components. We propose a novel approach using disentangled learning to make more efficient use of partially annotated datasets[10–12]. In our experiments, the proposed method is evaluated in comparison with three baselines to demonstrate its effectiveness.

2   Materials and methods

A disentangled strategy is implemented to train a single model on multiple partially annotated datasets. As a proof of concept, we simulate two partially annotated datasets from a fully annotated one. In our experiments, we utilize two common solutions to work with partially annotated datasets.

2.1   Dataset

The data used in this work stems from CT-ORG, which consists of computed tomography (CT) volumes from multiple clinical institutions. From these, we selected 28 volumes for training and 4 volumes for testing. The CT volumes are annotated with all five organ labels of interest: liver, lung, kidney, bone, and bladder. Partially annotated datasets are artificially generated from fully annotated datasets by simply neglecting parts of the

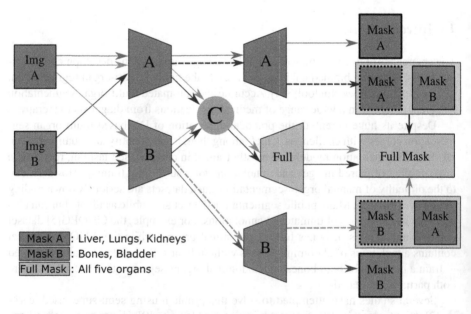

Fig. 1. Disentangled strategies of the proposed method. Four pathways are indicated using arrows in four colors and the disentangled network consists of two encoder networks and three decoder networks. The dashed arrows indicate the path with no optimization and the dashed data indicates the inference from the decoder block.

organ annotation. In particular, two subsets are created from the fully annotated dataset, one containing 14 CT volumes with liver, lungs and kidneys annotation, namely subset A, and the other containing 14 CT volumes with bones and bladder annotation, namely subset B.

2.2 Disentangled strategy

The proposed disentangled strategy is presented in Figure 1. During training, five networks are involved in total. Encoder A and B disentangle the input images from subset A and B accordingly, while decoder A and B generate the segmentation only in subset A and B. Decoder Full gathers the disentangled features from encoder A and B and generate the full segmentation mask of all five organ segmentation.

One key issue for training the decoder Full is the missing ground truth for the full segmentation mask. In our disentangled strategy, the missing segmentation masks in full ground truth is replaced with the intermediate prediction of one subset decoder, i.e. the input data from one subset is fed to the encoder/decoder of the other subset and the output is used to substitute for the ground truth.

To generate reasonably meaning full predictions which lead to a smoother training. For a smoother training of the decoder full, the encoder/decoder A and B is first pre-trained for 20 epochs. After pre-training the input batch is tagged with either subset A or B. When for example the input batch is from subset A, it is fed to encoder A and encoder/decoder A is trained first. Afterwards, the batch is fed to encoder B and the intermediate features from encoder A and B are concatenated as input to decoder full. Decoder B is not optimized when input batch is from subset A and it only outputs the alternated ground truth. When the input batch is from subset B, a similar process is followed.

2.3 Experimental setup

All trained networks in the experiments use the same segmentation model and training configuration, and we use 3D U-Net as the segmentation model[13]. Adam is optimizer, the learning rate is 5×10^{-4}, and a combination of dice loss and cross-entropy loss is applied as the loss function. We evaluated the model's performance with the dice score (DSC) and the intersection over union (IoU). Three baselines were defined in our experiments.

- Baseline 1 (Base1): A segmentation network is trained on 28 CT volumes with full annotations. Base1 represents the best-case condition, where all volumes are fully annotated.
- Baseline 2 (Base2): A segmentation network is trained on the mixture of subset A and B and no measure is done for partial annotation. Base2 represents the case when the networks is not aware of the partial annotation datasets and still trained for full organ segmentation.
- Baseline 3 (Base3): Two segmentation networks are separately well-trained for subset A and B and afterwards each of these networks is applied to compensate for the missing annotations in the other subset[14]. Base3 is one common strategy

Tab. 1. Segmentation performance and the training efficiency results of our proposed method and the baseline methods.

	DSC Avg.	IoU Avg.	Num of epochs Avg.
Base1	0.80	0.70	247
Base2	0.46	0.40	294
Base3	0.77	0.67	277
Our method	0.78	0.67	214

to utilize partially annotated datasets. However much more computation time and memory is required.

Furthermore, we extend the experiments by cross-validation to better evaluate the methods. After training, we tested each model using four volumes with full annotations.

3 Result

The segmentation results of the proposed method and the baseline methods are shown in Table 1. In addition to the average DSC and IoU, we also present the average number of epochs of the cross-validation models until the training converges. For Base3 the average epochs is aggregated from the training of all three models, and for our method the pre-training is included. From Table 1, it can be observed that Base1 achieves the highest

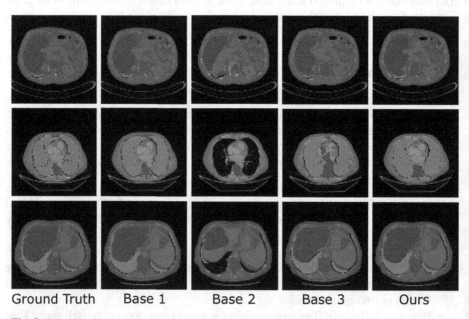

Ground Truth   Base 1   Base 2   Base 3   Ours

Fig. 2. Example slices of the organ segmentation in testing CT volumes. Liver, lung, bones and kidneys are each illustrated in blue, orange, purple and green color.

Tab. 2. Organ-wise segmentation results in DSC.

	Liver	Lung	Kidney	Bladder	Bone
Base1	0.86	0.92	0.71	0.57	0.81
Base2	0.42	0.50	0.27	0.11	0.39
Base3	0.85	0.92	0.60	0.52	0.77
Our method	0.87	0.94	0.61	0.52	0.77

Tab. 3. Organ-wise segmentation results in IoU.

	Liver	Lung	Kidney	Bladder	Bone
Base1	0.75	0.87	0.57	0.42	0.68
Base2	0.34	0.42	0.19	0.06	0.26
Base3	0.74	0.86	0.45	0.36	0.64
Our method	0.77	0.89	0.45	0.37	0.63

average DSC and IoU, followed by our method. In comparison of Base1, our method only shows a decrease of 0.02 in average DSC and 0.03 in average IoU. The segmentation performance of Base3 is very close to our proposed method, but the average number of training epochs is 29.4% more than our method. On the contrary, Base2 shows the worst segmentation performance, in addition to the highest average number of training epochs. As shown in Table 2 and 3 the organ-wise segmentation results of DSC and IoU all show the same trend as the average performance. Some example slices of the organ segmentation of the test CT volumes are shown in Figure 2.

4 Discussion

Our proposed method is trained from partially annotated datasets, which results in only a minimal drop in segmentation performance, compared with the baseline trained on fully annotated dataset. It also trains in a more efficient way compared with other common solutions to work with partially annotated datasets. Our work provides a novel strategy to leverage multiple segmentation datasets and to train a single model for all targets.

Two common solutions for training models using partially annotated datasets are implemented in the experiments. It is indicated that utilizing more available datasets can work as a work-around to increase the scale of dataset, and further improve the model performance. However, a simple mixing of partially annotated datasets leads to decreasing performance and efficiency of the model training. Training multiple models for each partial datasets can be a working solution, but the complexity increases with the increasing number of the involved datasets. The proposed strategy can be easily modified to multiple partially annotated datasets.

In our experiments, the partial annotations are simulated from a full annotated dataset, while the real-world datasets are more complex because of the different annotation groups and project regulations. Gathering the effort of annotation in the public segmentation datasets is still a challenging and open research question.

References

1. Aljabri M, AlGhamdi M. A review on the use of deep learning for medical images segmentation. Neurocomputing. 2022;506:311–35.
2. Hesamian M, Jia W, He X et al. Deep learning techniques for medical image segmentation: achievements and challenges. J Digit Imaging. 2019;32:582–96.
3. Lei Y, Fu Y, Wang T, Qiu RLJ, Curran WJ, Liu T et al. Deep learning in multi-organ segmentation. 2020.
4. Fu Y, Lei Y, Wang T, Curran WJ, Liu T, Yang X. A review of deep learning based methods for medical image multi-organ segmentation. Physica Medica. 2021;85:107–22.
5. Rister B, Yi D, Shivakumar K, Nobashi T, Rubin DL. CT-ORG, a new dataset for multiple organ segmentation in computed tomography. Sci. Data. 2020;7(1):381.
6. Ji Y, Bai H, Ge C, Yang J, Zhu Y, Zhang R et al. Amos: a large-scale abdominal multi-organ benchmark for versatile medical image segmentation. Proc NeuroIPS. 2022;35:36722–32.
7. Zhu X. Semi-supervised learning literature survey. Comput Sci. 2008;2.
8. Pan SJ, Yang Q. A survey on transfer learning. IEEE Trans Knowl Data Eng. 2010;22(10):1345–59.
9. Zhou ZH. A brief introduction to weakly supervised learning. Natl Sci Rev. 2018;5(1):44–53.
10. Zhou T, Ruan S, Canu S. A review: deep learning for medical image segmentation using multi-modality fusion. Array. 2019;3-4:100004.
11. Lyu Y, Liao H, Zhu H, Zhou SK. A^{3}DSegNet: anatomy-aware artifact disentanglement and segmentation network for unpaired segmentation, artifact reduction, and modality translation. 2021.
12. Yang Q, Guo X, Chen Z, Woo PYM, Yuan Y. D2-Net: dual disentanglement network for brain tumor segmentation with missing modalities. IEEE Trans Med Imaging. 2022;41(10):2953–64.
13. Ronneberger O, Fischer P, Brox T. U-Net: convolutional networks for biomedical image segmentation. Proc MICCAI. 2015:234–41.
14. Salimi Y, Shiri I, Mansouri Z, Zaidi H. Deep learning-assisted multiple organ segmentation from whole-body CT images. medRxiv. 2023.

Abstract: Generation of Synthetic 3D Data using Simulated MR Examinations in Augmented Reality

Aniol Serra Juhé[1,2], Daniel Rinck[2], Andreas Maier[1]

[1]Pattern Recogniton Lab, Friedrich-Alexander-Universität Erlangen-Nürnberg, Germany
[2]Siemens Healthcare GmbH, Erlangen, Germany
aniol.serra@fau.de

In the future, medical imaging devices such as computed tomography (CT) and magnetic resonance (MR) are expected to become increasingly autonomous. Therefore, design criteria and workflow of such devices will change substantially. Moreover, sensor data of the system are required to develop scene understanding algorithms to support and guide the user. Data availability might be a critical factor due to patient privacy issues, high cost of labelling data or impossibility to acquire it in dangerous situations. In this work, we present an approach to generate synthetic 3D point cloud data from a simulated MR examination experienced on the Microsoft Hololens2. The complete workflow of an MR examination using a virtual, autonomous MR scanner is reproduced in an AR scene. The user can interact with an avatar of the patient via voice commands, select a procedure in a GUI or position a coil. The user is recorded by a system of active stereo vision RGBD-cameras while interacting with AR elements. A registration routine of the AR scene and the RGBD-cameras is described, and accuracy measurements are provided. The real point clouds are fused with virtually generated point clouds from the AR scene. These point clouds are completely labelled and 3D bounding boxes of the objects as well as the rotation and translation of their corresponding CAD models are saved. Our approach can be used to generate synthetic depth data such as a real depth camera would see once the system – or even a system that does not yet physically exist - is built and installed on-site [1].

References

1. Juhé AS, Rinck D, Maier A. Generation of synthetic 3D data using simulated MR examinations in augmented reality. Proc IEEE. 2023:1–5.

Smoke Classification in Laparoscopic Cholecystectomy Videos Incorporating Spatio-temporal Information

Tobias Rueckert[1], Maximilian Rieder[1], Hubertus Feussner[2], Dirk Wilhelm[2], Daniel Rueckert[3,4], Christoph Palm[1,5]

[1] Regensburg Medical Image Computing (ReMIC), Ostbayerische Technische Hochschule Regensburg (OTH Regensburg), Regensburg
[2] Department of Surgery, Faculty of Medicine, Klinikum rechts der Isar, Technical University of Munich, Munich
[3] Artificial Intelligence in Healthcare and Medicine, Klinikum rechts der Isar, Technical University of Munich, Munich
[4] Department of Computing, Imperial College London, London
[5] Regensburg Center of Health Sciences and Technology, OTH Regensburg, Regensburg
tobias.rueckert@oth-regensburg.de

Abstract. Heavy smoke development represents an important challenge for operating physicians during laparoscopic procedures and can potentially affect the success of an intervention due to reduced visibility and orientation. Reliable and accurate recognition of smoke is therefore a prerequisite for the use of downstream systems such as automated smoke evacuation systems. Current approaches distinguish between non-smoked and smoked frames but often ignore the temporal context inherent in endoscopic video data. In this work, we therefore present a method that utilizes the pixel-wise displacement from randomly sampled images to the preceding frames determined using the optical flow algorithm by providing the transformed magnitude of the displacement as an additional input to the network. Further, we incorporate the temporal context at evaluation time by applying an exponential moving average on the estimated class probabilities of the model output to obtain more stable and robust results over time. We evaluate our method on two convolutional-based and one state-of-the-art transformer architecture and show improvements in the classification results over a baseline approach, regardless of the network used.

1 Introduction

Laparoscopic surgery has a number of advantages over conventional surgery, such as reduced surgical trauma, faster patient recovery, and a shortened hospital stay [1]. As the inside of the abdominal cavity is transmitted to an external monitor and is only visible on this display, a clear view at all times during the intervention is crucial for smooth progress and a satisfactory result. However, one challenge of such procedures is represented by the development of severe smoke due to surgeon activities, including the electronic coagulation of tissue. This presents difficulties for the surgical team due to the operating physicians's deteriorated field of view, which can significantly impair the success of an operation. A prerequisite for being able to react accordingly to this in downstream applications, like automated smoke evacuation or early-warning

© Der/die Autor(en), exklusiv lizenziert an
Springer Fachmedien Wiesbaden GmbH, ein Teil von Springer Nature 2024
A. Maier et al. (Hrsg.), *Bildverarbeitung für die Medizin 2024*,
Informatik aktuell, https://doi.org/10.1007/978-3-658-44037-4_78

systems, is the accurate and reliable recognition of smoke and its level of intensity in endoscopic video images. This can be realized by extracting visual features from the histogram of frames using Saturation Peak Analysis (SPA) [2, 3] or by approaches based on Convolutional Neural Networks (CNN) [2–6]. Employing semi-supervised learning methods has shown the potential to optimize the considerable amount of time and human resources required for image annotation by self-training a noisy student model [4], which can be improved by utilizing the temporal context within the network architecture and integrating a co-occurrence based undersampling strategy [5]. Current approaches further utilize components of CNN- and transformer-based architectures for smoke classification of laparoscopic frames [6]. However, the majority of existing work focuses on single-frame classification and ignores the temporal information inherent in unlabeled endoscopic video images, for which this paper provides two contributions:

- In addition to the spatial context, we utilize the temporal component by determining the optical flow (OF) between randomly sampled and preceding frames and provide the magnitude of the pixel-wise displacement as an additional input to the network.
- At evaluation time, we apply an exponential moving average (EMA) to the estimated class probabilities of the model output to ensure more stable and robust predictions for video frame classification due to the incorporation of temporal information.

2 Materials and methods

2.1 Dataset

We collected a dataset consisting of five videos recorded during real laparoscopic cholecystectomies, ranging from 29 to 51 minutes in duration. All videos were recorded at 25 frames per second (FPS) and have a resolution of 1920×1080 pixels. We used every 25th frame, which sums up to 11,377 images, and excluded 2,142 frames from that showing the area outside the abdominal cavity to protect the anonymity of the operating room staff, resulting in a total of 9,235 images. For each frame, there exists a manual annotation whether it belongs to a non-smoked, medium-smoked, or heavy-smoked scenery, and all labels were created by one medical computer scientist to ensure consistency across the dataset. Of the frames determined and annotated in this way, 5,929 are classified as non-smoked, 1,375 as medium-smoked, and 1,931 images correspond to the heavy-smoked category.

2.2 Baseline architectures

As a basis for our experiments, we use two CNN architectures belonging to the ResNet family [7], namely ResNet-18 and ResNet-34, as well as the SwinV2-T [8], a state-of-the-art transformer network for image classification. For both CNN and transformer-oriented architectures, we decided to use the variants with the lowest number of parameters, as we observed a fast adaptation of the networks to the training data and an early occurrence of overfitting in more complex models. With these architectures, the video images are processed on a per-frame basis and classified according to the above-mentioned categories.

2.3 Incorporation of spatio-temporal information

Given an RGB input image $x_i \in \mathbb{R}^{1 \times 3 \times H \times W}$ with $H \times W$ corresponding to the input resolution, and a one-hot encoded ground truth vector $y_i \in \mathbb{R}^{1 \times C}$ for $c \in C$ possible classes, we define a network as a function $N : \mathbb{R} \to \mathbb{R}$. The class predictions y_i' of a network can thus be obtained by $y_i' = \mathrm{argmax}(s_i)$, with $s_i = S(N(x_i))$ representing the probabilities for each class, determined by the softmax function $S : \mathbb{R}^C \to \mathbb{R}^C$ on basis of the raw outputs of the network $N(x_i)$. The argmax function then simply selects the class with the highest probability as the final prediction y_i' for x_i.

During training, we randomly select one sample x_j from the training dataset and determine, based on the frame number, the corresponding previous frame x_i, with $i = j - 1$. Based on these two consecutive images, we estimate the pixel-wise displacement $d_{i \to j} = F(x_i, x_j)$ using the optical flow algorithm [9], which can be written as a function $F = \mathbb{R}^2 \to \mathbb{R}$. The two channels of the result $d_{i \to j} \in \mathbb{R}^{1 \times 2 \times H \times W}$ provide information on the magnitude and direction of the displacement of the individual pixels. We convert the values of the magnitude channel to polar coordinates and divide all entries by the maximum magnitude to ensure that all values are within the interval $[0, 1]$. This maximum is determined before the training over the entire training dataset and corresponds to the largest displacement of a pixel in all images. The magnitude normalized in this way is then stacked to the RGB input of the network so that the transformed input has the form $x_j \in \mathbb{R}^{1 \times 4 \times H \times W}$. As the dimensions $H \times W$ of the RGB image and the magnitude channel are identical, no further adaptations are necessary here.

For validation, we use the exponential moving average as a further temporal component in order to make more stable and robust predictions for the current frame x_j based on previous results. For this purpose, the probability vector s_j of the individual classes c for the input frame x_j is weighted with a term α, and the prior term $\mathcal{E}_i$ consisting of results of previous EMA calculations is taken into account with the weight $1 - \alpha$. The modified prediction for the output y_j' based on this approach is

$$y_j' = \mathrm{argmax}(\underbrace{\alpha \cdot s_j + (1 - \alpha) \cdot \mathcal{E}_i}_{= \, s_j'}) \tag{1}$$

To maintain temporal consistency, the frames of the validation dataset are sampled in the appropriate order contrary to training, and the prior term $\mathcal{E}_i$ is updated with the aligned softmax vector s_j' subsequently to the processing of each sample.

2.4 Experiments and evaluation

We train the networks ResNet-18, ResNet-34, and SwinV2-T for two, four, and six epochs, respectively, resize all images to a resolution of 480×272 pixels, normalize the input RGB channels individually by their means and standard deviations, and use cross-entropy as our loss function. For all experiments, the Adam optimizer, a batch size of 50, a maximum learning rate of $1e^{-4}$, and a one-cycle scheduler strategy are used, which uses 30 % of the total training steps for the increase up to this value and then decreases cosine-shaped. All experiments are performed using the PyTorch framework [10], and

Tab. 1. F1-scores given in percent and standard deviations for the individual smoke intensity classes and for the overall results regarding the networks used. All results correspond to the averaged values across the five folds.

Experiment		Smoke Intensity (in %)			
Architecture	Method	S_{non}	S_{medium}	S_{heavy}	$S_{overall}$
	Baseline	91.25 ± 3.22	40.05 ± 15.93	82.28 ± 9.49	71.19 ± 8.54
ResNet-18	OF	91.82 ± 4.05	**43.13 ± 15.37**	83.06 ± 8.11	72.67 ± 7.56
	OF + EMA	**91.95 ± 3.76**	42.95 ± 15.91	**83.37 ± 8.20**	**72.76 ± 7.80**
	Baseline	89.11 ± 5.33	40.49 ± 15.11	81.93 ± 8.33	70.51 ± 8.69
ResNet-34	OF	91.40 ± 2.75	**43.17 ± 14.22**	83.52 ± 7.84	72.69 ± 7.37
	OF + EMA	**91.47 ± 2.71**	42.91 ± 14.12	**83.86 ± 7.74**	**72.74 ± 7.31**
	Baseline	92.24 ± 2.65	41.05 ± 15.82	82.21 ± 8.36	71.83 ± 7.24
SwinV2-T	OF	92.52 ± 2.44	43.33 ± 12.76	81.73 ± 8.50	72.52 ± 5.84
	OF + EMA	**92.73 ± 2.42**	**43.55 ± 13.01**	**82.31 ± 8.20**	**72.86 ± 5.91**

the implementation of the OF is based on the cuda accelerated Farneback algorithm [9] and the Nvidia Optical Flow SDK 2.0, both provided by OpenCV [11].

For the evaluation of our methods, we determine the F1-score once per epoch separately for each of the three classes based on the predictions and ground truth values of all images, and average the results over all classes. To obtain meaningful results, a five-fold cross-validation is performed in which each of the five videos is used once as the validation sequence and the others serve as the training dataset. We calculate the F1-score for each fold and average the individual values to obtain the final result.

3 Results

The quantitative, cross-validated results regarding the architectures used for each individual smoke intensity category as well as for the overall results are shown in Table 1. Our presented method including the magnitude of the pixel-wise shift using the OF was able to increase the baseline results averaged over all classes from 71.19 % to 72.67 %, 70.51 % to 72.69 %, and 71.83 % to 72.52 % for the three architectures, respectively. The additional employment of EMA led to further improvements up to 72.76 %, 72.74 %, and 72.86 %, respectively. In all experiments, the classification of non-smoked and heavy-smoked frames achieved a higher F1-score than the classification of medium-smoked frames. For the OF + EMA method, the α values 0.9, 0.8, and 0.8 were used for the ResNet-18, ResNet-34, and SwinV2-T networks, respectively. The developments of the F1-scores over the different α values in the interval $[0.1, 1.0]$ with 0.1 steps compared to the baseline and the OF method are shown in Figure 1, where an increase in the F1-score up to a certain point and a subsequent drop can be seen. Figure 2 shows the effect of different degrees of smokiness on the resulting OF, where it can be seen that increased smoke intensity leads to less homogeneous areas and contours and an increase in noise in the OF estimation. The color intensity-coded magnitude of the displacements shows higher values for non-smoked images concerning coherent structures such as moving instruments than for heavy-smoked images, and the majority of pixels of such structures are oriented in the same direction in non-smoked images, in contrast to the heavy-smoked modality.

4 Discussion

In this work, we proposed an approach to classify laparoscopic frames into three classes based on their smoke intensity utilizing temporal information. The use of OF-based pixel-wise displacement provides an efficient method to integrate the temporal context inherent in endoscopic video data into the training process of a network, with our results showing that the models benefit from the additional magnitude values provided. Our results further show that the used CNN-based and transformer-based architectures benefit equally from this approach, with no significant differences in the final F1-scores. Non-smoked and heavy-smoked video frames were classified considerably better than medium-smoked ones which can be attributed to the unbalanced number of class samples in the training data and the stronger discriminative features of the former two classes. In contrast to other approaches incorporating the temporal component, our method does not impose any requirements on the sampling strategy at training time, allowing the random selection of frames to be retained as part of the augmentation strategy. Applying EMA at validation time is a simple and efficient method to integrate prior results and obtain more stable and robust predictions, although our results show that the weighting of the prior term must be chosen with care.

Future work should extend this research by further analyzing the information that can be extracted from the OF and exploring ways to incorporate the temporal context into the smoke classification task.

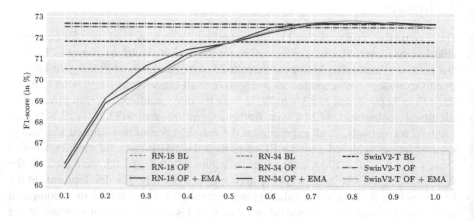

Fig. 1. F1-scores in percent corresponding to the respective α values for the Baseline (BL), OF, and OF + EMA methods for the two ResNet (RN) and the SwinV2-T architecture.

Fig. 2. Effect of smoke intensity on the OF estimation. The first row shows images with moving objects from the different smoke domains, with the estimated OF presented below, indicating the magnitude of the displacement of a pixel by its color intensity and its direction by the color value.

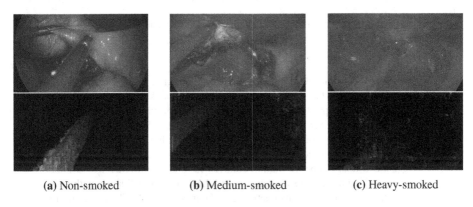

(a) Non-smoked   (b) Medium-smoked   (c) Heavy-smoked

Acknowledgement. Funding: This work was supported by the Bavarian Research Foundation [BFS, grant number AZ-1506-21], and the Bavarian Academic Forum [Bay-WISS].

References

1. Darzi A, Mackay S. Recent advances in minimal access surgery. Br Med J. 2002;324(7328):31–4.
2. Leibetseder A, Primus MJ, Petscharnig S, Schoeffmann K. Image-based smoke detection in laparoscopic videos. Comput Assist Robot Endosc Clin Image Based Proced. Springer, 2017:70–87.
3. Leibetseder A, Primus MJ, Petscharnig S, Schoeffmann K. Real-time image-based smoke detection in endoscopic videos. Proc ACM Multimedia. 2017:296–304.
4. Reiter W. Improving endoscopic smoke detection with semi-supervised noisy student models. Biomed Engineering. Vol. 6. (1). De Gruyter, 2020:20200026.
5. Reiter W. Co-occurrence balanced time series classification for the semi-supervised recognition of surgical smoke. Int J Comput Assist Radiol Surg. 2021;16(11):2021–7.
6. Wang H, Wang K, Yan T, Zhou H, Cao E, Lu Y et al. Endoscopic image classification algorithm based on poolformer. Front Neurosci. 2023;17.
7. He K, Zhang X, Ren S, Sun J. Deep residual learning for image recognition. Proc IEEE. 2016:770–8.
8. Liu Z, Hu H, Lin Y et al. Swin transformer v2: scaling up capacity and resolution. Proc IEEE. IEEE, 2022:12009–19.
9. Farnebäck G. Two-frame motion estimation based on polynomial expansion. Image Anal SCIA. Springer, 2003:363–70.
10. Paszke A et al. PyTorch: an imperative style, high-performance deep learning library. Adv Neural Inf Process Syst. Vol. 32. MIT Press, 2019.
11. Bradski G. The OpenCV library. J Softw Tools. 2000;120:122–5.

Learning High-resolution Delay-and-sum Beamforming

Christopher Hahne

Artificial Intelligence in Medical Imaging, ARTORG Center, University of Bern
christopher.hahne@unibe.ch

Abstract. Ultrasound (US) imaging is a versatile tool in modern healthcare diagnostics that often faces spatial resolution challenges. Although ultrasound localization microscopy (ULM) surpasses resolution constraints by fast perfusion scanning, it often relies on traditional delay-and-sum (DAS) beamformers. In response, we propose a differentiable DAS pipeline with a learnable apodization feature descriptor connected to a super-resolution network. Learning apodization weights and image super-resolution contributes to an improvement of B-mode image quality. Quantitative assessment on ULM data and validation with an *in vivo* dataset demonstrates the effectiveness of our approach. While this study employs ULM data, our findings provide insights that hold broader implications for computational beamforming.

1 Introduction

Within healthcare diagnostics, ultrasound (US) imaging is a non-invasive technology that allows us to peer inside the body's intricacies. At the core of US image reconstruction lies the process called delay-and-sum (DAS) beamforming, which is used for a broad range of today's medical diagnostics. When compared to other imaging modalities, however, US beamforming offers relatively low spatial resolution, governed by the physical wavelength. Given the critical role of detailed image resolutions for medical diagnosis, overcoming the diffraction limit is a key focus in US imaging research.

Ultrasound localization microscopy (ULM) emerges as a prominent solution for this challenge [1], making use of recent advances in plane wave emissions at high frame rates. In the celebrated study, researchers demonstrate the possibility to enhance the US image resolution via localization and tracking of contrast agents, known as microbubbles, traversing the perfused vascular system. Yet, most ULM frameworks employ traditional DAS beamformers to pinpoint individual microbubbles [2, 3], which may not fully exploit the potential of the US data. For instance, recent studies suggest to skip beamforming [4, 5], emphasizing the need to consider context-specific methods.

To that end, we devise, implement and validate a differentiable DAS pipeline accommodating learnable feature descriptors to facilitate an adaptive apodization prediction. Further, we install a super-resolution network to the trailing part of our DAS architecture. The motivation is that simultaneous learning of apodization weights and image super-resolution mutually benefit each other, ultimately enhancing the US image quality.

We assess the proposed architecture in a quantitative manner using available ULM data and demonstrate real-world performance using a separate *in vivo* dataset. While this study primarily focuses on ULM, we believe that the findings presented here have broader implications and benefits within the context of computational beamforming.

© Der/die Autor(en), exklusiv lizenziert an
Springer Fachmedien Wiesbaden GmbH, ein Teil von Springer Nature 2024
A. Maier et al. (Hrsg.), *Bildverarbeitung für die Medizin 2024*,
Informatik aktuell, https://doi.org/10.1007/978-3-658-44037-4_79

2 Materials and methods

Beamforming is a process encompassing both the angular steering of transmit waves (e.g., focused, isotropic or plane) and computational delay and summation upon signal reception. This methodology section embarks on algorithmic aspects of B-mode image reconstruction, serving as the foundation for learnable DAS module extensions.

Let $x(s,t,r) \in \mathbb{C}^{S \times T \times R}$ be an In-phase quadrature (IQ) signal from plane wave emissions $s \in \{1, 2, \ldots, S\}$ with $t \in \{1, 2, \ldots, T\}$ temporal samples for each receiving transducer $r \in \{1, 2, \ldots, R\}$. The planar DAS beamforming writes

$$X(t, \theta) = \int_0^S \int_0^R A(t, \theta, r) \, x(s, t - \tau(s, \theta, r), r) \, \exp\left(2\pi i f_0 \tau(s, \theta, r)\right) \, dr \, ds \quad (1)$$

where $X(t, \theta) \in \mathbb{C}^{T \times \Theta}$ denotes the B-mode image at steering directions θ, $2\pi i$ is the angular frequency with a carrier f_0 and $\tau(s, \theta, r)$ yields the time delay for each θ, s and r. The function $A(t, \theta, r)$ is often referred to as the *aperture function*, which manipulates received raw data after shifting and prior to summation. The apodization design plays a crucial role to enhance the beamformed image quality, which is typically characterized by the ability to reconstruct fine image details, suppress side lobes and reduce speckle noise or reverberation clutter. To address these artifacts and improve the B-mode image quality, (1) offers the following options to accommodate learnable weights:

1. Phase shift correction in $x(s, t, r)$ to address various speed of sounds in media [6]
2. Learning the apodization $A(t, \theta, r)$ for improved side lobe suppression [7]
3. Upsampling of $X(t, \theta)$ to yield $H(t, \theta)$, e.g. through learned pixel shuffling [8]

This study focuses on learning the apodization $A(t, \theta, r)$ and refined B-mode resolution in $H(t, \theta)$. Figure 1 illustrates the proposed learnable DAS. We choose the U-2-NetP [9] as a cutting-edge feature extractor for $A(t, \theta, r)$ and the mSPCN [3] to generate $H(t, \theta)$. For detailed information on convolutional layer design, please refer to the cited work.

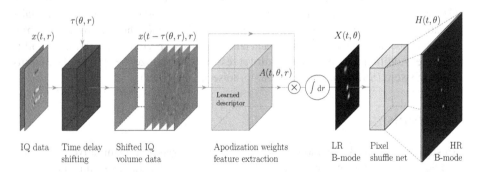

Fig. 1. Overview of the beamformer pipeline: We leverage sub-wavelength DAS beamforming from IQ data $x(t, r)$ as input to a differentiable super-resolution neural network. Our architecture enables learning of apodization weights $A(t, \theta, r)$ for each emission s to reconstruct a low resolution (LR) B-mode image $X(t, \theta)$ and a high resolution (HR) image $H(t, \theta)$ simultaneously.

Note that we use a binary aperture mask with f-number 1.9 regardless of $A(\cdot)$ to exclude signals $x(\cdot)$ at shallow reception angles prior to summation in (1). This binary steering mask is also used in the traditional DAS provided for comparison.

Let $\mathbf{H} \in [0, 1]^{RU \times RV}$ denote the ground-truth (GT) map containing scatterer locations at resolution scale R. Following the approach by Liu et al. [3], $\mathbf{H}$ is convolved with a bivariate Gaussian kernel with $\sigma = 2$. The training loss $\mathcal{L}_T$ then reads

$$\mathcal{L}_T = \lambda_y \|X(t, \theta) - \mathcal{D}(\mathbf{H}, R)\|_2^2 + \lambda_h \left(\|H(t, \theta) - \lambda_g \mathbf{H}\|_2^2 + \|H(t, \theta)\|_1 \right) \qquad (2)$$

where $\mathcal{D}(\cdot)$ takes care of anti-aliased downsampling with R to yield a B-mode image loss at the original resolution amplified by λ_y. The second term in $\mathcal{L}_T$ is the high-resolution loss scaled by λ_h, which contains an L_1 regularization term to prevent prediction of false positive scatterers. For better generalization, we normalize input IQ data $x(\cdot)$ to the $[-1, 1]$ range. We train for 40 epochs starting with a learning rate of 1e-3 and successively lower it after each epoch down to zero using the cosine annealing scheduler.

For a benchmark comparison, we employ the publicly available PALA dataset [2] that comes with *in silico* and *in vivo* sequences. We utilize *in silico* sequences 16 to 20 for training and validation, reserving the majority of sequences 0 to 15 for synthetic image rendering and testing of unseen data. Importantly, testing was independent and not used for hyperparameter tuning. Training occurs on an Nvidia RTX 3090 GPU with a batch size 16, while inference is executed on an RTX 2080 with a batch size 1 due to lower memory demands. We implement the proposed beamformer architecture with PyTorch utilizing GPU-accelerated parallelization. Similar to [2], singular value decomposition and a temporal bandpass are used to remove static reflections from the *in vivo* ULM data before entering the DAS network. The extraction of discrete point estimates in $H(t, \theta)$ is accomplished using non-maximum suppression (NMS) [5].

For quantitative assessment of the resolution accuracy, we calculate the root mean squared error (RMSE) between the estimated locations and the nearest GT position. For alignment with the PALA study [2], only RMSEs less than $\lambda/4$ are considered true positives and contribute to the total RMSE of all frames. In cases where the RMSE distance exceeds $\lambda/4$, the estimated is categorized as a false positive. Consequently, GT locations lacking an estimate within the $\lambda/4$ neighborhood are counted as false negatives. To quantify the MB detection capability, we employ the Jaccard Index, which takes into account both true positives and false negatives, providing a detection reliability measure. Additionally, for image quality assessment, we utilize the structural similarity index measure (SSIM) and peak-signal-to-noise-ratio (PSNR).

3 Results

To study our network's B-mode image quality, we carry out a quantitative assessment provided in Table 1. As baseline methods, we present the radial symmetry (RS) as used by the authors of the dataset [2] and the mSPCN [3]. The RMSE improvement of NMS-based $H(t, \theta)$ compared to RS is attributed to the high-resolution scale, which is offered by the integration of learned pixel shuffling [8]. Comparison with mSPCN can be regarded as an ablation study for the learned $A(t, \theta, r)$ since the proposed network

Tab. 1. Localization results from 15000 test frames of the PALA dataset [2] where networks are trained with $R = 8$ for fair comparison. Metrics are reported as mean±std. where applicable with units provided in brackets. Vertical arrows indicate direction of better scoring. T_D denotes the traditional DAS beamforming time interval for each frame, which amounts to 100 ms in here.

Method	RMSE [$\lambda/10$] ↓	Jaccard [%] ↑	SSIM [%] ↑	Params [#] ↓	Time [ms] ↓
DAS+RS [2]	1.179 ± 0.172	50.330	72.170	0	$T_D + 99$
DAS+mSPCN [3]	0.696 ± 0.097	85.406	92.829	453568	$T_D + 3$
$H(t, \theta)$	0.687 ± 0.089	93.900	96.750	2189664	205

incorporates mSPCN as a super-resolution module to predict $H(t, \theta)$. Table 1 reveals that the proposed method delivers a significant detection enhancement, as evidenced by an improved Jaccard index and a minor refinement of the RMSE accuracy. The SSIM score by accumulated $H(t, \theta)$ suggests that the substantial improvement in scatterer detection justifies the imposed memory and time requirements. This trade-off in time and accuracy can be a considerable choice for ULM and conventional online US screening.

Further, we analyze the quality of $X(t, \theta)$ in Figure 2 by investigating the presence of learned apodization weights. Figure 2b exhibits fine image details as a consequence of the effective side lobe reduction by $A(t, \theta, r)$. This side lobe suppression can be seen in a cross-sectional view of a single scatterer in Figure 2d. These observations are in line with a PSNR gain of about 10 dB when learning $A(t, \theta, r)$ instead of conventional DAS.

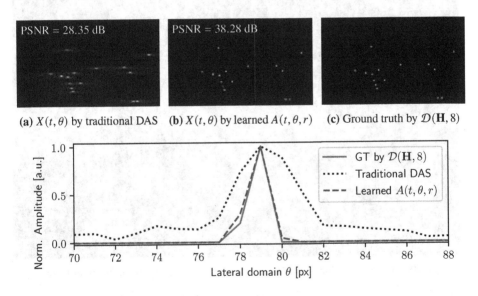

(a) $X(t, \theta)$ by traditional DAS   (b) $X(t, \theta)$ by learned $A(t, \theta, r)$ (c) Ground truth by $\mathcal{D}(\mathbf{H}, 8)$

(d) Cross-sectional view of (a), (b) and (c) at image row 47

Fig. 2. B-mode example depicting point scatterers in an unseen test frame (3 plane waves, 128 linear transducer array) of sequence 0, frame 0 from the *in silico* PALA dataset [2]. Comparison of (a), (b) and (c) shows the efficiency of $A(t, \theta, r)$ as validated by (d) and the PSNR (upper left).

Figure 3 shows results of the *in silico*-trained network applied to *in vivo* data containing a ULM acquisition of a rat brain [2]. The image is reconstructed by accumulating localizations from 73600 frames each processed by the proposed pipeline. This result underpins our architecture's ability to resolve fine image details in real-world scenarios. In particular, it demonstrates that learning apodization weights from simulation data is suitable for application to *in vivo* ULM data, successfully addressing the domain gap. Nonetheless, incorporating larger sets of training data with more diverse distributions is important for making a valuable contribution to the broader field of US imaging.

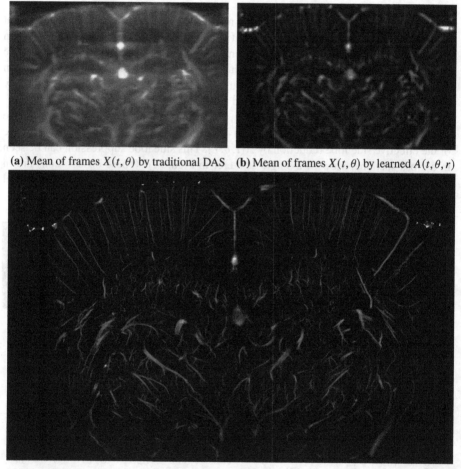

(a) Mean of frames $X(t, \theta)$ by traditional DAS   **(b)** Mean of frames $X(t, \theta)$ by learned $A(t, \theta, r)$

(c) NMS-based localizations from $H(t, \theta)$ at $R = 8$ with tracking by the Munkres linker [2]

Fig. 3. In vivo ULM example depicting the brain vascularity from rat-18 [2]. The images in (a) and (b) correspond to the mean over multiple frames $X(t, \theta)$ in the absence and presence of $A(t, \theta, r)$, respectively. The image in (c) employs NMS-based localizations in $H(t, \theta)$ at $R = 8$ together with a Munkres linker for temporal tracking [2]. The herein used US data comprises 92×800 frames with 3 compounded plane waves each captured by a linear transducer probe with 128 elements.

4 Discussion

The primary goal of this study is to advance high-resolution ultrasound (US) image formation by direct integration of learnable weights into the delay-and-sum (DAS) process. This research exhibits promise in generating B-mode images at sub-wavelength precision with improved side lobe suppression. The presented outcome offers novel insights into enhancing DAS processing, potentially overcoming the issue of low spatial resolution in the broader context of US imaging. However, it is essential to note that these findings are currently limited to an *in silico* and an *in vivo* dataset in the field of ultrasound localization microscopy (ULM). To broaden the applicability of the proposed architecture, we aim to incorporate datasets from diverse domains and parameters. Finally, the proposed differentiable DAS architecture and its corresponding PyTorch implementation serve as the base for the development of learning-based high-resolution beamformers.

Acknowledgement. This work is supported by the Hasler Foundation under project number 22027.

References

1. Errico C, Pierre J, Pezet S, Desailly Y, Lenkei Z, Couture O et al. Ultrafast ultrasound localization microscopy for deep super-resolution vascular imaging. Nature. 2015;527(7579):499–502.
2. Heiles B, Chavignon A, Hingot V, Lopez P, Teston E, Couture O. Performance benchmarking of microbubble-localization algorithms for ultrasound localization microscopy. Nat Biomed Eng. 2022;6(5):605–16.
3. Liu X, Zhou T, Lu M, Yang Y, He Q, Luo J. Deep learning for ultrasound localization microscopy. IEEE Trans Med Imaging. 2020;39(10):3064–78.
4. Hahne C, Sznitman R. Geometric ultrasound localization microscopy. Proc MICCAI. 2023:217–27.
5. Hahne C, Chabouh G, Couture O, Sznitman R. Learning super-resolution ultrasound localization microscopy from radio-frequency data. Proc IEEE IUS. 2023:1–4.
6. Simson W, Zhuang L, Sanabria SJ, Antil N, Dahl JJ, Hyun D. Differentiable beamforming for ultrasound autofocusing. Proc MICCAI 2023. Springer. 2023:428–37.
7. Chen Y, Liu J, Luo X, Luo J. ApodNet: learning for high frame rate synthetic transmit aperture ultrasound imaging. IEEE Trans Med Imaging. 2021;40(11):3190–204.
8. Shi W, Caballero J, Huszár F, Totz J, Aitken AP, Bishop R et al. Real-time single image and video super-resolution using an efficient sub-pixel convolutional neural network. Proc IEEE CVPR. 2016:1874–83.
9. Qin X, Zhang Z, Huang C, Dehghan M, Zaiane O, Jagersand M. U2-Net: going deeper with nested u-structure for salient object detection. Vol. 106. 2020:107404.

Neural Network-based Sinogram Upsampling in Real-measured CT Reconstruction

Lena Augustin, Fabian Wagner, Mareike Thies, Andreas Maier

Pattern Recognition Lab, Computer Science, Friedrich-Alexander-Universität
Erlangen-Nürnberg
lena.augustin@fau.de

Abstract. Computed tomography (CT) is one of the most popular non-invasive medical imaging modalities. A major downside of medical CT is the exposure of the patient to high-energy X-rays during image acquisition. One way to reduce the amount of ionising radiation is to record fewer projective views and then upsample the resulting subsampled sinogram. Post acquisition, this can be achieved through conventional sinogram interpolation algorithms or using neural networks. This paper compares the results of two upsampling network architectures with the results of conventional sinogram interpolation. We found that for subsampling factors two and four, the neural networks did not substantially improve the model predictions in terms of structured similarity and peak signal-to-noise ratio compared to conventional sinogram interpolation. This suggests that, for these subsampling factors and the given dataset, interpolation approximates the problem well enough.

1 Introduction

Computed tomography (CT) plays a crucial role in non-invasive medical imaging. It uses X-rays to acquire multiple projective views of the body from different angles and then combines these images to reconstruct a detailed volumetric representation of the internal structures of the body. As CT takes multiple images, the exposure to ionising radiation is considerably higher than with conventional X-ray imaging. For adult abdominal imaging, the type of data used in this work, the average effective radiation dose for CT imaging is 8 mSv, compared to 0.7 mSv for conventional X-ray [1]. In other words, the risk ratio of fatal radiation-induced cancer is 1:2,300 for CT and only 1:28,600 for conventional X-ray [1]. Therefore, minimising radiation exposure is in the interest of the patient's health.

One way to minimise patient dose is to use a so-called low-dose CT which reduces the patient's exposure time for all individual CT projections. However, this approach amplifies noise and introduces artefacts in the final reconstructed image, which decreases the diagnostic capabilities of the image and necessitates advanced pre- and post-processing [2].

Alternatively, fewer projection angles can be acquired to reduce patient dose. Here, the missing angles are typically interpolated during post-processing to limit streaking artefacts caused by missing information. Because of the advances in deep learning in the last couple of years, this processing step is now often conducted using neural networks. Common architectures for this task are U-Nets and convolutional neural networks (CNNs).

© Der/die Autor(en), exklusiv lizenziert an
Springer Fachmedien Wiesbaden GmbH, ein Teil von Springer Nature 2024
A. Maier et al. (Hrsg.), *Bildverarbeitung für die Medizin 2024*,
Informatik aktuell, https://doi.org/10.1007/978-3-658-44037-4_80

One of the first networks for upsampling sinograms was proposed by Lee et al. in 2017 [3]. They subsampled the sinogram by only taking every fourth angle and upsampled it using a simple CNN that only contains convolutional layers and ReLU activation functions. At the end, they add the processed input to the original input (residual connection). Using this approach, they received results that were considerably better than using linear or directional interpolation.

Some more recent works, such as the LU-Net designed by Li et al. [4] combine the traditional feed-forward approaches with recurrent neural networks (RNNs). This makes it possible to take into account that adjacent slices depend on each other. By combining a U-Net with an LSTM, Li et al. were able to significantly improve the results in both global and local metrics compared to only using a standard U-Net. In their approach, they placed an LSTM module in front of the convolutions in every downsampling step of the network but did not use any recurrent cells in the upsampling path.

Instead of just using the sinogram data, some works also use both the subsampled sinogram and the reconstructed image. One such method is the network proposed by Yu et al. [5]. To upsample the sinogram, they use an encoder-decoder architecture with a CNN as encoder and dual multi-layer perceptrons (one modulator MLP and one synthesiser MLP) as decoder. Then, they reconstruct the image using filtered backprojection. But, as the reconstructed image can still contain some artefacts, they also designed a CNN that removes those artefacts after the reconstruction. This ensures that the image the radiologist sees, i. e. the reconstruction, is as clear as possible.

This paper presents a CNN and a U-Net for upsampling sinograms. Contrary to both the CNN proposed by Lee et al. [3] and the LU-Net designed by Li et al. [4], we use real sinogram data, making our results more realistic than those obtained using phantom data. The goal of this work is to investigate whether the networks can upsample the real-data subsampled sinograms such that reconstructions matching at least the quality of full-dose scans can be computed.

2 Materials and methods

We designed two different upsampling networks, a CNN and a U-Net, and trained them on real sinograms that were subsampled by factors two and four. [1] Both networks are residual networks that take an interpolated version of the sinogram as input. This section presents details about the data we used, the layout of the networks, and the training procedure.

2.1 Dataset & data pre-processing

For our work, we use full-dose abdominal CT data from the Low-dose CT image and projection dataset by McCollough et al. [6]. Using real data ensures that our results are as realistic as possible. As the data was recorded using a helix CT, it is first transformed to fan beam CT using the library helix2fan developed by Wagner et al. [7].

In total, we use ten full abdominal patient scans: four for training, one for validation, and five for testing. After removing incomplete slices, each of the training and validation

---

[1] Code available at https://github.com/LenaAugustin/upsampling-in-real-measured-ct-reconstruction

scans consists of 156 slices acquired in 2304 angular steps with a 736 pixel wide detector. These scans serve as the ground truth, the subsampled scans are obtained by only taking the data from every n^{th} angle where n is the subsampling factor. Each reconstructed scan consists of 156 slices of size 512×512. Some of the test scans have slightly fewer slices because fewer slices were recorded.

Figure 1 shows one of the sinograms, its subsampled version, one slice of the reconstruction of the subsampled sinogram and one slice of the target reconstruction. It can be clearly seen that reconstructing a subsampled sinogram leads to considerable artefacts in the resulting image.

2.2 Network architecture

Figure 2 describes how the data is processed: After the aforementioned preprocessing where incomplete slices are removed, the subsampled sinograms are interpolated. This provides the network with a good initial guess of the missing values and thus considerably increases the training speed. To interpolate the sinograms, we used spline interpolation with an order of three. The individual interpolated sinogram slices are then fed to the network, where they are processed. Subsequently, the individual slices are stacked and then reconstructed using the differentiable filtered back projection algorithm developed by Matteo Ronchetti [8].

Details about the layout of the networks can be found in Figure 3 and Figure 4, respectively. The CNN consists of 22 convolutional layers. As the interpolated sinograms have the same shape as the target sinogram, we keep the width and height constant

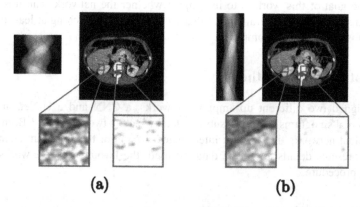

(a) **(b)**

Fig. 1. Example for a subsampled sinogram with subsampling factor 4 and its reconstruction (a) and the corresponding full-size sinogram and its reconstruction (b).

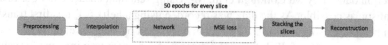

Fig. 2. Data processing pipeline.

throughout the network and only change the number of channels. This ensures that we preserve as much information as possible.

The U-Net consists of four downsampling and four upsampling steps with two convolutions in between each step. To lose as little information as possible, we keep the number of detector positions constant and only down-/upsample the angular dimension, as this is the dimension that was subsampled.

2.3 Training the networks

For training our networks, we used four scans for training and one for validation. Contrary to many previous works in the field, including the CNN proposed by Lee et al. [3], we feed the whole sinogram slices to the network instead of splitting them into small patches. This enables our network to consider non-local structures. As the network input is very large, we used a batch size of one. To calculate the loss, we used the mean squared error between the target sinogram and the upsampled sinogram. Both networks were trained with subsampling factors $n = 2$ and $n = 4$, i.e. the subsampled sinograms consisted of every second and every fourth angle, respectively. All four resulting networks were trained for 50 epochs with stochastic gradient descent as optimiser. The CNNs use a learning rate of 10^{-4}, the U-Nets use a learning rate of $5 \cdot 10^{-4}$. The networks were trained using PyTorch Lightning [9].

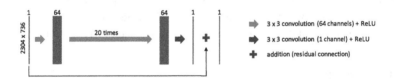

Fig. 3. Layout of the CNN.

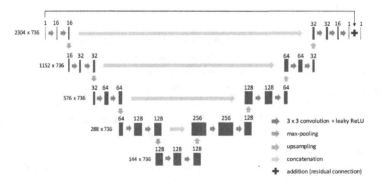

Fig. 4. Layout of the U-Net.

Tab. 1. Comparison of SSIM and PSNR values for both network architectures and both subsampling factors and interpolated images.

	Mean SSIM ± SD	Mean PSNR ± SD	Min. & max. SSIM	Min. & max. PSNR
CNN; n = 2	0.7029 ± 0.0095	39.3766 ± 0.2378	0.6657; 0.7437	37.5016; 41.9160
U-Net; n = 2	0.7049 ± 0.0163	39.4019 ± 0.2380	0.6675; 0.7447	38.2917; 41.9502
Interp.; n = 2	0.7033 ± 0.0250	39.1214 ± 1.5429	0.6672; 0.7430	37.4027; 41.9155
CNN; n = 4	0.4681 ± 0.0165	36.9680 ± 0.2927	0.4155; 0.5358	35.6307; 39.5145
U-Net; n = 4	0.4680 ± 0.0161	36.9627 ± 0.2944	0.4159; 0.5363	35.6386; 39.5174
Interp.; n = 4	0.4675 ± 0.0393	36.9143 ± 1.4716	0.4150; 0.5345	35.4973; 39.5139

3   Results

To evaluate the performance of the networks, we calculated the structural similarity index measure (SSIM) and the peak signal-to-noise ratio (PSNR) between the reconstructed network output and the reconstructed ground truth and compared them to the SSIM and PSNR of the interpolated images. For each of the five test scans, we averaged the result over all slices of the respective scan. The results are listed in Table 1.

The results show that all networks achieved similar performances in terms of SSIM and PSNR to interpolating the images. In all cases, the mean SSIM differs only in the third decimal digit. All networks very slightly increased the mean PSNR of the images, especially for $n = 2$, and reduced the already very small within-scan standard deviation of SSIM and PSNR. An important factor to consider when interpreting the mean SSIM of the test sets is that it differs largely between the scans (Tab. 1, column 3).

4   Discussion

All in all, the results suggest that the networks were not able to extract a substantial amount of information from the dataset and that interpolation thus approximates the problem well enough. This is indicated by three key observations: Firstly, the loss is very small from the beginning and barely changes, indicating that interpolation provides a result that is already close to the optimal solution with respect to the calculated loss. Secondly, the SSIM between the reconstructed network output and the reconstructed interpolated images is very high (e. g. 0.9986 for the U-Net with $n = 2$). Thirdly, when passing the training sets through the trained model, the resulting SSIM is very close to that of the test sets (e. g. 0.7198 for the U-Net with $n = 2$). This shows that the networks did not overfit and that the results were not caused by dissimilarities between the test sets and the training data.

Consequently, for the small subsampling factors used in this paper, the small improvements to the SSIM and PSNR generally do not justify the additional computational load imposed by using neural networks instead of conventional interpolation.

The most important element of the networks is the residual connection. Without it, the network performs considerably worse. For the CNN with $n = 2$, the non-residual network completely loses the sinogram information, resulting in a prediction that resembles a white circle on a black background and a mean test set SSIM of -0.0025. The U-Net performs considerably better, but still only reaches an SSIM of 0.5135. Contrary to the behaviour of the residual network, the non-residual network training starts with a high loss that decreases quickly.

The rather low SSIM suggests that there is still room for improvement. One way to obtain better results could be to use an RNN instead of a standard feedforward network. This would take into account that the slices depend on each other. Also, as the used filtered backprojection algorithm is differentiable, the reconstruction could be incorporated into the training. This way, it would be possible to directly optimise the reconstruction. Other steps to improve the quality of the overall image include post-processing the reconstruction and pre-processing the sinogram before it is reconstructed.

A limitation of the networks is that they were only trained and evaluated on abdominal CT data. It should thus be checked how the networks perform with CT data of different regions of the body. Additionally, due to computational constraints, the models were trained with a small batch size of one, which potentially decreases their capacity to learn complex patterns. Furthermore, the networks were trained on a very limited dataset, consisting of only four scans, which might hinder the model's ability to generalise.

5   Conclusion

This paper presented a residual CNN and a residual U-Net for upsampling real sinograms. The results show that the SSIM and PSNR of the reconstructed prediction did not substantially improve over the SSIM and PSNR of the reconstructed conventionally interpolated sinograms for both subsampling factors two and four. This suggests that, for the given data, interpolation approximates the problem well enough. Further research can investigate higher subsampling factors and more complex network architectures.

References

1. Giordano B, Grauer J, Miller C, Morgan T, Rechtine G et al. Radiation exposure issues in orthopaedics. JBJS. 2011;93(12):e69.
2. Ma Y, Wei B, Feng P, He P, Guo X, Wang G. Low-dose CT image denoising using a generative adversarial network with a hybrid loss function for noise learning. IEEE Access. 2020;8:67519–29.
3. Lee H, Lee J, Cho S. View-interpolation of sparsely sampled sinogram using convolutional neural network. Proc SPIE. Vol. 10133. 2017:617–24.
4. Li S, Ye W, Li F. LU-Net: combining LSTM and u-net for sinogram synthesis in sparse-view SPECT reconstruction. Math Biosci Eng. 2022;19(4):4320–40.
5. Yu M, Han M, Baek J. A convolutional neural network based super resolution technique of CT image utilizing both sinogram domain and image domain data. MProc SPIE. Vol. 12032. 2022:564–9.
6. McCollough C, Chen B, Holmes D, Duan X, Yu Z, Yu L et al. Low dose CT image and projection data. 2020.
7. Wagner F, Thies M, Pfaff L, Aust O, Pechmann S, Maul N et al. On the benefit of dual-domain denoising in a self-supervised low-dose CT setting. Proc IEEE ISBI. 2023:1–5.
8. Ronchetti M. TorchRadon: Fast Differentiable Routines for Computed Tomography. 2020.
9. Falcon W, The PyTorch Lightning Team. PyTorch Lightning. Version 1.4. 2019.

Data Consistent Variational Networks for Zero-shot Self-supervised MR Reconstruction

Florian Fürnrohr[1], Jens Wetzl[2], Marc Vornehm[1,2], Daniel Giese[2,3], Florian Knoll[1]

[1]Computational Imaging Lab, Friedrich-Alexander-Universität Erlangen-Nürnberg, Germany
[2]Magnetic Resonance, Siemens Healthcare GmbH, Erlangen, Germany
[3]Institute of Radiology, University Hospital Erlangen, Germany
florian.fuernrohr@fau.de

Abstract. Variational Networks are a common approach in deep learning-based accelerated MR reconstruction. Due to their architecture, they may however fail in enforcing data consistency. We propose an adjustment to the Variational Network, integrating an optimization block that ensures consistency with the measured k-space points. We show the superiority of the method for zero-shot self-supervised 3D reconstruction quantitatively on retrospectively undersampled knee-data, and qualitatively in prospectively undersampled MR angiography images.

1 Introduction

Magnetic resonance imaging (MRI) is an indispensable clinical tool, providing images with excellent soft tissue contrast and high diagnostic value. However, data acquisition is inherently slow and prone to motion corruption. Parallel imaging is a widespread technique for accelerating MRI, but forms an ill-posed problem at high acceleration factors. Deep learning techniques have successfully been used to solve this reconstruction problem, but typically require a fully sampled ground truth. In many cases acquisition of high resolution data in a fully sampled manner is problematic. For instance in cardiac imaging, due to heart motion, data acquisition is only possible at specific phases within the cardiac cycle, culminating in infeasible scan times. Recently, Yaman et al. [1] proposed a self-supervised technique that enables learning-based reconstruction without fully sampled data. Since this method still requires a large amount of training data, it was extended to a zero-shot approach for scan-specific accelerated MR reconstruction [2]. This not only overcomes the limitation of having to acquire a large dataset for training, but also addresses generalization concerns of database-trained models.

Reconstruction is done via unrolled networks [3, 4], which incorporate the physics of the data acquisition by unrolling conventional iterative algorithms for a fixed number of iterations. The variational network (VN) [4, 5] is an established method consisting of multiple cascades, each representing an update step in a gradient descent optimization scheme. Each cascade contains a refinement (R) block, consisting of a convolutional neural network (CNN) operating in image space, and a data consistency (DC) block, regulating the deviation from the measurements in k-space.

In this study, we carry out self-supervised reconstruction of 3D MR angiography and investigate whether iterative optimization via conjugate gradient (CG) within the network can enhance data consistency, as we have observed solutions with deviations from the measured data.

2 Materials and methods

The recovery of an image $\mathbf{x}$ from undersampled k-space measurements $\mathbf{y}_\Omega$ in accelerated MRI can be formulated as the inverse problem

$$\arg\min_{\mathbf{x}} \|\mathbf{y}_\Omega - \mathbf{E}_\Omega \mathbf{x}\|_2^2 + \mathcal{R}(\mathbf{x}) \qquad (1)$$

where $\mathbf{E}_\Omega$ is the forward encoding operator, consisting of coil sensitivity profiles, the Fourier transform, and a masking operator for the undersampling pattern Ω. $\mathcal{R}(\cdot)$ is a regularizer enabling incorporation of prior information into the reconstruction. In compressed sensing (CS), the compressibility of MR images is exploited by preferring solutions that are sparse in some transform domain [6]. Typical choices for $\mathcal{R}(\cdot)$ in CS are total variation and the L_1-norm of the wavelet transform (L1-W). Deep learning approaches aim to learn the regularizer $\mathcal{R}(\cdot)$ via a neural network.

2.1 Zero-Shot SSDU

Yaman et al. proposed self-supervision via data undersampling (SSDU) [1], enabling training without a fully sampled reference. As the acquisition of a large database of undersampled MR measurements is time-consuming, instance-specific reconstruction of a single MR scan is beneficial. This also counteracts generalization problems of pretrained models, while being agnostic to varying acceleration rate, sampling pattern, or field strength. Therefore, SSDU was extended to zero-shot SSDU (ZS-SSDU) [2], enabling scan-specific reconstruction. To avoid overfitting, early stopping based on a validation loss is performed. As there are no separate scans available to build a validation set in ZS-SSDU, the validation loss is computed on a subset (Γ) of the measured k-space data. Together with a multi-mask setting [7], which can be seen as a data augmentation technique, the k-space is split into three disjoint sets $\Omega = \Theta_k \sqcup \Lambda_k \sqcup \Gamma, k \in \{1, \ldots, K\}$. Training is then performed by

$$\min_{\theta} \frac{1}{K} \sum_{k=1}^{K} \mathcal{L}\left(\mathbf{y}_{\Lambda_k}, \mathbf{E}_{\Lambda_k}\left(f\left(\mathbf{y}_{\Theta_k}, \mathbf{E}_{\Theta_k}; \theta\right)\right)\right) \qquad (2)$$

where $\mathcal{L}(\cdot)$ defines a loss in k-space, f is the unrolled network for reconstruction, and θ are the trainable parameters of the model.

2.2 Variational network

The Variational Network [4, 5] is an unrolled network, performing physic-guided reconstruction while being able to adapt to scan-specific variations in a data-driven manner. It updates the k-space iteratively, starting from the zero-filled k-space $\mathbf{k}_0$, until a fixed number of cascades T, finally transforming $\mathbf{k}_T$ from k-space to image space via the adjoint $\mathbf{E}^H$ of the forward operator $\mathbf{E}$. Each cascade consists of a data consistency term (DC) and a refinement or regularization term (R). The update rule for cascade n is given by

$$\mathbf{k}_{n+1} = \mathbf{k}_n - \underbrace{\lambda_n \mathbf{M}(\mathbf{k}_n - \mathbf{k}_0)}_{\text{DC}} + \underbrace{\mathbf{E} \circ \text{CNN}(\mathbf{E}^H \mathbf{k}_n)}_{\text{R}} \qquad (3)$$

where λ_n is a learnable data consistency weight, $\mathbf{M}$ is the masking operator, and $\text{CNN}(\cdot)$ is a convolutional neural network with trainable parameters.

2.3   Proposed data consistent variational network

The DC in (3) constitutes one gradient decent step into the direction of a solution consistent with the measured data $\mathbf{k}_0$. In a classical iterative scheme this operation is performed several times, leading to data consistency. In a VN, the update is only unrolled to a fixed number of steps, often very few. Also the expressive power of the CNN in the refinement term R might push the current estimate of the k-space $\mathbf{k}_n$ to a totally different place in the loss landscape, diminishing the influence of the single DC step. Furthermore, the step size in the DC term is learnable, making it possible to learn ineffective DC steps. This might lead to inconsistent solutions, especially in the self-supervised setting, where the loss is not provided with ground truth reference of the measured points.

We therefore propose to enforce consistency with the acquired measurements by solution of a numerical optimization problem that punishes large deviations from the measured data, while being regularized to stay close to the current estimate $\mathbf{x}_n = \mathbf{E}^H \mathbf{k}_n$

$$\mathbf{x}_{\tilde{n}} = \arg\min_{\mathbf{x}} \|\mathbf{M}\mathbf{E}\mathbf{x} - \mathbf{k}_0\|_2^2 + \mu_n \|\mathbf{x} - \mathbf{x}_n\|_2^2 \qquad (4)$$

The regularization parameter μ_n can be fixed or learned during training. The data consistency subproblem (4) can be solved using conjugate gradient descent (CG), where we set a fixed number of CG steps. This way, we introduce numerical optimization into the VN without additional parameters except for one scalar parameter per cascade if μ_n is learned. We propose to solve (4) only in the last step of the VN, while still retaining the DC term in (3). The proposed network structure is illustrated in Fig. 1.

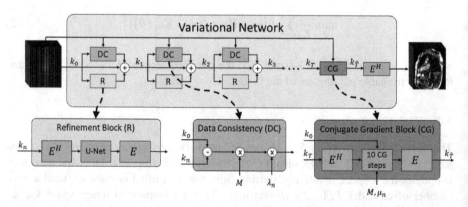

Fig. 1. Network structure. The Variational Network is unrolled for a fixed number of cascades T. Each cascade consists of a data consistency (DC) and a refinement (R) block. The output of the last cascade is fed into an conjugate gradient block (CG), that performs 10 optimization steps.

Tab. 1. Quantitative results on retrospectively undersampled knee data. Structural similarity (SSIM) and peak signal-to-noise ratio (PSNR) for three different reconstruction methods: L1-wavelet compressed sensing (L1-W-CS), the Variational Network without conjugate gradient block (VN w/o CG), and the Variational Network with conjugate gradient block (VN w/ CG).

	SSIM [%]			PSNR [dB]		
	L1-W-CS	VN w/o CG	VN w/ CG	L1-W-CS	VN w/o CG	VN w/ CG
8x	79.6 *	75.2 *	84.1	31.6	28.1 *	31.9
12x	78.9 *	73.9 *	83.3	31.0	27.9 *	31.7

*statistically significant (p-value < 0.05) difference to proposed VN w/ CG

2.4 Experiments

For evaluation we reconstructed data from 3D high-resolution MR acquisitions in the zero-shot self-supervised manner described in (2). As a baseline method, we computed L_1-wavelet regularized compressed sensing (L1-W-CS) reconstructions. For all other experiments, we used a VN with five cascades, as CNN in (3) we chose an U-Net with 3D convolutions. We set a mixed $L_1 - L_2$ loss $\mathcal{L}(\cdot)$ in (2). We performed reconstructions of each scan using the VN without a CG block (VN w/o CG), and using the proposed approach with a CG optimization block (4) after the last cascade (VN w/ CG). There were no differences in network architecture and parameterization apart from integrating the CG block. Coil sensitivities were pre-computed using ESPIRiT [8].

For quantitative comparison, we used 15 samples of the Stanford Fullysampled 3D FSE Knee dataset [9], as fully sampled scans of the heart are difficult to obtain. We then retrospectively undersampled the data with factors $R = 8$ and $R = 12$, using a variable-density poisson distribution with a fully sampled k-space center of size 24×24. Structural similarity (SSIM) and peak signal-to-noise ratio (PSNR) were computed and independent two sample t-tests for statistical significance were performed.

For prospective evaluation, five healthy volunteers were scanned at 1.5T (MAG-NETOM Sola, Siemens Healthineers AG, Erlangen, Germany). Written informed consent was obtained prior to data acquisition. Imaging was performed with resolution of $1.2 \times 1.2 \times 1.2$ mm^3, fully sampled k-space center of size 24×24, and acceleration factor of $R \approx 11$. One experienced expert performed a rating of the different reconstructions,

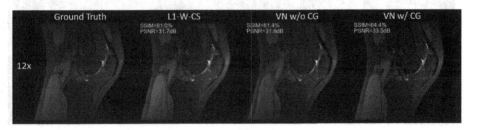

Fig. 2. Exemplary reconstructions of retrospectively undersampled data. Form left to right: fully sampled ground truth, reconstructions using L1-wavelet compressed sensing, the Variational Network without CG, and the Variational Network with CG.

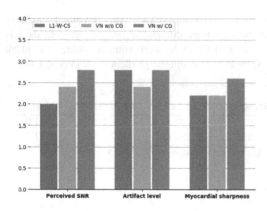

Fig. 3. Expert rating of prospectively acquired 3D angiography. Reconstructions were rated in terms of perceived SNR, artifact level and myocardial sharpness. Evaluation scale 1: poor, 2: fair, 3: good, 4: excellent.

grading perceived SNR, artifact level, and myocardial sharpness on a four point scale form poor to excellent.

3 Results

For the retrospective knee data, mean SSIM and PSNR are presented in Tab. 1. Exemplary reconstructions for $R = 12$ are depicted in Fig. 2. Expert ratings of prospectively acquired 3D angiography data were performed using all three methods and are displayed in Fig. 3. An example scan of the heart is shown in Fig. 4.

4 Discussion

The quantitative results of Tab. 1 show a clear performance increase of the proposed model compared to the baseline CS model, as well as to the standard VN w/o CG. The VN w/ CG scores highest values in SSIM and PSNR for both acceleration factors. Reconstructions in Fig. 2 show the same trend. Visually we observe the VN w/o CG

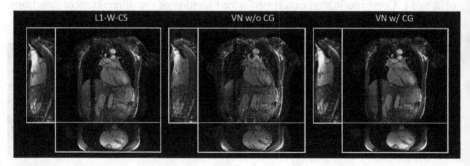

Fig. 4. Exemplary reconstructions of prospectively acquired angiography. L1-wavelet compressed sensing reconstructions are displayed on the left, the results for Variational Network without CG in the middle, and reconstructions of the Variational Network with CG on the right.

results in blurrier and the L1-W-CS in more noisy reconstructions than the proposed VN w/ CG. The expert rating of the prospective cardiac images (Fig. 3), shows an increasing trend in perceived SNR. The noise level of the CS approach is worst, followed by the VN w/o CG, both outperformed by the VN w/ CG, demonstrating the capability of the VN for noise suppression. Comparing the methods in terms of artifact level, the VN w/o CG overall performed worst, while the baseline CS method and the VN w/ CG perform similar. Large deviations from the measurements can introduce artifacts in the reconstructions. This is visible in the example in Fig. 4, where the reconstruction of the VN w/o CG suffers from noticeable artifacts, while the other approaches appear artifact-free. Myocardial sharpness is an important part of the diagnostic value of a cardiac image. While the VN w/o CG fails to improve myocardial sharpness compared to CS, the proposed method shows highest ratings in that field.

Overall, the proposed method outperformed both other methods in quantitative metrics on retrospective data, while also showing superior performance on prospective data. It was able to reconstruct 3D MRA with high quality, using scan-specific training without fully sampled reference. Future work will focus on reducing reconstruction times for ZS-SSDU, which are currently prohibitive for clinical translation.

References

1. Yaman B, Hosseini SAH, Moeller S, Ellermann J, Uğurbil K, Akçakaya M. Self-supervised learning of physics-guided reconstruction neural networks without fully sampled reference data. Magn Reson Med. 2020;84(6):3172–91.
2. Yaman B, Hosseini SAH, Akçakaya M. Zero-shot self-supervised learning for MRI reconstruction. ArXiv. 2021.
3. Aggarwal HK, Mani MP, Jacob M. MoDL: Model-based deep learning architecture for inverse problems. IEEE Trans Med Imaging. 2018;38(2):394–405.
4. Hammernik K, Klatzer T, Kobler E, Recht MP, Sodickson DK, Pock T et al. Learning a variational network for reconstruction of accelerated MRI data. Magn Reson Med. 2018;79(6):3055–71.
5. Sriram A, Zbontar J, Murrell T, Defazio A, Zitnick CL, Yakubova N et al. End-to-end variational networks for accelerated MRI reconstruction. Med Image Comput Comput Assist Interv. Springer. 2020:64–73.
6. Lustig M, Donoho DL, Santos JM, Pauly JM. Compressed sensing MRI. IEEE Signal Process Mag. 2008;25(2):72–82.
7. Yaman B, Gu H, Hosseini SAH, Demirel OB, Moeller S, Ellermann J et al. Multi-mask self-supervised learning for physics-guided neural networks in highly accelerated magnetic resonance imaging. NMR Biomed. 2022;35(12):e4798.
8. Uecker M, Lai P, Murphy MJ, Virtue P, Elad M, Pauly JM et al. ESPIRiT: an eigenvalue approach to autocalibrating parallel MRI: where SENSE meets GRAPPA. Magn Reson Med. 2014;71(3):990–1001.
9. Epperson K, Sawyer AM, Lustig M, Alley M, Uecker M. Creation of fully sampled MR data repository for compressed sensing of the knee. Proc Sec Mag Reson Techn. 2013.

Deep Image Prior for Spatio-temporal Fluorescence Microscopy Images
DECO-DIP

Lina Meyer[1,2,3], Lena-Marie Woelk[1,2,3], Christine E. Gee[4], Christian Lohr[5],
Sukanya A. Kannabiran[6], Björn-Philipp Diercks[6], René Werner[1,2,3]

[1]Institute of Applied Medical Informatics, University Medical Center Hamburg-Eppendorf
(UKE), Hamburg, Germany
[2]Department of Computational Neuroscience, UKE, Hamburg, Germany
[3]Center for Biomedical Artificial Intelligence (bAIome), UKE, Hamburg, Germany
[4]Institute of Synaptic Physiology, UKE, Hamburg, Germany
[5]Division of Neurophysiology, Institute of Zoology, University of Hamburg, Hamburg, Germany
[6]Department of Biochemistry and Molecular Cell Biology, UKE, Hamburg, Germany
r.werner@uke.de

Abstract. Image deconvolution and denoising is a common postprocessing step
to improve the quality of biomedical fluorescence microscopy images. In recent
years, this task has been increasingly tackled with the help of supervised deep
learning methods. However, generating a large number of training pairs is, if at all
possible, often laborious. Here, we present a new deep learning algorithm called
DECO-DIP that builds on the Deep Image Prior (DIP) framework and does not
rely on training data. We extend DIP by incorporating a novel loss function that,
in addition to a standard L^2 data term, contains a term to model the underlying
image generation forward model. We apply our framework both to synthetic
data and Ca^{2+} microscopy data of biological samples, namely Jurkat T-cells and
astrocytes. DECO-DIP outperforms both classical deconvolution and the standard
DIP implementation. We further introduce an extension, DECO-DIP-T, which
explicitly utilizes the time dependence in live cell microscopy image series.

1 Introduction

Fluorescence microscopy is a powerful technique that allows imaging of biological
specimens with high specificity and contrast. It is, however, subject to degradation
effects, such as diffraction-limited blur and noise [1]. The former is caused by the finite
aperture of the objective lens, which acts as a low-pass filter and spreads the light from
each point source in the specimen into a characteristic shape the point spread function
(PSF). Deconvolution aims to reverse the convolution between the true specimen and
the PSF to restore a sharper image. In addition, the image acquisition process leads to
image noise of two main types: signal-dependent Poisson noise and signal-independent
Gaussian noise. To reduce the noise level, denoising methods can be applied.

There are countless methods available for deconvolution and denoising, ranging
from classical methods, such as Wiener filtering and the Richardson-Lucy algorithm
[2, 3] to advanced approaches. The latter are currently often based on supervised deep
learning (DL) [4, 5]. Conventional methods require either a known or an estimated PSF

© Der/die Autor(en), exklusiv lizenziert an
Springer Fachmedien Wiesbaden GmbH, ein Teil von Springer Nature 2024
A. Maier et al. (Hrsg.), *Bildverarbeitung für die Medizin 2024*,
Informatik aktuell, https://doi.org/10.1007/978-3-658-44037-4_82

and often involve iterative optimization procedures, while DL methods, which can be more run-time efficient in inference mode, usually require large amounts of training data and computational resources.

Ulyanov, Vedaldi, Lempitsky proposed a new deep learning method called deep image prior (DIP) that is not training data-driven but uses the structure of a neural network as a (regularization) prior for solving inverse problems like denoising and superresolution [6]. Originally developed for the natural image domain, the method has meanwhile been adapted for structured illumination microscopy (SIM) [7] and enhanced with the idea of temporal consistency through recursive deep image prior video (RDPV) [8].

Here, we combine both extensions and modify them to suit fluorescence microscopy imaging by incorporating an imaging forward model, namely a convolution with the PSF, into the network and exploit knowledge about time dependence in live cell imaging data. Our algorithm, called DECO-DIP (DECOnvolution Deep Image Prior) is compared against two conventional methods, richardson-lucy (RL) and TD ER [9], and standard DIP for three different datasets: synthetic data to allow for an objective quantitative evaluation and two real-world data sets, Jurkat T-cell and astrocyte Ca^{2+} fluorescence microscopy imaging data.

2 Materials and methods

The source code and example image data are provided publicly available at github. com/IPMI-ICNS-UKE/DECO-DIP.

2.1 Imaging data

2.1.1 Synthetic data. The synthetic data set consists of videos with randomly moving dots imitating localized fluorophore signals. The degradation of real fluorescence microscope images was imitated by convolution with a PSF, assuming Poisson noise with variance of the signal divided by 0.05, and Gaussian noise with variance σ^2 between 0.001 and 0.1.

2.1.2 Genetically encoded Ca^{2+} indicator for optimal imaging (R-GECO) tagged to lysosomal TPC2 in Jurkat T cells. Jurkat T cells were transiently transfected with two pore channel 2 (TPC2) fused to GECO-1.2. Images were acquired with a 100x objective fitted in a super-resolution spinning disc microscope with a resolution of 65 nm per pixel. The acquisition time for a single frame was 150 ms and a 561 nm laser was adopted to excite TPC2-R.GECO.1.2, the emission wavelength was detected at 606/54 nm.

2.1.3 Confocal Ca^{2+} imaging in astrocytes in situ. The genetically encoded Ca^{2+} indicator jGCaMP7b was subcloned into an AAV-PhP.eB vector under the control of the GFAP promoter. Imaging set-up was a confocal fluorescence microscope (16x objective, NA 0.8, 226 nm/pixel resolution) in acute mouse brain slices of the olfactory bulb using a 488 nm laser for excitation (emission filter 515/15) at a frame rate of 1 Hz.

2.2 Deep image prior and implemented variants

Denoising and deconvolution are inverse problems that can be formulated as an energy minimization problem of the type

$$x^* = \arg\min_x E\,(x, x_o) + R\,(x) \tag{1}$$

with x_0 as degraded input image, x the sought output image, $E\,(x, x_o)$ the task-dependent data term, and $R(x)$ a regularizer. Ulyanov, Vedaldi, Lempitsky [6] proposed to drop the explicit regularization and to replace Eq. 1 by

$$\theta^* = \arg\min_\theta E\,(f_\theta\,(z)\,, x_o)\,,\quad x^* = f_{\theta^*}\,(z) \tag{2}$$

with θ as the initially random parameters of a neural network that acts as an implicit regularizer and the code z, which is a fixed randomly initialized tensor. The implicit regularization is achieved by stopping the training before convergence, as the network fits faster to natural-looking rather than noisy signals.

In the simplest case, the data term is an L^2 distance. We modify this similarly to Burns, Liu [7], who incorporated a forward model for structured illumination microscopy (SIM) reconstruction into the loss function. Here, we implemented the following modified loss function, which is a combination of a standard L^2-norm loss and a loss term that includes the convolution of the sought output image with the PSF of the imaging process

$$E(x, x_0) = (1 - \alpha)\,\|f_\theta(z) - x_0\|^2 + \alpha\,\|f_\theta(z) * h - x_0\|^2 \tag{3}$$

where h denotes the point spread function. The parameter α controls the weighting of the two loss terms. We call this modification of the standard DIP algorithm DECO-DIP.

In addition, we introduce DECO-DIP-T, an extension that exploits the temporal dimension of image sequences. The information about adjacent frames is incorporated via forward and backward steps. In the forward step, we apply RDPV [8] by initializing the network with optimized weights from the previous frame and iterating through the frames chronologically. The backward step is the application of RDPV in reverse chronological order starting with the network for the last frame (optimized during the forward step). The final results are the outputs of the networks during the backward step.

2.3 Experiments

The performance of DECO-DIP was tested on datasets 1 and 2 and compared to the standard RL deconvolution (scikit-image implementation) and the original DIP. The PSF was calculated using the implementation by Woelk et al. [9]. The used parameters can be found in the github repository. For all DIP experiments, we used an U-net structure with varying depths d. We used between $N = 500$ and $N = 1000$ iterations and a learning rate LR = 0.01. For the synthetic data, the performance was evaluated by the structural similarity index SSIM of the original and the reconstructed images.

The performance of DECO-DIP-T was evaluated on datasets 1 and 3 and compared to DECO-DIP and time-dependent entropy-based restoration (TD ER) [9]. For the first image of an image sequence, we used the standard DIP parameters. Subsequent images were learned using a smaller number of iterations N_V and learning rate LR_V due to the use of the pre-fitted network.

3 Results

All experiments were run on a NVIDIA RTX A4000 GPU. DIP restoration times varied, ranging from about 30 seconds to several minutes, depending on image size and the number of iterations.

3.1 Synthetic data

The results of the different restoration approaches for an example image of the synthetic set are shown in Figure 1(a). The parameters for each method were optimized to maximize SSIM. The RL result shows significant background noise and a blurred signal after a single iteration. Additional iterations sharpen the signal, but amplify the background noise and introduce ringing artifacts. The original DIP outputs an image with substantially less noise than RL. DECO-DIP with depth $d = 8$ further reduces background noise and sharpens the signal. (DECO-)DIP with depth $d = 6$ illustrates a decreased performance with decreased network depth.

Numerical results in Figure 1(b) confirm the visual impression. Across varying levels of Gaussian noise, DECO-DIP with $d = 8$ generates images with the highest SSIM values, outperforming RL deconvolution and the original DIP. While the original DIP is better for low noise levels, the RL deconvolution is more effective for higher noise levels ($\sigma^2 \lesssim 0.01$), although not as good as DECO-DIP with $d = 8$. The shallower networks with $d = 6$ produce smaller SSIM values than their deeper counterparts.

3.2 Application to low exposure live cell data

Figure 2 illustrates the reconstruction results for dataset 2. The RL algorithm yields clearer signals when compared to the original input data, but still contains substantial

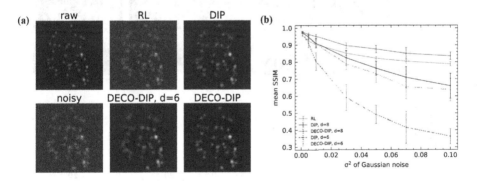

Fig. 1. (a) Example results for the synthetic data set with Gaussian noise variance $\sigma^2 = 0.01$. First row: raw image (ground truth), restoration results for RL (one iteration) and DIP ($d = 8$, $N = 750$). Second row: noisy (input) image and DECO-DIP results ($d = 6$ and $d = 8$, both with $\alpha = 0.7$ and $N = 500$). (b) Mean SSIM of result and original image averaged over 20 randomly generated synthetic images as a function of σ^2 of the Gaussian noise for RL (orange), DIP (blue) with $d = 6$ (dashed) and $d = 8$ (solid) and DECO-DIP (green) with $d = 6$ (dashed) and $d = 8$ (solid).

background noise. Both DIP and DECO-DIP effectively remove background noise, with DECO-DIP producing a better-reconstructed signal than DIP.

Figure 3 shows examples of DECO-DIP-T for the synthetic and the astrocyte datasets in comparison to DECO-DIP and TD ER. TD ER produces a good reconstruction but retains some background noise. The DECO-DIP image has less background noise but contains some artifacts. The DECO-DIP-T result represents the best reconstruction of the signal with the least amount of background noise. The raw image of the synthetic data can be found in Figure 1(a).

4 Discussion

We demonstrated that DIP with an optimized loss function, incorporating prior knowledge about the imaging process in terms of the microscope PSF, outperforms the original DIP as well as the RL algorithm in reconstructing fluorescence microscopy images. The time-dependent version DECO-DIP-T further reduces background noise and enhances the signal reconstruction.

However, reconstruction with DECO-DIP takes about half a minute to several minutes and a GPU is needed. Moreover, the parameters have to be tuned for the specific dataset. Thus, the choice between DECO-DIP and faster, easy-to-use standard algorithms like RL depends on time, hardware, and reconstruction performance constraints.

In the future, we plan to improve the performance of DECO-DIP by further modifications of the loss function such as sparsity constraints or explicit regularizers. Exploring potentially better suited network architectures is also a promising direction.

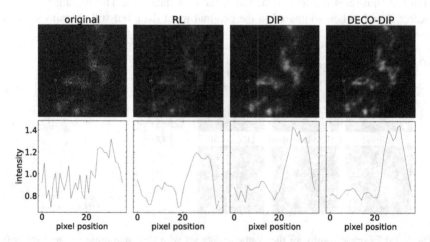

Fig. 2. Results for T-cell images captured at a low 150 ms exposure time. From left to right: raw image, RL (5 iterations), DIP ($N = 750$, $d = 8$), and DECO-DIP ($N = 1000$, $\alpha = 0.95$, $d = 8$). The first row contains a zoomed-in region of interest of the original image. The second row shows the intensity profile along the red line (top to bottom) in the images above.

Fig. 3. Illustration of the performance of DECO-DIP-T. (a) Left to right: raw image and results for TD ER, DECO-DIP, and DECO-DIP-T for synthetic data (first row) and astrocytes (second row). (b) Detail of astrocyte results (bottom row in (a)). Parameters for dataset 1: TD ER: $\lambda = 0.1$, $\lambda_T = 0.1$, DECO-DIP: $N = 500$, $\alpha_{PSF} = 0.7$, $d = 8$, DECO-DIP-T: $N = 500$, $N_V = 38$, $\alpha_{PSF} = 0.7$, $d = 8$. Parameters for dataset 3: TD ER: $\lambda = 0.05$, $\lambda_T = 0.05$, DECO-DIP: $N = 2000$, $\alpha_{PSF} = 0.99$, $d = 8$, DECO-DIP-T: $N = 2000$, $N_V = 90$, $\alpha_{PSF} = 0.99$, $d = 8$.

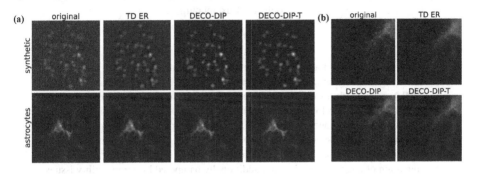

Acknowledgement. This work was funded by the Deutsche Forschungsgemeinschaft (DFG, German Research Foundation) grant number 335447717; SFB 1328, project A02 to B.-P.D. and R.W. and project A07 to C.E.G. and C.L.

References

1. Ettinger A, Wittmann T. Methods in Cell Biology. Ed. by Waters JC, Wittman T. Vol. 123. Academic Press, 2014:77–94.
2. Richardson WH. Bayesian-based iterative method of image restoration. J Opt Soc Am. 1972;62(1):55.
3. Lucy LB. An iterative technique for the rectification of observed distributions. Astron J. 1974;79:745.
4. Weigert M, Schmidt U, Boothe T, Müller A, Dibrov A, Jain A et al. Content-aware image restoration: pushing the limits of fluorescence microscopy. Nat Methods. 2018;15(12):1090–7.
5. Wang H, Rivenson Y, Jin Y, Wei Z, Gao R, Günaydın H et al. Deep learning enables cross-modality super-resolution in fluorescence microscopy. 2019;16(1):103–10.
6. Ulyanov D, Vedaldi A, Lempitsky V. Deep image prior. Int J Comput Vis. 2020;128:1867–88.
7. Burns Z, Liu Z. Untrained, physics-informed neural networks for structured illumination microscopy. Opt Lett. 2023;31(5):8714–24.
8. Cascarano P, Comes MC, Mencattini A, Parrini MC, Piccolomini EL, Martinelli E. Recursive deep prior video: a super resolution algorithm for time-lapse microscopy of organ-on-chip experiments. en. Med Image Anal. 2021;72:102124.
9. Woelk LM, Kannabiran SA, Brock VJ, Gee CE, Lohr C, Guse AH et al. Time-dependent image restoration of low-SNR live-cell Ca2 fluorescence microscopy data. Int J Mol Sci. 2021;22(21):11792.

Unified Retrieval for Streamlining Biomedical Image Dataset Aggregation and Standardization

Raphael Maser, Meryem Abbad Andaloussi, François Lamoline, Andreas Husch

Imaging AI Group, Luxembourg Centre for Systems Biomedicine, University of Luxembourg, Belvaux, Luxembourg
andreas.husch@uni.lu

Abstract. Advancements in computational power and algorithmic refinements have significantly amplified the impact and applicability of machine learning (ML), particularly in medical imaging. While ML in general thrives on extensive datasets to develop accurate, robust, and unbiased models, medical imaging faces unique challenges, including a scarcity of samples and a predominance of poorly annotated, heterogeneous datasets. This heterogeneity manifests in varied acquisition conditions, target populations, data formats and structures. Data acquisition of large datasets is often additionally hampered by compatibility issues of source specific downloading tools with high-performance computing (HPC) environments. To address these challenges, we introduce the unified retrieval tool (URT), a tool that unifies the acquisition and standardization of diverse medical imaging datasets to the brain imaging data structure (BIDS). Currently, downloads from the cancer imaging archive (TCIA), OpenNeuro and Synapse are supported, easing access to large-scale medical data. URT's modularity allows the straightforward extension to other sources. Moreover, URT's compatibility with Docker and Singularity enables reproducible research and easy application on HPCs.

1 Introduction

Although machine learning (ML) is not a recent invention, the rapid increase of compute power in the last decade has led to increasingly sophisticated ML models, not only in language models [1, 2] but also in the realm of computer vision and medical imaging [3–6]. These large ML models typically require huge amounts of diverse, high-quality data, ideally capturing multiple domains provided in a compatible format. One step towards this goal is the brain imaging data structure (BIDS) [7], which provides a standardized dataset structure, simplifying large-scale training on massive data collections. URT expands this concept by unifying access to diverse sources of data in a simple command-line tool and integrating automatic BIDS conversion of added datasets.

1.1 Background

Given an input space $U \subset \mathbb{R}^{n_u}$ and an output space $Y \subset \mathbb{R}^{n_y}$, an ML model is an approximator of any Borel-measurable function mapping from U to Y. The robustness and representativeness of the approximation relies on quantity and quality of training samples, see e.g. [2, 6]. Although data collection poses a general problem, medical imaging is especially affected by data scarcity [8]. Several reasons exist for this lack of data, in particular: 1) comparably small numbers of available patients, 2) various forms of restricted access, and 3) the challenge of consistent annotation/ground-truth [9]. First, datasets used for non-medical computer vision tasks are usually of a much larger scale. For instance the extremely popular ImageNet dataset [10] includes a total of 14 million images. That is no comparison with the scale of most medical datasets that are limited by the number of available patients. Second, medical data are frequently subject to ethical restrictions, complex data-protection procedures or other similar concerns, leading to limited access for researchers. Third, there is considerable difficulty in annotating medical images and acquiring ground-truth. Traditionally, annotation has been reliant on trained medical experts and there is considerable variability in annotations among different physicians [8, 11]. Indeed, low inter-rater agreement among experts emerges rather frequently. For instance, [12] reported that each annotation in their study was determined by averaging the assessments of four junior ophthalmologists and then verified by a senior ophthalmologist.

All the aforementioned difficulties also imply a higher cost for gathering medical data. However, large, high-quality datasets are a requirement for training reliable ML models. As [8] puts it: "[...] reaching better generalization in medical imaging may require assembling significantly larger datasets, while avoiding biases [...]".

1.2 Problem

Collecting and aggregating large-scale datasets from heterogeneous sources is complicated, especially in HPC environments. One technical limitation is the incompatibility of required download tools with HPC environments. Some tools rely on GUI's, which do not work by default when connecting per SSH, others require root permissions for installation that are not available to HPC users. A further limitation is a lack of standardization in dataset structure. This renders the training of ML models aggregating multiple datasets difficult, as a conversion to a common structure is required first. Therefore, there is a need for tools that provide a unified interface for automatic download and standardization of large dataset collections in a reproducible way while being fully compatible with HPC environments. Finally, reproducibility and tracking of dataset sources are key to avoid quality problems. In particular, accidental data duplicates, as they were for example found in public X-Ray imaging collections for COVID-19, where complex inclusion relationships of datasets sometimes lead to multiple inclusions of the same data [13], have to be strictly avoided.

1.3 Relevance of the BIDS standard

BIDS is a first step towards standardizing the structure of medical imaging formats for research, with a focus on brain scans, which could be leveraged to ease the large-scale training of ML models with data from different source domains. Imaging data is usually not standardized, which makes large-scale training and modification of the data collection time-consuming [9]. Brain data is typically available in DICOM or NifTI format with varying degrees of metadata availability and there is no universally accepted structure for storing the data. Oftentimes imaging modalities are not clear-cut which requires a high effort of the practitioner before any model training can happen. BIDS provides a flexible framework for standardizing image collections in a common structure and format. This makes datasets not only more accessible but also interchangeable, i.e. it simplifies and accelerates the possibility of large-scale and multi-modal training.

2   Materials and methods

URT takes the approach of BIDS one step further by unifying multiple data sources and providing the ability to download and convert an arbitrary number of supported datasets to BIDS automatically. Creating large data collections often entails a significant time investment. This time-consuming task creates a barrier to the development of more advanced ML models in medical imaging. URT aims at unifying and automating this process in a single tool written in Python.

2.1   Architecture of URT

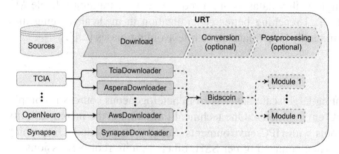

Fig. 1. Graphical summary of the URT architecture

Figure 1 illustrates the URT architecture. It is split into three main parts: download, conversion and postprocessing. Depending on the source and type of the data, URT will choose the correct downloader for that task and initiate the download. Afterwards, the dataset can be converted automatically to BIDS, as long as the required mapping specification is available in URT (more details in 2.1.2). URT also supports automated postprocessing via the integrated modules, the user can define the modules as needed. Both, conversion and postprocessing, are optional. Note that nonsupported datasets can be easily added by specifying the source and required downloader, as well as the mapping for the BIDS conversion (if the conversion is desired). Modularity is one of the key features of URT, allowing users to add new downloaders and postprocessing modules if needed. This flexibility ensures that URT can evolve and adapt to new data formats. In addition, to enhance efficiency when handling multiple datasets, the URT tool enables batch processing, allowing for the sequential download and conversion of each dataset provided in a list without user interaction. Currently supported sources and downloaders are presented in the following section.

2.1.1   Sources and downloaders. URT currently integrates three sources: The cancer imaging archive (TCIA) [14], OpenNeuro [15] and Synapse[1]. TCIA offers two different

---

[1]http://www.synapse.org

ways of downloading data, depending on the type of data. Both sources and their respective downloaders are indicated in Figure 1.

For datasets in the DICOM format, TCIA provides downloads via its TCIA Rest API, which is supported through the "TciaDownloader" class in URT. To ensure data integrity the downloader automatically checks for partial downloads and corrupted files using MD5 hashes. Datasets in the NifTI format on TCIA are not available through the API but only as IBM Aspera Faspex package. Thus the "AsperaDownloader" class supports Aspera downloads in URT by calling the IBM Aspera CLI tool[2] internally.

OpenNeuro data is available on an AWS S3 instance and is supported by the "Aws-Downloader ", which uses the AWS CLI download tool[3]. Synapse datasets are supported by implementing the official Python package[4] in the "SynapseDownloader". All these downloaders have in common that they put emphasis on fault-tolerance for achieving a maximum of robustness. If some source requires user authentication (for datasets with restricted access), credentials can be stored in URT.

URT depends on a definition file containing the metadata required for the download. It usually contains the original format of the data, the source URL and the downloader which should be used. Integrating a new dataset is straightforward by providing this information. If the data originates from a new source not supported by the existing tools, URT facilitates the addition of a new downloader.

2.1.2   Conversion to BIDS structure. BIDS is a data organization format for neuroimaging experiments. To convert neuroimaging datasets to BIDS, we use the bidscoin library, [16] which contains bidsmapper and bidscoiner. We create a bidsmap, which is a mapping between the metadata, paths, and filenames of the original dataset and its BIDS standardized counterpart for each dataset. For that, the bidsmapper takes a specific template bidsmap, scans the data in its original format and creates a study bidsmap, which is used by the bidscoiner to finally convert the data. Both steps are fully integrated into URT, given that the template bidsmap and arguments for bidscoin are defined. User-defined bidsmaps can also be incorporated into URT if necessary. However, creating bidsmaps requires some domain knowledge of the respective dataset to create a template bidsmap matching the specific dataset structure. Once the data is converted, it is stored as 3D NifTI files in the BIDS folder structure and thus manageable by libraries like PyBIDS.

2.2   Ensuring reproducibility

Due to the large number of different programming languages and package sources, reliable dependency management cannot be achieved by using virtual environments alone. The main code, as well as the TCIA API integration, are written in Python, however Aspera CLI, necessary for the download of some datasets, is only available as Ruby Gem and the newest official version of AWS CLI is available via package managers of the respective distribution (e.g. yum). In order to avoid dependency conflicts

---

[2]https://github.com/IBM/aspera-cli
[3]https://aws.amazon.com/cli
[4]https://pypi.org/project/synapse-downloader/

as well as complicated setups on the user side, URT is available as Docker image. By encapsulating the dependencies in a container, URT is easy to use, lightweight and provides reproducible results across different machines.

2.3 Application in high-performance-computing environments

A strong emphasis was put on the compatibility with high-performance-computing (HPC) environments. Using Docker directly on HPCs is usually not allowed. The docker daemon managing the execution of Docker container requires root access, which poses security risks in a multi-user computing environment. Instead, Singularity is often used as a drop-in replacement. The URT Docker image is fully compatible with Singularity, even without using the "fakeroot" option (which is not supported by every system). Given the substantial size of some datasets and the extensive number of files in DICOM datasets (3D images stored as a series of 2D files), URT can process and compress the data on a temporary storage drive before transferring it to the target directory. This is especially advantageous in HPC environments, where the maximum number of files is often limited by inode limits.

3   Results

The unified retrieval tool (URT) was developed to address the unique challenge posed by the medical imaging field in terms of data acquisition and standardization. URT is containerized using Docker and Singularity, leading to independence of the underlying systems architecture and reproducible results. It is simple to use, even in HPC environments. All downloaders are fault tolerant and provide integrity checks of the downloaded data. Once template bidsmaps are provided for a given dataset the automatic download and conversion is possible without user interaction. URT is provided open source on GitHub[5].

4   Discussion

URT is a first step towards a unique tool for the acquisition and standardization of medical image datasets from diverse sources. It is a valuable asset for researchers as it provides a HPC compatible way of robust data download and conversion. It simplifies downloading and standardizing heterogeneous datasets from different sources and avoids the dependency management typically associated with these tasks, enabling the creation of reproducible dataset collections. The authors believe that URT will save a significant amount of time to researchers and increase reproducibility. Future work will include integrating additional relevant downloader modules to URT, while additional bidsmaps for novel datasets could be provided by community. Furthermore, adding a graphical user interface while retaining full HPC compatibility is foreseen.

---

[5]https://github.com/LuxImagingAI/URT

Acknowledgement. The authors thank Ben Bausch for insightful discussions. FL is a Quilvest Research Fellow under a donation by Quilvest S.A.; AH and RM are supported by the Luxembourg National Research Fund grant #150220234 (BIML-19/FNR-DFG); MAA is a fellow of the University of Luxembourg Institute for Advanced Studies. HPC experiments presented in this report were carried out using the HPC facilities of the University of Luxembourg [17].

References

1. Brown T, Mann B, Ryder N, Subbiah M, Kaplan JD, Dhariwal P et al. Language models are few-shot learners. Adv Neural Inf Process Syst. 2020;33:1877–901.
2. Kaplan J, McCandlish S, Henighan T, Brown TB, Chess B, Child R et al. Scaling laws for neural language models. arXiv preprint arXiv:2001.08361. 2020.
3. Tan M, Le Q. Efficientnet: rethinking model scaling for convolutional neural networks. Proc PMLR. PMLR. 2019:6105–14.
4. Dosovitskiy A, Beyer L, Kolesnikov A, Weissenborn D, Zhai X, Unterthiner T et al. An image is worth 16x16 Words: transformers for image recognition at scale. Proc ICLR. 2021.
5. Xie Z, Zhang Z, Cao Y, Lin Y, Wei Y, Dai Q et al. On data scaling in masked image modeling. Proc IEEE CVPR. 2023:10365–74.
6. Zhai X, Kolesnikov A, Houlsby N, Beyer L. Scaling vision transformers. Proc IEEE CVPR. 2022:12104–13.
7. Gorgolewski KJ, Auer T, Calhoun VD, Craddock RC, Das S, Duff EP et al. The brain imaging data structure, a format for organizing and describing outputs of neuroimaging experiments. Sci Data. 2016;3(1):160044.
8. Varoquaux G, Cheplygina V. Machine learning for medical imaging: methodological failures and recommendations for the future. NPJ Digit Med. 2022;5(1):48.
9. Willemink MJ, Koszek WA, Hardell C, Wu J, Fleischmann D, Harvey H et al. Preparing medical imaging data for machine learning. Radiol. 2020;295(1):4–15.
10. Deng J, Dong W, Socher R, Li LJ, Li K, Fei-Fei L. ImageNet: a large-scale hierarchical image database. Proc IEEE ICCV. Ieee. 2009:248–55.
11. Schilling MP, Ahuja N, Rettenberger L, Scherr T, Reischl M. Impact of annotation noise on histopathology nucleus segmentation. Cur Direct Biomed Eng. Vol. 8. (2). De Gruyter. 2022:197–200.
12. Gavrielides MA, Kinnard LM, Myers KJ, Peregoy J, Pritchard WF, Zeng R et al. A resource for the assessment of lung nodule size estimation methods: database of thoracic CT scans of an anthropomorphic phantom. Opt Express. 2010;18(14):15244–55.
13. Garcia Santa Cruz B, Bossa MN, Sölter J, Husch AD. Public Covid-19 X-ray datasets and their impact on model bias: a systematic review of a significant problem. Med Image Anal. 2021;74:102225.
14. Clark K, Vendt B, Smith K, Freymann J, Kirby J, Koppel P et al. The cancer imaging archive (TCIA): maintaining and operating a public information repository. J Digit Imaging. 2013;26:1045–57.
15. Markiewicz CJ, Gorgolewski KJ, Feingold F, Blair R, Halchenko YO, Miller E et al. The OpenNeuro resource for sharing of neuroscience data. eLife. 2021;10:e71774.
16. Zwiers MP, Moia S, Oostenveld R. BIDScoin: a user-friendly application to convert source data to brain imaging data structure. Front Neuroinform. 2022;15:65.
17. Varrette S, Bouvry P, Cartiaux H, Georgatos F. Management of an academic HPC cluster: the UL experience. Proc IEEE HPCS. 2014:959–67.

Abstract: Object Detection for Breast Diffusion-weighted Imaging

Dimitrios Bounias[1,2], Michael Baumgartner[1,3,4], Peter Neher[1,5,6], Balint Kovacs[1,2],
Ralf Floca[1,7], Paul F. Jaeger[4,8], Lorenz A. Kapsner[9], Jessica Eberle[9],
Dominique Hadler[9], Frederik Laun[9], Sabine Ohlmeyer[9],
Klaus H. Maier-Hein[1,2,3,5,6,10], Sebastian Bickelhaupt[9]

[1]Medical Image Computing (MIC), German Cancer Research Center (DKFZ), Heidelberg
[2]Medical Faculty, Heidelberg University
[3]Faculty of Mathematics and Computer Science, Heidelberg University
[4]Helmholtz Imaging, German Cancer Research Center (DKFZ), Heidelberg
[5]German Cancer Consortium (DKTK), Partner Site Heidelberg
[6]Pattern Analysis and Learning Group, Heidelberg University Hospital
[7]Heidelberg Institute of Radiation Oncology (HIRO), Heidelberg
[8]Interactive Machine Learning Group, German Cancer Research Center (DKFZ), Heidelberg
[9]Institute of Radiology, Uniklinikum Erlangen, FAU
[10]National Center for Tumor Diseases (NCT), Heidelberg University Hospital and DKFZ
dimitrios.bounias@dkfz-heidelberg.de

Diffusion-weighted imaging (DWI) is a rapidly emerging unenhanced MRI technique in oncologic breast imaging. This IRB approved study included n=818 patients (with n=618 malignant lesions in n=268 patients). All patients underwent a clinically indicated multiparametric breast 3T MRI examination, including a multi-b-value DWI acquisition (50,750,1500). We utilized nnDetection, a state-of-the-art self-configuring object detection model, with certain breast cancer-specific extensions to train a detection model. The model was trained with the following extensions: (i) apparent diffusion coefficient (ADC) as additional input, (ii) random bias field, random spike, and random ghosting augmentations, (iii) a size-balanced data loader to ensure that the fewer large lesions were given an equal chance to be picked in a mini-batch and (iv) replacement of the loss function with a size-adjusted focal loss, to prioritize finding primary lesions while disincentivizing small indeterminate false positives. The model was able to achieve an AUC of 0.88 in 5-fold cross-validation using only the DWI acquisition, and compares favorably against multireader performance metrics reported for screening mammography in large studies in the literature (0.81, 0.87, 0.81). It also achieved 0.70 FROC for primary lesions, indicating a relevant localization ability. This study shows that AI has the ability to complement breast cancer screening assessment in DWI-based examinations. This work was originally published at RSNA 2023 [1].

References

1. Bounias D, Baumgartner M, Neher P, Kovacs B, Floca R, Jaeger PF et al. AI for Diffusion-weighted Breast MRI. RSNA. 2023.

Abstract: Semi-automatic White Matter Tract Segmentation using Active Learning

attRACTive

Robin Peretzke[1,2], Klaus Maier-Hein[1,2,3,4,5,6,7], Jonas Bohn[1,4,8],
Yannick Kirchhoff[1,6,7], Saikat Roy[1,7], Sabrina Oberli-Palme[1], Daniela Becker[9,10],
Pavlina Lenga[9], Peter Neher[1,4]

[1]German Cancer Research Center (DKFZ) Heidelberg, Division of Medical Image Computing, Germany
[2]Medical Faculty Heidelberg, Heidelberg University, Heidelberg, Germany
[3]National Center for Tumor Diseases (NCT), NCT Heidelberg, a partnership between DKFZ and university medical center Heidelberg
[4]Pattern Analysis and Learning Group, Heidelberg University Hospital, Heidelberg, Germany
[5]HIDSS4Health - Helmholtz Information and Data Science School for Health, Karlsruhe/Heidelberg, Germany
[6]Faculty of Mathematics and Computer Science, Heidelberg University, Heidelberg, Germany
[7]Faculty of Bioscience, Heidelberg University, Heidelberg, Germany
[8]Department of Diagnostic and Interventional Radiology, Faculty of Medicine, Technical University of Munich, Munich, Germany
[9]Department of Neurosurgery, Heidelberg University Hospital, Heidelberg, Germany
[10]IU, International University of Applied Sciences, Erfurt, Germany
robin.peretzke@dkfz-heidelberg.de

Accurately identifying white matter tracts in medical images is essential for various applications, including surgery planning. Supervised machine learning models have reached state-of-the-art solving this task automatically. However, these models are primarily trained on healthy subjects and struggle with strong anatomical aberrations, e.g. caused by brain tumors. This limitation makes them unsuitable for tasks such as preoperative planning, wherefore time-consuming and challenging manual delineation of the target tract is employed. We propose semi-automatic entropy-based active learning for quick and intuitive segmentation of tracts from tractography consisting of millions of streamlines. The method is evaluated on 21 openly available healthy subjects from the Human Connectome Project and an internal dataset of ten neurosurgical cases. With only a few annotations, this approach enables segmenting tracts on tumor cases comparable to healthy subjects (dice = 0.71), while the performance of automatic methods dropped substantially (dice = 0.34). The method named attRACTive is implemented in the software MITK Diffusion. Manual experiments on tumor data showed higher efficiency than traditional ROI-based segmentation [1].

References

1. Peretzke R. atTRACTive: Semi-automatic white matter tract segmentation using active learning. Proc IEEE. 2023:237–46.

Abstract: Metal Inpainting in CBCT Projections using Score-based Generative Model

Siyuan Mei, Fuxin Fan, Andreas Maier

Pattern Recognition Lab, Friedrich-Alexander-Universität Erlangen-Nürnberg, Germany
siyuan.mei@fau.de

During orthopaedic surgery, the insertion of metallic implants or screws is often performed under mobile C-arm systems. However, due to the high attenuation of metals, severe metal artifacts occur in 3D reconstructions, which degrade the image quality significantly. Therefore, many metal artifacts reduction (MAR) algorithms have been developed to reduce the artifacts. In this work, a score-based generative model is trained on simulated knee projections to learn the score function of the perturbed data distribution, and the inpainted images are obtained by removing the noise during the conditional sampling process [1]. Specifically, the backbone of the score-based neural network is a simple U-Net which is conditioned on a time variable while the perturbation kernel utilizes the variance exploding form. A hyperparameter sweep is conducted to confirm the optimal hyperparameters in the sampling process, revealing that a signal-to-noise ratio of 0.4 and a number of discretization steps equal to 1000 achieve the best trade-off between efficiency and accuracy. Finally, the result implies that the inpainted images by the proposed unsupervised method have more detailed information and semantic connection to the bones or soft tissue, achieving the lowest mean absolute error of 0.069 and the highest peak-signal-to-noise ratio of 43.07 compared with the inverse distance weighting interpolation method and the mask pyramid network. Besides, the score-based generative model can also recover projections with large circular and rectangular masks, showing its generalization in inpainting tasks.

References

1. Mei S, Fan F, Maier A. Metal inpainting in CBCT projections using score-based generative model. Proc IEEE ISBI. 2023:1–5.

Abstract: Physics-informed Conditional Autoencoder Approach for Robust Metabolic CEST MRI at 7T

Junaid R. Rajput[1,2], Tim A. Möhle[1], Moritz S. Fabian[1], Angelika Mennecke[1], Jochen A. Sembill[3], Joji B. Kuramatsu[3], Manuel Schmidt[1], Arnd Dörfler[1], Andreas Maier[2], Moritz Zaiss[1]

[1]Institute of Neuroradiology, University Hospital Erlangen, Erlangen, Germany
[2]Pattern Recognition Lab Friedrich-Alexander-University Erlangen-Nürnberg
[3]Department of Neurology, University Hospital Erlangen-Nürnberg, Erlangen Germany
junaid.rajput@fau.de

Chemical exchange saturation transfer (CEST) is an MRI technique used to identify solute molecules through proton exchange. The CEST spectrum reveals various metabolite effects, which are extracted using Lorentzian curve fitting. However, the effectiveness of the separation of CEST effects is compromised by the inhomogeneity of the B_1 saturation field and noise in the acquisition. These inconsistencies result in variations within the associated metabolic maps. The existing B_1 correction methods necessitate a minimum of two sets of CEST spectra. From these, a B_1-corrected CEST spectrum at a fixed B_1 level is interpolated, effectively doubling the acquisition time. In this study, we investigated the use of an unsupervised physics-informed conditional autoencoder (PICAE) to efficiently correct B_1 inhomogeneity and isolate metabolic maps while using a single CEST scan. The proposed method uses two autoencoders. Conditional autoencoder (CAE) for B_1 correction of the CEST spectrum at arbitrary B_1 levels and Physical Informed Autoencoder (PIAE) for Lorentzian line fitting. CAE consists of fully connected layers whose latent space and input are both conditioned at the B_1 level, eliminating the need for a second scan. PIAE uses a fully connected neural network as an encoder and a Lorentzian distribution generator as a decoder. This not only facilitates model interpretation, but also overcomes the shortcomings of traditional curve fitting, in particular its susceptibility to noise. The PICAE-CEST maps showed improved visualization of tumor features compared to the conventional method. The proposed method yielded at least 25% higher structural similarity index (SSIM) compared to the T_1-weighted reference image enhanced with the exogenous contrast agent gadolinium in the tumor ring region. In addition, the contrast maps exhibited lower noise and greater homogeneity throughout the brain compared to the Lorentzian fit of the interpolation-based B_1-corrected CEST spectrum [1].

References

1. Rajput JR, Möhle TA, Fabian MS, Mennecke A, Sembill JA, Kuramatsu JB et al. Physics-informed conditional autoencoder approach for robust metabolic CEST MRI at 7T. Proc MICCAI. Springer, 2023:449–58.

© Der/die Autor(en), exklusiv lizenziert an
Springer Fachmedien Wiesbaden GmbH, ein Teil von Springer Nature 2024
A. Maier et al. (Hrsg.), *Bildverarbeitung für die Medizin 2024*,
Informatik aktuell, https://doi.org/10.1007/978-3-658-44037-4_87

Comparing Image Segmentation Neural Networks for the Analysis of Precision Cut Lung Slices

Mohan Xu[1], Susann Dehmel[1], Lena Wiese[1,2]

[1]Fraunhofer Institute for Toxicology and Experimental Medicine, Hannover, Germany
[2]Institute of Computer Science, Goethe University Frankfurt, Frankfurt a. M., Germany
mohan.xu@item.fraunhofer.de

Abstract. Bronchodilators serve as a pivotal intervention for ameliorating symptoms associated with Inflammatory and allergic lung diseases. The objective assessment of bronchodilator efficacy is critical for therapeutic optimization. Measuring airflow volume through precision cut lung slices (PCLS) imaging at varying time intervals provides a quantitative means to assess airway patency. To enhance the efficiency of this evaluation process, our study extends the existing image segmentation workflow to encompass a wider range of neural networks. Extensive experiments have been conducted across varied data preprocessing methods and loss functions. Furthermore, we contrast the performance differences between single and ensemble models, alongside a visual comparative analysis of their detailed variances in image segmentation. This refined workflow not only surpasses previous experimental results but also enhances the accuracy of lung treatment programs, offering a broader array of choices for future image segmentation tasks.

1 Introduction

Bronchodilators relax bronchial smooth muscle, dilate the bronchi, and alleviate airflow limitations. They constitute a vital therapeutic tool for managing inflammatory and allergic lung diseases. Evaluating the effectiveness of various bronchodilators can be achieved by measuring the airflow capacity of PCLS. During image acquisition, factors such as petri dish movement, changes in illumination conditions, out-of-focus images, or obscured airways can adversely impact the image quality of PCLS [1], affecting the accuracy of assessment results. Hence, this study focuses on the precise and efficient segmentation and calculation of airway areas in images of varying quality.

Deep learning, as a branch of machine learning, boasts remarkable capabilities in pattern recognition and feature learning, making it highly applicable in medical image analysis. Within the realm of medical image analysis, image segmentation stands as a crucial application, giving rise to a plethora of neural networks that exhibit outstanding performance. The skip-connection structure, introduced in [2, 3], establishes connections between the encoder and decoder, harnessing information at multiple levels. Furthermore, it seamlessly integrates shallow and deep features to bridge potential semantic gaps. Atrous convolution, as discussed in [4, 5], enhances the receptive field of feature map points without introducing additional parameters. PSPNet [6] achieves rapid segmentation results while maintaining high-quality image segmentation. Linknet [7] and FPN [8] share similarities with Unet in their architectures. However, Linknet adopts the resnet structure for its encoder block, while FPN accomplishes feature fusion

© Der/die Autor(en), exklusiv lizenziert an
Springer Fachmedien Wiesbaden GmbH, ein Teil von Springer Nature 2024
A. Maier et al. (Hrsg.), *Bildverarbeitung für die Medizin 2024*,
Informatik aktuell, https://doi.org/10.1007/978-3-658-44037-4_88

by up-sampling feature maps at varying scales. In PAN [9], the FPA module significantly expands the receptive field, while the GAU module extracts global context from high-level features, guiding the weighting operation of low-level features. MAnet [10], similar to the Unet structure, seeks to capture spatial dependencies between pixels on a global scale and channel dependencies among arbitrary feature maps through multi-scale semantic feature fusion.

Utilizing the bronchoconstriction dataset collected from PCLS, [11] employed Unet for image segmentation across four categories: background, airway, blood vessel, and airway boundary. This approach significantly accelerates image segmentation compared to manual methods. [1] expanded the scope of user-oriented web applications to include Unet, PSPNet, LinkNet, and FPN, constructing a comprehensive end-to-end image analysis framework. This study introduces new data preprocessing methods, neural network architectures and loss functions building upon prior research, ultimately yielding superior outcomes across a spectrum of evaluation metrics. Moreover, we conduct a comparison of segmentation performance between single and ensemble models, demonstrating that the ensemble approach enhances the model's ability to discriminate image details without incurring extra training costs.

2 Materials and methods

2.1 Dataset and experimental setup

Inverted microscopes and digital video cameras were employed to capture images of the airway region in PCLS samples contained in petri dishes, which had been treated with bronchodilators. The experimental design encompassed a wide range of variations in compounds, doses and samples, resulting in a total of 420 different experimental setups. The bronchoconstriction dataset, comprising 420 images, consists of images captured under various experimental conditions. Each image includes components such as background, airway, airway boundary, and possible blood vessels. In this study, we employed 9 popular image segmentation networks defined in the segmentation models pytorch [1], which include Unet, Unet++, Deeplabv3, Deeplabv3+, FPN, Linknet, PSPNet, PAN, and MAnet. The training process for these models utilized an SGD optimizer, trained for 80 epochs with a learning rate of 0.1. Early Stopping was implemented with a threshold set to 20 epochs. To ensure the comparability of experimental results, we adopted the dataset partitioning approach from references [1, 11] and conducted 10-fold cross-validation.

2.2 Proposed workflow

In this section, we detail the enhanced workflow for image segmentation. Figure 1 illustrates the process wherein a given input image, along with its corresponding ground truth, is subjected to a preprocessing step before being fed into a neural network for training. Following this, the neural network's output is processed through a softmax function prior to the computation of the loss function against the ground truth. Distinct

---

[1]https://github.com/qubvel/segmentation_models.pytorch

colors in the output image represent the various components of the PCLS. Furthermore, images can undergo testing using either a single neural network or ensemble neural networks by adjusting the respective weights.

The preprocessing step encompasses resize, online data augmentation and normalization. To enhance the dataset, which was resized to 512x512, we employed 6 methods from the albumentations library [12] for online data augmentation of the training set, as illustrated in Fig. 1(a-f). These data augmentation methods can be applied independently or in combination to the images, with the application likelihood and intensity modifiable through parameter adjustments. Normalization serves to equalize the variations among disparate data volumes and to optimize the data distribution, thereby accelerating the convergence of the model.

The nine neural networks utilized for the image segmentation task comprise an encoder, a decoder, and a segmentation head. The encoder is charged with extracting both global and local features from the image. We selected the pretrained *resnet101* model as the encoder to expedite model convergence. The decoder incrementally enhances the resolution of the feature maps through up-sampling or deconvolution, integrating them with feature maps from various stages of the encoder. Positioned subsequent to the decoder, the segmentation head guarantees that the output channel count of the network corresponds to the number of categories to be predicted. Images are tested by using trained neural networks with varying weights, adhering to the condition: $\sum_{i=1}^{n} w_i = 1$. When testing is conducted on a single model, the weight assigned to that model is set to 1, while the weights for all other models are set to 0.

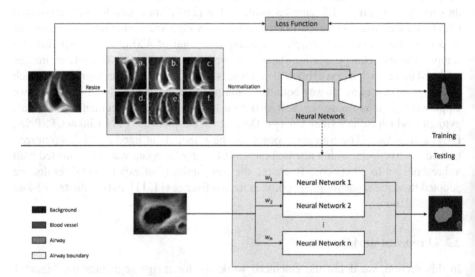

Fig. 1. Image segmentation workflow based on bronchoconstriction dataset, where a-f correspond to 6 data augmentation methods: Flip, BrightnessContrast, GridDistortion, OpticalDistortion, CLAHE and RandomGamma. The annotations in the lower-left indicate the categories associated with the various colored regions in the predictions.

Tab. 1. Comparative analysis of Unet performance with various data augmentation methods.

	Original	a	a+b	a+c	a+d	a+e	a+e+f
IoU	94.95	95.40	95.30	94.87	94.63	95.48	95.55
Dice	97.37	97.61	97.56	97.32	97.19	97.66	97.71
ASD	5.02	3.00	2.82	3.35	3.62	2.95	2.80

Tab. 2. Comparative analysis of Unet performance with various loss functions.

	Cross entropy loss	Focal loss	Dice loss	Tversky loss
IoU	94.95	92.44	94.66	94.79
Dice	97.37	96.01	97.20	97.27
ASD	5.02	5.75	6.89	5.39

The loss function, a vital indicator of model performance in deep learning, assesses the degree of divergence between the model's predictions and the actual values. During the training of neural networks, we examined the model's performance across four loss functions: cross-entropy loss, focal loss, dice loss, and tversky loss, comparing the variances in outcomes to identify the most effective loss function.

3 Results

To determine the optimal data augmentation and loss function combinations, we conducted a series of experiments using Unet. The effects of the 6 data augmentation methods, as identified in Figure 1, are presented in Table 1. Notably, the inclusion of the horizontal and vertical flip methods significantly enhanced the model's performance. The implementation of the Flip method resulted in improvements of 0.45% in IoU and 0.24% in Dice coefficients, along with a decrease of 1.98 in the average surface distance (ASD). Subsequent experiments, building upon the Flip method, determined that a combination of Flip, CLAHE, and Gamma augmentations (a+e+f) yielded the highest performance on the bronchoconstriction dataset. Concerning loss functions, Table 2 presents a comparative analysis of their impact on model performance when no data augmentation is applied. The model utilizing cross entropy loss surpassed other loss functions across all metrics. Relative to the least effective loss function, the cross entropy loss registered enhancements of 2.51% in IoU, 1.26% in Dice, and 0.73 in ASD.

Table 3 presents the performance outcomes derived from 10-fold cross-validation of nine neural networks, utilizing a consistent random seed. The enhanced workflow demonstrates superior performance over previous work in terms of IoU and Dice coefficients, particularly for the Unet architecture, which exhibits improvements of 1.94% and 1.11%, respectively. Furthermore, additional architectures such as Unet++, MAnet, PAN, Deeplabv3, and Deeplabv3+ were employed for image segmentation tasks within the bronchoconstriction dataset. Of these, Deeplabv3+ achieved the most favorable results across all three evaluation metrics. In the ensemble experiments, we compared three ensemble strategies (Ensemble 1 contains Deeplabv3+ and Unet++; Ensemble 2 contains Deeplabv3+, Unet++, Unet, FPN and Deeplabv3; Ensemble 3 contains Deeplabv3+,

Tab. 3. Comparative analysis of neural network performance: our work versus previous work.

	Previous work [1]		Our work		
	IoU	Dice	IoU	Dice	ASD
Unet	93.14	96.34	95.08±0.32	97.45±0.17	3.74±0.44
PSPNet	92.95	96.27	93.14±0.45	96.38±0.24	4.03±0.55
Linknet	93.43	96.52	94.92±0.40	97.36±0.21	5.09±1.32
FPN	94.16	96.91	95.00±0.26	97.41±0.14	3.44±0.36
Unet++		-	95.14±0.47	97.47±0.25	3.73±0.53
MAnet		-	94.96±0.27	97.38±0.15	3.55±0.37
PAN		-	94.65±0.56	97.22±0.27	3.65±0.78
Deeplabv3		-	95.00±0.28	97.40±0.15	3.63±0.43
Deeplabv3+		-	95.18±0.43	97.50±0.23	3.11±0.45
	Ensemble 1		95.42±0.29	97.63±0.16	3.08±0.29
	Ensemble 2		95.55±0.20	97.70±0.11	2.79±0.13
	Ensemble 3		95.53±0.21	97.69±0.11	2.79±0.16

Unet++, Unet, FPN, Deeplabv3 and MAnet). Each assigning equal weights to the models. The findings reveal that while the ensemble approach surpasses Deeplabv3+ in terms of overall performance, indiscriminately increasing the number of models does not guarantee improved image segmentation results. Figure 2 illustrates the performance of the single and ensemble models in segmenting background, airway and airway boundary.

4   Discussion

In this study, we executed a series of experiments on the bronchoconstriction dataset, extending the existing workflow across four dimensions: data processing methods, neural network architectures, loss functions, and evaluation metrics. These experiments aimed to identify the optimal training strategy. The results indicate that the enhanced workflow surpasses its predecessors in performance and offers a range of options for improving the performance of image segmentation tasks. Within the ensemble strategy, the assignment of model weights accurately reflects each model's contribution to overall performance. Notably, merely increasing the number of models while reducing the weights of existing models does not positively impact model performance.

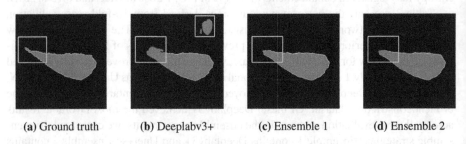

(a) Ground truth   (b) Deeplabv3+   (c) Ensemble 1   (d) Ensemble 2

Fig. 2. Comparative visualization of image segmentation on single and ensemble models.

Given that images in the bronchoconstriction dataset featuring the blood vessel category comprise merely 7.4% of the dataset, the influence of category imbalance on model performance cannot be overlooked. In view of this, future work will address this imbalance issue to improve the segmentation of minority categories within the dataset.

Acknowledgement. This work was supported by the Fraunhofer Internal Programs under Grant No. Attract 042-601000.

References

1. Wiese L, Höltje D. NNCompare: a framework for dataset selection, data augmentation and comparison of different neural networks for medical image analysis. Proc IEEE. 2021:1–7.
2. Ronneberger O, Fischer P, Brox T. U-net: convolutional networks for biomedical image segmentation. Proc MICCAI. 2015:234–41.
3. Zhou Z, Rahman Siddiquee MM, Tajbakhsh N, Liang J. Unet++: A nested U-net architecture for medical image segmentation. Proc MICCAI. 2018:3–11.
4. Chen LC, Papandreou G, Schroff F, Adam H. Rethinking atrous convolution for semantic image segmentation. arXiv preprint arXiv:1706.05587. 2017.
5. Chen LC, Zhu Y, Papandreou G, Schroff F, Adam H. Encoder-decoder with atrous separable convolution for semantic image segmentation. Proc ECCV. 2018:801–18.
6. Zhao H, Shi J, Qi X, Wang X, Jia J. Pyramid scene parsing network. Proc IEEE. 2017:2881–90.
7. Chaurasia A, Culurciello E. Linknet: exploiting encoder representations for efficient semantic segmentation. Proc IEEE. 2017:1–4.
8. Lin TY, Dollár P, Girshick R, He K, Hariharan B, Belongie S. Feature pyramid networks for object detection. Proc IEEE. 2017:2117–25.
9. Khosravan N, Mortazi A, Wallace M, Bagci U. Pan: projective adversarial network for medical image segmentation. Proc MICCAI. 2019:68–76.
10. Li R, Zheng S, Zhang C, Duan C, Su J, Wang L et al. Multiattention network for semantic segmentation of fine-resolution remote sensing images. IEEE. 2021;60:1–13.
11. Steinmeyer C, Dehmel S, Theidel D, Braun A, Wiese L. Automating bronchoconstriction analysis based on U-net. EDBT/ICDT Workshops. 2021.
12. Buslaev A, Iglovikov VI, Khvedchenya E, Parinov A, Druzhinin M, Kalinin AA. Albumentations: fast and flexible image augmentations. Information. 2020;11(2).

Comparison of Deep Learning Image-to-image Models for Medical Image Translation

Zeyu Yang[1,2], Frank G. Zöllner[1,2]

[1]Computer Assisted Clinical Medicine, Medical Faculty Mannheim, Heidelberg University, Mannheim, Germany
[2]Mannheim Institute for Intelligent Systems in Medicine, Medical Faculty Mannheim, Heidelberg University, Mannheim, Germany
Zeyu.Yang@medma.uni-heidelberg.de

Abstract. We conducted a comparative analysis of six image-to-image deep learning models for the purpose of MRI-to-CT image translation comprising resUNet, attUnet, DCGAN, pix2pixGAN with resUNet, pix2pixGAN with attUnet, and the denoising diffusion probabilistic model (DDPM). These models underwent training and assessment using the SynthRAD2023 Grand Challenge dataset. For training, 170 MRI and CT image pairs (patients) were employed, while a set of 10 patients was reserved for testing. In summary, the pix2pixGAN with resUNet achieved the highest scores (SSIM = 0.81±0.21, MAE = 55.52±3.50, PSNR = 27.19±6.29). The DDPM displayed considerable potential in generating CT images that closely resemble real ones in terms of detail and fidelity. Nevertheless, the quality of its generated images exhibited notable fluctuations. Consequently, further refinement is necessary to stabilize its output quality.

1 Introduction

Magnetic resonance imaging (MRI) and computed tomography (CT) represent two of the most prevalent medical imaging modalities. Owing to their distinctive attributes, the integration of MRI and CT in multimodal imaging is a common practice in the clinical domain [1]. Currently, CT and MRI scans are conducted separately, incurring not only substantial costs but also introducing non-rigid misalignment issues between the resultant images. Given these challenges, medical image synthesis is a promising approach to mitigate this issue [2]. This method establishes a mapping function that transforms a known source image into an unknown target image. Recently, deep learning approaches have illustrated significant potential for this purpose, yielding substantial advantages for diverse applications, such as noise reduction, artifact removal, image segmentation, and registration [3–5].

We propose a comparative analysis of various image-to-image models for the transformation of images between CT and MRI modalities. Our investigation includes six distinct models, namely, resUNet, attUnet, DCGAN, pix2pixGAN with resUNet, pix2pixGAN with attUnet, and the diffusion model (Denoising Diffusion Probabilistic Model, DDPM).

© Der/die Autor(en), exklusiv lizenziert an
Springer Fachmedien Wiesbaden GmbH, ein Teil von Springer Nature 2024
A. Maier et al. (Hrsg.), *Bildverarbeitung für die Medizin 2024*,
Informatik aktuell, https://doi.org/10.1007/978-3-658-44037-4_89

2 Materials and methods

2.1 Patient data

We acquired a total of 180 datasets of paired MRI and CT volumes from the Syn-thRAD2023 challenge [6]. The data is compiled from multiple centers and is divided into 170 training samples and 10 test cases. For details on the data set please refer to [6].

2.2 Image pre-processing

To get the paired images, several pre-processing steps were performed by the challenge organizer [6]. Briefly, the process involves converting DICOM to compressed NIfTI, performing rigid registration between CT and MR/CBCT images, anonymizing the data, segmenting the patient outline (provided as a binary mask), and finally, cropping the MR/CBCT, CT, and mask images to remove the background and reduce file size. Furthermore, we standardized the size of all images to 512×512, and performed intensity min-max normalization to a range of $[0, 1]$.

2.3 Network architecture

A total of six distinct models were trained and assessed within this study. These models encompass two variants of the Unet architecture: Unet incorporating residual connections (referred to as resUnet) [7] and Attention Unet (abbreviated as attUnet) [8]. Additionally, three generative adversarial network (GAN) frameworks were included: deep convolutional GAN (DCGAN), pix2pix-GAN with resUnet, and pix2pix-GAN with attUnet. Furthermore, one diffusion model (the denoising diffusion probabilistic model, DDPM) was implemented.

The resUnet and attUnet models were derived from the MONAI platform [9]. The ResUnet was configured with a channel sequence of (8, 16, 32, 64, 128), corresponding strides of (2, 2, 2, 2), a total of 2 residual units, and a *Sigmoid* activation function. The attUnet used the same channel sequence and strides as the resUnet, but introduced a distinctive feature by incorporating attention gates (AGs) to filter the information propagated through the skip connections within each output layer [8].

The DCGAN model was implemented as described by Radford et al. [10]. It employes a discriminator architecture comprising strided convolution layers and a generator structured around a series of four fractionally-strided convolutions. Given our specific objective of image translation from MRI to CT, we replaced the generator with an attUnet, maintaining the same architectural framework as previously described. The objective of integrating this model is to evaluate whether incorporating a discriminator would enhance the performance of the Unet network.

The pix2pix-GAN framework was based on Isola et al. [11]. We substituted the original pix2pix-Unet generator with the attUnet and resUnet architectures, which were constructed in accordance with the previously mentioned specifications. These modified Unet structures were then integrated with the discriminator of the pix2pix GAN model.

Moreover, due to the observed limitations of the UNet and GAN models in generating satisfactory image details, particularly for small tissue structures, we investigated the conditional denoising diffusion probabilistic model (DDPM) [12]. It features a diffusion-model-Unet designed with a channel sequence of (64, 128, 256, 256). At each level, two residual blocks were incorporated, and the final layer was enhanced with an attention layer with eight attention heads, each with 32 channels. To address the specific task of image translation from MRI to CT, the source MRI image was appended to the noisy image as an extra channel. Consequently, this modification resulted in a 2-channel input configuration for the Unet component within the diffusion model.

2.4 Network training

We trained each model for 200 epochs. The DCGAN, pix2pix-GANs and diffusion model were trained using their standard settings [10–12]. For the Unets, an initial learning rate of 0.0002, Adam optimizer with $\beta_1 = 0.5$ and $\beta_2 = 0.999$, and Mean Squared Error (MSE) loss was used.

2.5 Evaluation

The obtained synthetic CT images (sCT) were compared to original CT using three metrics: Mean absolute error (MAE), Structural similarity index (SSIM), and Peak signal-to-noise ratio (PSNR). MAE measures the average absolute difference between the generated image and the ground truth image. A lower MAE indicates that the generated image is closer to the ground truth image in terms of pixel-level differences. SSIM evaluates the structural similarity between the generated image and the ground truth image, taking into account factors like luminance, contrast, and structure. SSIM values range from -1 to 1, with 1 indicating a perfect similarity. PSNR (Peak Signal-to-Noise Ratio) measures the ratio between the maximum possible power of a signal (the pixel values of the original image) and the power of the noise (the difference between the original and generated image). A higher PSNR value is generally associated with better image quality.

3 Results

3.1 Strategy for hyperparameter tuning

For tuning the hyperparameter, the training dataset, was split into a training set (150 patients) and a tuning set (20 patients). Hyperparameters were iteratively optimized using MAE, PSNR, and SSIM. The hyperparameters adjusted during this tuning process included the learning rate, the update interval for the discriminator, the number of channels, the stride of convolutional layers, the choice of loss function, the type of activation function, the inclusion or exclusion of an activation layer, and the lambda parameter for the pix2pix-GAN model.

3.2 Validation phase results

Table 1 presents quantitative results by each implemented model. Among all the models, the pix2pix-resUNet model achieved the best results on the validation set, as indicated by

Tab. 1. Quantitative evaluation of the six models on ten unseen datasets. Value are given as mena±stadard deviation.

mean±std	resUnet	attUnet	DCGAN	pix2pix-res	pix2pix-att	ddpm
SSIM	0.70±0.12	0.58±0.25	0.37±0.03	0.81±0.21	0.75±0.15	0.62±0.27
MAE	65.86±3.48	87.16±2.40	1893.96±80.75	55.52±3.50	79.18±3.06	166.10±8.25
PSNR	24.19±4.26	24.19±4.42	3.61±0.33	27.19±6.29	21.23±4.00	12.76±6.89

an average SSIM of 0.81±0.21, an average MAE of 55.52±3.50, and an average PSNR of 27.19±6.29. The resUnet and attUnet models are capable of attaining a relatively high PSNR, but a lower performance in terms of SSIM.

The DCGAN model achieved the poorest results, with a lowest mean SSIM and a lowest mean PSNR, indicating a significant dissimilarity from the original image. Additionally, representative examples of two slices from a patient are depicted in Figure 1. Our findings demonstrate that the DDPM model achieves the highest SSIM score, the highest PSNR and lowest MAE score in case A. Subjective observations further

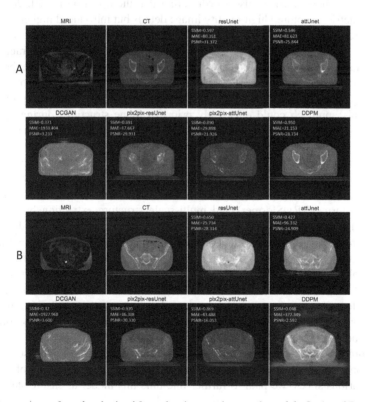

Fig. 1. Comparison of results obtained from the six neural network models. In A and B, two slices of the same patient are depicted. Metrics including SSIM, MAE, and PSNR are displayed at the top left of each generated image.

support the notion that DDPM excels in preserving image detail and fidelity. In contrast, the result of case B in Figure 1 indicates that DDPM could also introduce a substantial amount of noise, while pix2pix-resUnet surpasses it with the highest SSIM, PSNR, and lowest MAE scores in this scenario. It appears that the denoising process applied by DDPM to this specific slice may have been ineffective or incomplete.

4 Discussion

In this study, we compared six deep learning image-to-image models for the transformation of images between CT and MRI modalities. The pix2pix-resUnet model stood out for its quantitative performance on a 10-patient validation set, though it fell short in replicating fine details compared to actual CT images. In contrast, the DCGAN model produced images of the worst quality. This outcome can be attributed to the absence of a comparative evaluation between the generated and real images in its loss function. To address this limitation, the Pix2Pix-GAN model incorporates a reconstruction loss—specifically, a Mean Squared Error (MSE) function in our case—into the generator's loss component. It is also worth noting that the diffusion model, despite lower average metrics, captured high-quality image details but introduced higher noise levels.

The representation of bone structures in the GAN-based approaches was relatively poor, likely due to the fact that these structures occupy only a small fraction of the entire image. To address this issue, future work will concentrate on enhancing the depiction of bone structures. One potential solution is the application of a weighted Mean Squared Error (weightedMSE) loss function, which would incorporate a bone mask. This approach could effectively prioritize bone structures during the training process, potentially leading to more accurate and detailed representation in the generated images.

Comparing with the leaderboards of the challenge, our results haven't matched the SynthRAD2023 leader's SSIM of 0.89±0.03, MAE of 29.61±1.78, and PSNR of 29.61±1.79. This gap may be due to their Unet with advanced residual dilated swin transformer (RDSformer) and multi-scale structure extraction branches (MSE branches) between the convolution layers of the CNN-based encoder in the Unet. The implementation of these two distinct methods has significantly enhanced the ability of the Unet to capture both global and long-range spatial information and to extract structures at multiple scales [13]. We also trail behind the fourth-place's 2.5D pix2pix-GAN (SSIM of 28.80±1.60, MAE of 62.76±13.06, PSNR of 0.87±0.03). They utilized a 2.5D methodology, feeding five consecutive data slices into the network along the channel dimension, which yielded significantly improved detail and image quality compared to our 2D method [14].

Future research will focus on refining GAN-based models by multi-scale structure extraction, and employing a 2.5D network. Given the promising results of our DDPM across various slices, we plan to further fine-tune this model to ensure stability in its outputs.

Disclaimer. The authors declare that they have no conflict of interest.

Acknowledgement. This research project is part of the Research Campus M2OLIE and fundedby the German Federal Ministry of Education and Research (BMBF) within the Framework "Forschungscampus: public-private partnership for Innovations" under the funding code 13GW0388A.

References

1. Lyu Q, Wang G. Conversion between CT and MRI images using diffusion and score-matching models. 2022;(arXiv:2209.12104).
2. Kearney V, Ziemer BP, Perry A, Wang T, Chan JW, Ma L et al. Attention-aware discrimination for MR-to-CT image translation using cycle-consistent generative adversarial networks. Radiol Artif Intell. 2020;2(2):e190027.
3. Strittmatter A, Schad LR, Zöllner FG. Deep learning-based affine medical image registration for multimodal minimal-invasive image-guided interventions: a comparative study on generalizability. Z Med Phys. 2023;23.
4. Raj A, Tollens F, Hansen L, Golla AK, Schad LR, Nörenberg D et al. Deep learning-based total kidney volume segmentation in autosomal dominant polycystic kidney disease using attention, cosine loss, and sharpness aware minimization. Diagnostics. 2022;12(5):1159.
5. Bauer DF, Russ T, Waldkirch BI, Tönnes C, Segars WP, Schad LR et al. Generation of annotated multimodal ground truth datasets for abdominal medical image registration. Int J CARS. 2021;16(8):1277–85.
6. Thummerer A, Bijl E van der, Galapon A, Verhoeff JJC, Langendijk JA, Both S et al. SynthRAD 2023 grand challenge dataset: generating synthetic CT for radiotherapy. Med Phys. 2023;50(7):4664–74.
7. Ronneberger O, Fischer P, Brox T. U-net: convolutional networks for biomedical image segmentation. Proc MICCAI. 2015:234–41.
8. Oktay O, Schlemper J, Folgoc LL, Lee M, Heinrich M, Misawa K et al. Attention U-net: learning where to look for the pancreas. Medical Imaging Deep Learning. Ed. by Ginneken B van, Welling M. Vol. 1. 2018.
9. Cardoso MJ, Li W, Brown R, Ma N, Kerfoot E, Wang Y et al. MONAI: an open-source framework for deep learning in healthcare. 2022;(arXiv:2211.02701).
10. Radford A, Metz L, Chintala S. Unsupervised representation learning with deep convolutional generative Adversarial Networks. Proc ICLR. 2016.
11. Isola P, Zhu J, Zhou T, Efros AA. Image-to-image translation with conditional adversarial networks. Proc IEEE CVPR. Los Alamitos, CA, USA, 2017:5967–76.
12. Ho J, Jain A, Abbeel P. Denoising ciffusion probabilistic models. Proc IEEE. (NIPS'20). Vancouver, BC, Canada: Curran Associates Inc., 2020.
13. Chen Z, Zheng K, Li C, Yiwen Z. A hybrid network with multi-scale structure extraction and preservation for MR-to-CT synthesis in SynthRAD2023. SynthRAD2023. 2023.
14. Alain-Beaudoin A, Savard L, Bériault S. Paired MR-to-sCT translation using conditional GANs: an application to MR-guided radiotherapy. SynthRAD2023. 2023.

3D Deep Learning-based Boundary Regression of an Age-related Retinal Biomarker in High Resolution OCT

Wenke Karbole[1,2], Stefan B. Ploner[1,2], Jungeun Won[2], Anna Marmalidou[3], Hiroyuki Takahashi[3], Nadia K. Waheed[3], James G. Fujimoto[2], Andreas Maier[1]

[1]Pattern Recognition Lab, FAU Erlangen-Nürnberg, Germany
[2]Department for Electrical Engineering and Computer Science and Research Laboratory of Electronics, Massachusetts Institute of Technology, Cambridge, MA
[3]Department of Ophthalmology, New England Eye Center, Boston, MA
wenke.karbole@fau.de

Abstract. Vision is essential for quality of life, but is threatened by vision-impairing diseases like age-related macular degeneration (AMD). A recently proposed biomarker potentially to distinguish normal aging from AMD is the gap visualized between the retinal pigment epithelium (RPE) and the Bruch's membrane. Due to lack of automated processing, to date, this gap was only described sparsely in histologic data or on optical coherence tomography (OCT) B-scans. By segmenting the posterior RPE boundary automatically for the first time, we enable fully-automatic quantification of the thickness of this gap in vivo across whole volumetric OCT images. Our novel processing pipeline leverages advancements in motion correction, volumetric image merging, and high resolution OCT. A novel 3D boundary regression network named depth map regression network (DMR-Net) estimates the gap thickness in the volume. As 3D networks require full-volume ground truth boundary labels, which are labor-intensive, we developed a novel semi-automatic labeling approach to refine existing labels based on the visibility of the gap with minimal user input. We demonstrate thickness maps across a wide age range of healthy participants (23 – 79 years). The median absolute error in the test set is 0.161 µm, which is well below the axial pixel spacing (0.89 µm). For the first time, our results allow spatially resolved analysis to investigate pathologic deviations in normal aging and AMD.

1 Introduction

Vision, the primary sense through which we navigate our daily lives, is central to how we comprehend the world around us. The ability to process visual information relies on the healthy functioning of our eyes, a complex organ that undergoes progressive changes as we age. One example of changes in ocular aging happens at the usually only few micrometers thick gap between the retinal pigment epithelium (RPE) and Bruch's Membrane (BrM). It appears as dark hyporeflective gap (Hypor.Gap) in high resolution optical coherence tomography (OCT) images of young, healthy individuals (Fig. 1). Over time, as part of the normal aging process, this band becomes thinner and, eventually, non-resolvable, which makes exact localization of the posterior end of the RPE (pRPE) impossible. This feature gains particular significance in pathologies such as age-related macular degeneration (AMD), a leading cause of blindness globally. In

AMD, thickening of the Hypor.Gap can be observed in early stages of the disease, due to the accumulation of basal laminar deposits [1]. To be able to distinguish pathologic effects from normal aging, at first, a thorough understanding of the Hypor.Gap and its transformation with age is needed in healthy individuals.

Various retinal layers were previously segmented in OCT images. Along with their popularity in medical image segmentation, U-net-shaped networks were used to segment OCT images. A layer segmentation-specific approach is to regress the boundaries, which allows to achieve subpixel accuracy [2]. He et al. included a boundary regression module in a 2D U-net. 3D convolutions were not used due to sparse scans, and are problematic due to motion-induced distortion between scan lines (B-scans) of the raster-scanned images. The Hypor.Gap was not segmented automatically to date because of challanges with segmenting the pRPE: a high-resolution OCT device is required, the gap thickness of only few pixels is susceptible to noise, and its visibility varies locally. While a semi-automatic approach based on classical machine learning techniques was applied to individual B-scans [1], it was too time consuming to be applied to dense volumes.

This study presents a novel fully-automated approach for the estimation of the Hypor.Gap's thickness across dense volumetric images. High resolution OCT enables visibility of the gap in the first place. Volume merging enhances data quality and allows more fine-grained results. Motion-correction compensates image distortions, enabling reliable 3D image processing to further improve robustness. Utilizing these advances, a semi-automatic method for estimating the local gap visibility was developed. It allows boundary label refinement with minimal necessary user input for entire volumes, enabling the creation of ground truth data sufficient for 3D network training. Finally, the proposed 3D depth map regression network (DMR-Net) enables fully-automatic volumetric thickness estimation with a subpixel accuracy.

2 Materials and methods

The OCT dataset covers a broad demographic spectrum, including ages from 23 to 79 years (exact case counts per group in Fig. 5). For every subject, six consecutive volumetric scans were acquired over a 6 × 6 mm field centered around the fovea, with isotropic 500 × 500 A-scan sampling. The high resolution OCT device [3] and factor-2 spectral upsampling in axial direction result in a pixel spacing of 0.89 µm axial and 12 µm transverse. For better contrast between the hyperreflective RPE and BrM layers and the hyporeflective gap, algorithms are directly applied to the image intensities, without the logarithm transform that is commonly used in OCT. The dataset for the training of the DMR-Net consists of 42 volumes, and the quantitative evaluation was performed on a held-out test set of four cases with available ground truth. Age-dependent spatial variation was also analyzed qualitatively based on the predicted results in a larger cohort of 51 healthy subjects, all not contained in the network training process.

Initial labels for the pRPE and the BrM center were created by the 2D nnU-net based approach of Lin et al. [4] for each of the six scans individually (Fig. 1). Using the approaches of Ploner et al., the six volumetric images were motion-corrected [5], illumination equalized [6], and merged. Using the same motion estimates, the initial layer depth maps were corrected for axial displacement and merged analogously. For memory-efficient network training and inference, the volumetric data was flattened and cropped to the 245 pixels above and 10 pixels below the BrM, and 490×490 pixels in the transverse directions, to exclude data gaps that were revealed by the motion correction. The flattening enhances the visibility of the gap and simplifies pRPE segmentation.

The merged pRPE labels had sufficient precision in areas with a visible gap. Visual inspection revealed that, when no gap is visible, the not localizable pRPE was estimated at a distance to the BrM which resembled the typical distance in the visible areas. In order to refine the labels to better match the visual impression of a gap being resolved or not, the initial pRPE labels were assigned the BrM position if a gap was not visible (and therefore the pRPE not localizeable), which results in a Hypor.Gap thickness of zero. The general procedure for the ground truth refinement is visualized as a flowchart in Fig. 1. The visibility algorithm assesses each A-scan of the merged volume: For BrM, the maximal intensity value in a 3-voxel range around the boundary is selected, and for the pRPE, the minimal intensity value of the three voxels below the boundary is selected (Fig. 1 left). Then, the algorithm calculates a ratio of these intensities to estimate the visibility. A ratio close to 1 (yellow) implies little difference, i. e., no visible gap. Since the A-scan-wise calculated ratios are noisy, we apply Gaussian filtering followed by thresholding, creating a binary visibility map (Fig. 1 middle). This threshold is the only parameter that required user adjustment, and a single global value was sufficient to achieve a result that matched human perception across the whole volume. Figure 1 right visualizes the modified pRPE boundary in areas with no visible gap.

For automated thickness estimation, we propose an architecture called depth map regression network (DMR-Net), designed to process the BrM-flattened volumes and predict the pRPE depth positions, represented as a 2D map of continuous values (Fig. 2). The transformation from 3D to 2D poses a regression task. The DMR-Net is based on a 3D U-net architecture, and integrates the soft-argmax module proposed by He et al. [2]. The soft-argmax transforms the U-net output features by computing a weighted sum of depth positions along each A-scan, using the softmax output as weights for the respective locations. The resulting continuous value specifies the pRPE boundary's location

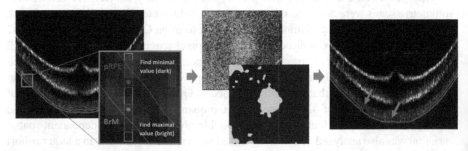

Fig. 1. Intensity-based ground truth refinement of the pRPE (orange) and BrM (blue): By A-scan-wise calculation of the ratio of the brightest and darkest voxel around both initial boundaries (left), a visibility map (purple: visible, yellow: invisible) is created (middle, back), denoised and thresholded (middle, front). If the gap is considered invisible, the pRPE is placed on top of BrM indicating a Hypor.Gap thickness of zero (right).

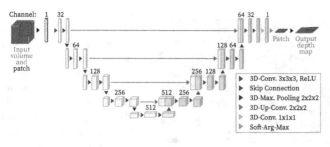

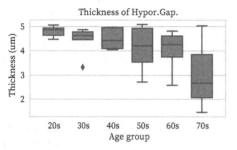

Fig. 2. Architecture of the proposed depth map regression network (DMR-Net) for predicting precise retinal layer boundaries. Dark grey blocks represent input/output data; light grey blocks show channel size.

Fig. 3. Estimated thicknesses of the hyporeflective gaps for different age groups. A declining trend in thickness is apparent with increasing age is apparent.

(depth) with sub-pixel accuracy, providing a precise surface localization than voxel-level segmentation as performed by standard U-net architectures. The gap thickness is then computed by subtracting the constant location the BrM was flattened to.

For training, the ADAM optimizer was used with learning rate and weight decay set to 1e-4, and mean squared error loss. The model was trained on 42 volumes using a 5-fold cross-validation procedure and is configured to run for a maximum of 400 epochs, including task-specific data augmentation (left/right flipping, brightness, contrast and image blur variations) and early stopping.

3 Results

We conducted a quantitative evaluation on four randomly selected hold-out test cases. This evaluation involved calculating the median absolute error in the axial direction for each case and then averaging these values across all cases. The resulting average error was 0.161 µm. This is significantly lower than the axial pixel spacing of the volumes, which is 0.89 µm, demonstrating that the DMR-Net effectively achieves subvoxel-level accuracy. Furthermore, the median absolute errors for each of the four test cases were all below 0.25 µm, indicating a consistently low variation between the cases.

The estimated thickness of the hyporeflective gap in age groups is shown in Fig. 3. While the median thickness for the groups from the 20's to 60's is consistently close to 5 µm and just slowly declining, a clear drop is apparent in subjects of age 70 and older.

Fig. 4 presents an exemplary case of a 64 years old subject. The top shows a B-scan around the foveal region, indicating the capability of a network to recognize the hyporeflective gap characteristic of this area. Notably, the gap is unresolved in the center (parafovea) yet discernible in the outer parts (perifovea). The network's prediction is shown by the red line that traces this feature, which is also depicted in the en-face depth

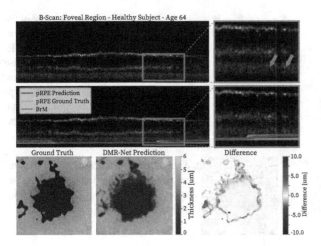

Fig. 4. Top: B-scan from central region with and without labels flattened to BrM (blue). pRPE network prediction (red) and ground truth (gray). Blue arrows (top right) point to visible Hypor.Gap. Bottom: Ground truth and predicted en-face depth maps (left) representing the Hypor.Gap thickness across the whole volume, and difference between ground truth and prediction (right).

maps at the bottom of the figure. Here, values near zero in the parafovea represent the network's prediction of an unresolved gap. The transition between the visible and non-visible areas is more gradual in the network prediction than in the ground truth. This is evident in the difference plot (bottom), where differences between the network prediction and ground truth are most prominent on the edge of the visible area. This transition is a particularly challenging region for label generation since a precise transition point is hard to identify, introducing uncertainty in the labels. Despite these challenges, the network's output remains closely aligned with the ground truth, mainly with deviations less than a micrometer – corresponding to less than the width of a pixel. Such minor discrepancies affirm the network's performance and qualitative evaluation confirms the output to be a reasonable solution in capturing the intricate details of the feature.

Fig. 5 illustrates the predicted thickness maps averaged per age group, offering a nuanced view of the spatial variation in Hypor.Gap thickness with aging. It reveals a consistently thick gap in younger subjects, evidenced by lighter shades. As age progresses, there is a visible trend towards darker shades in the maps, implying a general decrease in the gap's thickness. Notably, all age groups exhibit a thinner region in the parafoveal area, becoming more pronounced with age and suggesting to be a common feature of age-related change. Despite these variations, the foveal region in the very center consistently exhibits a thicker hyporeflective gap across all ages.

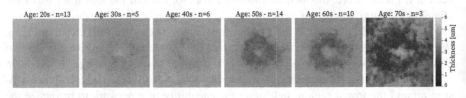

Fig. 5. Average thickness maps for each age group. Left eyes were mirrored to achieve consistent nasal (left side in the figures) and temporal orientation (right).

4 Discussion

We fully-automatically quantified the Hypor.Gap thickness across a 6×6 mm field using dense, high-resolution OCT volumes in subjects that cover a wide age-range. Our study results confirm the formerly described declining thickness trend with age [1].

We expand on previous results by – for the first time – providing dense en-face thickness estimations for the Hypor.Gap in vivo, which enable the analysis of spatial dependencies of the feature. Specifically, this allows spatial correlation with established spatially varying retinal characteristics, such as the cone-to-rod ratio, which is assumed to play a critical role in AMD. A median error under 0.25 pixels shows the network's subvoxel-precision capability. However, resolving the thin, faint Hypor.Gap, near the device's resolution limit is challenging such that the thickness values in this study are estimates, especially those below this limit of the device (2.7 µm) rather indicate the feature's resolvability and visibility. Poor scan quality, like shadowing or blurring, may degrade results. A challenge in analyzing faint features like the Hypor.Gap is the reliability of the ground truth. Human labeling of such ambiguous data leads to high inter- and intra-reader variance. Therefore, applying a neural network becomes particularly beneficial since vast amounts of high-dimensional data collectively contribute to the model fitting and can reduce variance inherent in manual annotations.

We are currently expanding our AMD dataset for future comparison and will enhance clinical insights by organizing the en-face results using the clinically established ETDRS grid.

Acknowledgement. DFG project 508075009, NIH projects R01EY011289-36 and R01EY034080-01A1.

References

1. Chen S, Abu-Qamar O, Kar D, Messinger JD, Hwang Y, Moult EM et al. Ultrahigh resolution OCT markers of normal aging and early AMD. Ophthalmol Sci. 2023;3(3):100277.
2. He Y, Carass A, Liu Y, Jedynak BM, Solomon SD, Saidha S et al. Structured layer surface segmentation for retina OCT using fully convolutional regression networks. Med Image Anal. 2021;68:101856.
3. Lee B, Chen S, Moult EM, Yu Y, Alibhai AY, Mehta N et al. High-speed, ultrahigh-resolution spectral-domain OCT with extended imaging range using reference arm length matching. Transl Vis Sci Technol. 2020;9(7):12–2.
4. Lin J. DL-enabled Accurate Bruch's Membrane Segmentation in Ultrahigh-resolution SD- and Ultrahigh-Speed SS-OCT. MA thesis. Massachusetts Institute of Technology, 2021.
5. Ploner S, Chen S, Won J, Husvogt L, Breininger K, Schottenhamml J et al. A spatiotemporal model for precise and efficient fully-automatic 3D motion correction in OCT. MICCAI. Springer. 2022:517–27.
6. Ploner S, Won J, Schottenhamml J, Girgis J, Lam K, Waheed N et al. A spatiotemporal illumination model for 3D image fusion in optical coherence tomography. IEEE ISBI. 2023.

Accelerating Artificial Intelligence-based Whole Slide Image Analysis with an Optimized Preprocessing Pipeline

Fabian Hörst[1,2], Sajad H. Schaheer[1], Giulia Baldini[1], Fin H. Bahnsen[1], Jan Egger[1,2],
Jens Kleesiek[1,2,4,5]

[1]Institute for AI in Medicine, University Hospital Essen (AöR), Essen, Germany
[2]Cancer Research Center Cologne Essen, University Hospital Essen (AöR), Essen, Germany
[4]German Cancer Consortium (DKTK, Partner site Essen), Heidelberg, Germany
[5]Department of Physics, TU Dortmund University, Dortmund, Germany
fabian.hoerst@uk-essen.de

Abstract. As the field of digital pathology continues to advance, the computer-aided analysis of whole slide images (WSI) has become an essential component for cancer diagnosis, staging, biomarker prediction, and therapy evaluation. However, even with the latest hardware developments, the processing of entire slides still demands significant computational resources. Therefore, many WSI analysis pipelines rely on patch-wise processing by tessellating a WSI into smaller sections and aggregating the results to retrieve slide-level outputs. One commonality among all these algorithms is the necessity for WSI preprocessing to extract patches, with each algorithm having its own requirements such as sliding window extraction or extracting patches at multiple magnification levels. In this paper, we present a novel Python-based software framework that leverages NVIDIA's cuCIM library and parallelization to accelerate the preprocessing of WSIs, named PathoPatch. Compared to existing frameworks, we achieve a substantial reduction in processing time while maintaining or even improving the preprocessing capabilities. The code is available under https://github.com/TIO-IKIM/PathoPatcher.

1 Introduction

Whole slide images (WSIs) have revolutionized the field of pathology, enabling the use of computer-aided image processing techniques for the field of pathology. The integration of machine learning (ML) and digital pathology represents a paradigm shift in the pathological workflow. Traditional methods of pathology, relying on manual assessment of glass slides under a microscope, are now extended by computer-aided systems that have the potential to automate clinical diagnoses, predict therapy response, and biomarker discovery. WSIs are stored as pyramidal images with internal tiling, where the image is divided into a grid of smaller tiles, allowing for efficient representation and retrieval of image data at multiple resolutions. Nevertheless, the high resolution at which WSIs are acquired leads to large image sizes, commonly exceeding dimensions of $100,000 \times 100,000$ pixels (px). Hence, analyzing WSI using ML is mainly based on patch-wise slide examination. In the context of patch-wise processing, a WSI is dissected into smaller sections, which are subsequently used as input for the respective ML algorithm. Few works specifically focus on WSI preprocessing; instead, it is imple-

© Der/die Autor(en), exklusiv lizenziert an
Springer Fachmedien Wiesbaden GmbH, ein Teil von Springer Nature 2024
A. Maier et al. (Hrsg.), *Bildverarbeitung für die Medizin 2024*,
Informatik aktuell, https://doi.org/10.1007/978-3-658-44037-4_91

mented as a necessary step in the "extract, transform, load (ETL)" algorithm pipeline without optimization. For instance, the work by Chen et al. [1] (CLAM) introduces preprocessing as part of algorithm development. Another solution is Deep-Histopath (D-Histo) [2], initially tailored for a conference challenge and subsequently extended for broader usage, albeit lacking annotation support. As an algorithm-agnostic solution, PathFlowAI (PathAI) [3] is widely used, but it is designed as an end-to-end solution with model integration rather than a standalone preprocessing tool. Several works have been published as Python frameworks, including SliDL [4], FAU-DLM [5], histolab [6], and TIAToolBox (TIA) [7].

In this paper, we introduce a flexible Python-based WSI preprocessing pipeline that has been optimized for speed and adaptability, which we name PathoPatch. We compare PathoPatch to existing solutions, such as the widely used TIAToolbox [7]. Our results demonstrate that our framework significantly improves preprocessing speed and functionality compared to existing solutions, reducing runtime by up to 80 %. Due to its OpenSlide [8] support, our framework is designed to handle WSI from many scanning manufacturers with different (proprietary) file formats.

2   Material and methods

2.1   Software requirements

Efficient WSI preprocessing demands specific software capabilities, spanning both functional and technical aspects. The software should support adaptable patch sizes and overlap (sliding window), along with magnification/pixel resolution selection, and multiresolution extraction. Tissue detection is crucial to prevent the extraction of non-tissue patches. Annotations should guide the process when specific tissue types or structures are of interest. Loading these annotations is essential for selective patch extraction and segmentation algorithms. Another important pipeline component is stain normalization to standardize the color appearance across multiple slides. To enhance the quality of the extracted patches, the software should include mechanisms for marker removal. On the technical side, image processing speed is crucial, particularly when dealing with large WSIs, which can contain over 100,000 patches depending on magnification and patch size. The selection of files for processing should be flexible, avoiding a folder-centric approach (e.g., CLAM), to mitigate redundant file storage. Given the widespread use of Python in algorithm implementations, the software should be designed as a Python framework that seamlessly integrates with users' deep learning (DL) codebases. Alternatively, it should provide a command-line interface (CLI) for parameter configuration.

2.2   Technical overview

Our solution, named PathoPatch, is a Python-based software built on top of common image-manipulating libraries, including OpenSlide [8] for WSIs, OpenCV [9] and scikit-image [10]. The software consists of five sequential components: Slide checking, tissue detection, patch extraction, optional post-processing, and storage. Users can interact with PathoPatch via a command-line interface, where they can configure essential preprocessing parameters such as patch size, overlap, pixel resolution, annotations, and post-processing operations. These configurations can also be specified in a configuration file. During slide and input checking, the software examines WSI consistency and required metadata. PathoPatch supports loading segmentation annotations from ".json / .geojson" files, compatible with common WSI annotation/viewing software. As the first image processing step, tissue detection is performed on a downsampled slide preview using otsu-thresholding [11]. Additionally, a tissue mask can be supplied as a polygon annotation. Based on this, the software allows for the extraction of all patches from the tissue masks, post-processing them in parallel, and storing them as independent image files. Alternatively, users can choose to extract patches from specific annotation classes within the tissue area. If available, polygonal annotations are converted into patch-matching segmentation masks for training segmentation networks. Notably, PathoPatch supports patch extraction from different pyramid levels simultaneously, offering context patches with a broader field-of-view. Optional postprocessing includes stain normalization using the Macenko method [12] and patch checking (e.g., filter out patches with marker). PathoPatch's modular structure allows for pipeline customization and extension.

A fundamental advantage of PathoPatch is its fast and parallelized patch extraction. To further accelerate this process, NVIDIA's Compute Unified Device Architecture Clara Image (cuCIM) library [13], which utilizes graphics processing unit (GPU) based image processing with CUDA-accelerated capabilities, is used. cuCIM provides an OpenSlide-compatible application interface and an adaptable caching mechanism, although it does not encompass all the functionalities of OpenSlide. Therefore, we extended the cuCIM application interface. Compared to OpenSlide, cuCIM significantly improves the patch-extraction speed, mainly due to the caching mechanisms. As it is not guaranteed that the extracted patches align with the internal WSI tiling of pyramidal levels, tiles need to be accessed multiple times, leading to a surplus of I/O operations. The caching mechanism mitigates this issue by storing previously loaded WSI tiles in the host's random access memory (RAM). PathoPatch automatically uses either OpenSlide or cuCIM based on the available hardware.

2.3 Experimental setup

In addition for comparing PathoPatch with existing frameworks based on functionality, we conducted experiments to compare patch extraction runtime. Specifically, we examined the impact of multiprocessing and the choice of the slide interface backend (OpenSlide (Version 3.4.1) vs. cuCIM v23.06.00)). We collected an internal WSI cohort (".svs", 240 px internal tiling) and processed these WSIs using a standardized configuration, including a patch size of 256 px (no overlap), extraction at ×40 magnification, and no postprocessing. The resulting number of patches allowed us to categorize the WSIs into five groups based on the number of patches they generated. This enabled us to compare WSIs of various tissue dimensions. Each group consisted of 10 WSIs. For each WSI, we systematically varied the number of processes (1, 2, 4, 8, and 16) and the choice of the backend (OpenSlide or cuCIM), conducting five runs for each configuration. The runtimes were then averaged over these five experiments. Notably, for the large WSIs (23414-53414 and >53414 patches), we just evaluated the impact of OpenSlide and cuCIM with 8/16 processes, as the runtime for fewer processes was impractical. To

Tab. 1. Comparison of preprocessing frameworks. Requirements are separated into image options for patching parameters, components, interfaces, and implementation. The abbrevations Seg., Sel., OS and CU stand for Segmentation, Selection, OpenSlide and cuCIM.

Requirements	CLAM [1]	D-Histo [2]	PathAI [3]	FAU [5]	SliDL [4]	TIA [7]	Our
Select Patch Size	✓	✓	✓	✓	✓	✓	✓
Select Patch Overlap	✓	✓	✓	-	✓	✓	✓
Select Resolution	✓	-	✓	✓	✓	✓	✓
Multi-Resolution	-	-	✓	-	-	-	✓
Tissue Detection	✓	✓	✓	✓	✓	✓	✓
Stain Normalization	-	✓	✓	-	-	✓	✓
Load Annotations	-	-	✓	Just ROI	✓	-	✓
Exclude Seg.	-	-	✓	-	✓	-	✓
Marker Removal	-	✓	-	-	-	-	✓
CLI	✓	-	✓	-	-	✓	✓
Flexible WSI Sel.	-	-	-	✓	-	✓	✓
Multi-Processing	-	✓	✓	✓	✓	-	✓
Backend	OS	OS	OS	OS	pyvips	OS/OWN	OS/CU

provide a comparison with existing solutions, we also conducted runtime experiments using the TIAToolbox (Version 1.4.0) framework. We compared our performance to both the original single-threaded implementation of TIAToolbox and a multi-threaded extension integrated by us. As the runtime was very high for TIAToolbox, we limited the TIAToolbox experiments to three WSIs for each patch number class (5 runs), comparing PathoPatch on these three WSIs. We assigned all experiments the same computing capacity (24 CPU cores, 32 GB RAM, NVIDIA A100 GPU with 80 GB RAM for each experiment, SSD Storage).

3 Results

3.1 Functionality

Table 1 provides a comparison of major frameworks for WSI preprocessing. Notably, PathoPatch and PathAI are the only ones that meet all patching requirements. Multi-resolution extraction is not supported by any of the remaining frameworks, as it's an edge use case just affecting multi-resolution models. Most frameworks lack support for loading annotations, necessary for segmentation algorithms, except for PathAI, SliDL, and PathPatch. All frameworks include at least OpenSlide as the backend, with TIA-Toolbox offering the most backend flexibility. Marker removal is supported only by Deep-Histopath. We support marker removal with tissue annotation, mask filtering, and patch-wise DL filtering. During development, we tried marker removal based on the filters, but they proved to be not robust enough for our purposes. Functionally, PathFlowAI is similar to PathoPatch, focusing more on direct analytical applications with integrated models, while PathoPatch can be used as a standalone software. While histolab is a versatile and extensible Python framework, and it is essential to recognize its strengths, it was not considered as a standalone solution in our evaluation and excluded from Table 1. Histolab offers a range of features that can be integrated into specific workflows, making it a valuable resource for users seeking a customizable solution. However, for our specific use case and the need for a standalone solution, we found that PathoPatch and PathFlow AI better align with our requirements, providing comprehensive support for various functionalities.

3.2 Runtime

The runtime results for the OpenSlide vs. cuCIM comparison with PathoPatch are depicted (Fig. 1). The cuCIM implementation indeed demonstrates a speedup in comparison to OpenSlide. When considering the number of processes used, the optimum number seems to be eight processes. While with fewer processes, the runtime is higher and fluctuates more, with eight processes a nearly constant throughput can be achieved. Comparatively, increasing the number of processes from one to eight with OpenSlide backend results in a runtime decrease of 71.9% on average, which can be further reduced by approximately 26.3% on average by using cuCIM. In comparison with TIAToolbox (Fig. 2), our framework proves to be significantly faster with both cuCIM and the OpenSlide backend. The speedup increases as more patches are extracted. Compared to TIAToolbox with only one process (not shown), our measurements show a remarkable runtime decrease of 79.9%. Our speed advantage, even in the presence of OpenSlide, is likely attributed to our optimized communication between patch extraction and storing.

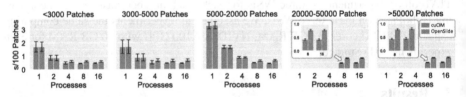

Fig. 1. Patch extraction runtime comparison between the OpenSlide and cuCIM implementation of PathoPatch, separated by number of processes used and patch amount per WSI. Runtime is measured by seconds per 100 patches, with standard deviation indicated by error bars (black).

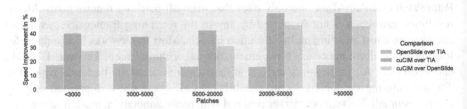

Fig. 2. Runtime decrease comparison between PathoPatch and TIAToolbox when using 8 parallel processes (average). OpenSlide and cuCIM stand for PathoPatch with respective backends.

4 Discussion

In this work, we introduced PathoPatch, a modular Python-based software framework designed for WSI preprocessing. Due to its modular architecture. By incorporating NVIDIA cuCIM and leveraging multiprocessing, we significantly accelerated the preprocessing time. While we have successfully integrated all the mentioned requirements into our software, the automatic removal of markers remains a complex challenge. In future versions, we plan to address this challenge by incorporating a DL model that can extract marker annotations from thumbnails rather than relying on hand-crafted annotations or patch-wise assessment like currently. Traditional methods for marker removal solely based on image filters have proven to be insufficient during our development. As part of our future development, we will also extend the automatic software testing.

Acknowledgement. This work received funding from "KITE" (Plattform für KI-Translation Essen) from the REACT-EU initiative (https://kite.ikim.nrw/, EFRE-0801977) and the Cancer Research Center Cologne Essen (CCCE).

References

1. Lu MY, Williamson DF, Chen TY, Chen RJ, Barbieri M, Mahmood F. Data-efficient and weakly supervised computational pathology on whole-slide images. Nat Biomed Eng. 2021;5(6):555–70.
2. Dusenberry M, Hu F, Jindal N, Eriksson D. Deep-histopath. https://github.com/CODAIT/deep-histopath. 2019.
3. Levy JJ, Salas LA, Christensen BC, Sriharan A, Vaickus LJ. PathFlowAI: A high-throughput workflow for preprocessing, deep learning and interpretation in digital pathology. Pac Symp Biocomput. 2020;25:403–14.
4. Berman AG, Orchard WR, Gehrung M, Markowetz F. SliDL: a toolbox for processing whole-slide images in deep learning. PLoS One. 2023;18(8):e0289499.
5. Neuner C, Jabari S, Vilz S. WSI processing pipeline. https://github.com/FAU-DLM/wsi_processing_pipeline. 2023.
6. Marcolini A, Bussola N, Arbitrio E, Amgad M, Jurman G, Furlanello C. histolab: a Python library for reproducible digital pathology preprocessing with automated testing. SoftwareX. 2022;20(101237).
7. Pocock J, Graham S, Vu QD, Jahanifar M, Deshpande S, Hadjigeorghiou G et al. TIAToolbox as an end-to-end library for advanced tissue image analytics. Commun Med. 2022;2(1).
8. Goode A, Gilbert B, Harkes J, Jukic D, Satyanarayanan M. OpenSlide: A vendor-neutral software foundation for digital pathology. J Pathol Inform. 2013;4(1):27.
9. Bradski G. The opencv library. Dr. Dobb's Journal of Software Tools. 2000.
10. van der Walt S, Schönberger JL, Nunez-Iglesias J, Boulogne F, Warner JD, Yager N et al. scikit-image: image processing in python. PeerJ. 2014;2:e453.
11. Otsu N. A Threshold Selection Method from Gray-Level Histograms. IEEE Trans Syst Man Cybern. 1979;9(1):62–6.
12. Macenko M, Niethammer M, Marron JS, Borland D, Woosley JT, Guan X et al. A method for normalizing histology slides for quantitative analysis. Proc IEEE Int Symp Biomed Imaging. 2009:1107–10.
13. NVIDIA. cuCIM. https://github.com/rapidsai/cucim. 2023.

Abstract: Transient Hemodynamics Prediction using an Efficient Octree-based Deep Learning Model

Noah Maul[1,2], Katharina Zinn[1], Fabian Wagner[1], Mareike Thies[1],
Maximilian Rohleder[1,2], Laura Pfaff[1,2], Markus Kowarschik[2], Annette Birkhold[2],
Andreas Maier[1]

[1]Pattern Recognition Lab, Friedrich-Alexander-Universität Erlangen-Nürnberg, Germany
[2]Siemens Healthcare GmbH, Forchheim, Germany
noah.maul@fau.de

Patient-specific hemodynamics assessment has the potential to support diagnosis and treatment of neurovascular diseases. Currently, conventional medical imaging modalities are not able to accurately acquire high-resolution hemodynamic information that would be required to assess complex neurovascular pathologies. Alternatively, computational fluid dynamics (CFD) simulations can be applied to tomographic reconstructions to obtain clinically relevant hemodynamic quantities. However, enormous computational resources and expert knowledge would be required to execute CFD simulations, which are usually not available in clinical environments. Recently, deep-learning-based methods have been proposed as CFD surrogates to improve computational efficiency. Nevertheless, the prediction of high-resolution transient CFD simulations for complex vascular geometries poses a challenge to conventional deep learning models. In this work, we present an architecture that is tailored to predict high-resolution (spatial and temporal) velocity fields for complex synthetic vascular geometries. For this, an octree-based spatial discretization is combined with an implicit neural function representation to efficiently handle the prediction of the 3D velocity field for each time step. The presented method is evaluated for the task of cerebral hemodynamics prediction before and during the injection of contrast agent in the internal carotid artery (ICA). Compared to CFD simulations, the velocity field can be estimated with a mean absolute error of $0.024\,\mathrm{m\,s^{-1}}$, whereas the run time reduces from several hours on a high-performance cluster to a few seconds on a consumer graphical processing unit [1].

References

1. Maul N, Zinn K, Wagner F, Thies M, Rohleder M, Pfaff L et al. Transient hemodynamics prediction using an efficient octree-based deep learning model. Proc Med Imaging. Springer Nature Switzerland, 2023:183–94.

Abstract: Utility-preserving Measure for Patient Privacy

Deep Learning-based Anonymization of Chest Radiographs

Kai Packhäuser, Sebastian Gündel, Florian Thamm, Felix Denzinger, Andreas Maier

Pattern Recognition Lab, Friedrich-Alexander-Universität Erlangen-Nürnberg, Germany
kai.packhaeuser@fau.de

Robust and reliable anonymization of chest radiographs constitutes an essential step before publishing large datasets of such for research purposes. The conventional anonymization process is carried out by obscuring personal information in the images with black boxes and removing or replacing meta-information. However, such simple measures retain biometric information in the chest radiographs, allowing patients to be re-identified by a linkage attack. Therefore, there is an urgent need to obfuscate the biometric information appearing in the images. We propose the first deep learning-based approach (PriCheXy-Net) to targetedly anonymize chest radiographs while maintaining data utility for diagnostic and machine learning purposes. Our model architecture is a composition of three independent neural networks that, when collectively used, allow for learning a deformation field that is able to impede patient re-identification. Quantitative results on the ChestX-ray14 dataset show a reduction of patient re-identification from 81.8 % to 57.7 % (AUC) after re-training with little impact on the abnormality classification performance. This indicates the ability to preserve underlying abnormality patterns while increasing patient privacy. Lastly, we compare our proposed anonymization approach with two other obfuscation-based methods (Privacy-Net, DP-Pix) and demonstrate the superiority of our method towards resolving the privacy-utility trade-off for chest radiographs. This work has previously been published at MICCAI 2023 [1]. Code is available at https://github.com/kaipackhaeuser/PriCheXy-Net.

References

1. Packhäuser K, Gündel S, Thamm F, Denzinger F, Maier A. Deep learning-based anonymization of chest radiographs: a utility-preserving measure for patient privacy. Proc MICCAI. 2023:262–72.

Autorenverzeichnis

Printed in the United States
by Baker & Taylor Publisher Services